Atlas of Musculoskeletal Imaging

Atlas of Musculoskeletal Imaging

Thomas Lee Pope, Jr., M.D., F.A.C.R.
Professor of Radiology and Orthopaedics
Medical University of South Carolina
Charleston, South Carolina

Stephen Loehr, M.D.
Division of Radiologic Sciences
Wake Forest University
The Bowman Gray School of Medicine
Winston-Salem, North Carolina

Contributing author:
Chris Hagenstad, M.D.
House Officer
Medical College of Virginia
Richmond, Virginia

2000

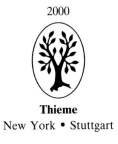

Thieme
New York • Stuttgart

Thieme New York
333 Seventh Avenue
New York, NY 10001

Executive Editor: Jane Pennington, Ph.D.
Editorial Director: Avé McCracken
Assistant Editor: Jinnie Kim
Director, Production & Manufacturing: Anne Vinnicombe
Production Editor: Xenia Golovchenko
Marketing Director: Phyllis Gold
Sales Manager: Ross Lumpkin
Chief Financial Officer: Seth S. Fishman
President: Brian D. Scanlan
Cover Designer: Marsha Cohen
Compositor: PRD Group
Printer: Edwards Brothers

Library of Congress Cataloging-in-Publication Data

Pope, Thomas Lee.
    Atlas of musculoskeletal imaging/Thomas L. Pope, Jr. and Stephen Loehr.
        p.   cm.
    Includes bibliographical references (p.   ) and index.
    ISBN 0-86577-695-4 (hardcover)
    1. Musculoskeletal system—Magnetic resonance imaging.   I. Loehr, Stephen.
    II. Title.
    RC925.7.P67   1998
    616.7'07548—dc21
    DNLM/DLC
    for Library of Congress   98-27858
                                                                        CIP

Important note: Medical knowledge is ever-changing. As new research and clinical experience broaden our knowledge, changes in treatment and drug therapy may be required. The authors and editors of the material herein have consulted sources believed to be reliable in their efforts to provide information that is complete and in accord with the standards accepted at the time of publication. However, in view of the possibility of human error by the authors, editors, or publisher of the work herein, or changes in medical knowledge, neither the authors, editors, publisher, nor any other party who has been involved in the preparation of this work, warrants that the information contained herein is in every respect accurate or complete, and they are not responsible for any errors or omissions or for the results obtained from use of such information. Readers are encouraged to confirm the information contained herein with other sources. For example, readers are advised to check the product information sheet included in the package of each drug they plan to administer to be certain that the information contained in this publication is accurate and that changes have not been made in the recommended dose or in the contraindications for administration. This recommendation is of particular importance in connection with new or infrequently used drugs.

Some of the product names, patents, and registered designs referred to in this book are in fact registered trademarks or proprietary names even though specific reference to this fact is not always made in the text. Therefore, the appearance of a name without designation as proprietary is not to be construed as a representation by the publisher that it is in the public domain.

Printed in the United States of America

5 4 3 2 1

TNY ISBN 0-86577-695-4
GTV ISBN 3-13-108061-2

Dedication

This book is dedicated to my dad and hero, the late Thomas Pope, Sr.; to my family, Roger (and Cathy) and Florence Pope; and especially to my emotional support, my wife, Lou and my sons David and Jason. Without all of them, life would be much less tolerable.

Thomas Lee Pope, Jr., M.D., F.A.C.R.

I dedicate this work to my loving wife, Laura; to Dr. C. Douglas Maynard; and to the Department of Radiology at Wake Forest University Medical Center for their encouragement, support, and patience during completion of this project.

Stephen Loehr, M.D.

Contents

Foreword

Anatomy is important. In musculoskeletal radiology, as in real estate, it is location, location, location. Where the property is located or where the lesion is located makes all the difference in the world. In real estate, location is the major determinant of property value, whereas in the interpretation of musculoskeletal imaging, location is a major determinant in the recognition of the true nature of a lesion and a key to the development of an appropriate differential diagnosis. Where a lesion is goes a long way to telling you what it is. And by knowing precisely where it is and what is around it, the surgeon can devise an approach to the lesion and knows what to watch out for along the way. There is simply no substitute for knowledge of anatomy.

Very few radiologists involved in cross-sectional imaging, even specialists in skeletal radiology, know human anatomy so well that they can confidently interpret magnetic resonance imaging and computer tomography without feeling the need to refer to an anatomic atlas of some sort from time to time. This is particularly true when faced with an examination of an infrequently examined joint. And even more so when the area of interest is at a distance from a joint. Because of the heightened role of cross-sectional imaging in the assessment of soft tissue abnormalities (i.e., tumors, infections, and the like), such examinations are much more frequent than in the past and, indeed, in some medical centers have become an everyday occurrence. Therefore, there is a frequent need to refer to an anatomic atlas to aid in the interpretation of these examinations.

So you go to the bookcase seeking information in order to properly identify the appropriate muscles, tendons, and fascial planes, and determine the critical relationships of the lesion in question to the surrounding nerves and vascular structures. After taking down an atlas to look up the important anatomy, you often find it to be devoid of information regarding anatomy along the shaft of long bones away from the joints. Unfortunately the anatomical diagrams and accompanying images are limited to the joints and there is no illustration of the anatomy in between. This portion of the anatomy is left to your imagination!

Or maybe you are lucky enough to find an illustration of the anatomy you seek, only to realize that the illustration is of the opposite extremity—that is, the side opposite the one you are interested in, the side opposite that in which the lesion in question is located. All illustrations are limited to a single extremity, say the right extremity, and it just so happens that you are faced with a lesion in the left extremity. There is, of course, a 50/50 chance that this will occur. You are out of luck and posed with the requirement of "mirror-image thinking." You have to reverse the image in your mind to determine the anatomy on the side you are interested in, the side opposite that displayed in the atlas. This is not always easy; realizing, of course, that if you are not careful you could make a mistake.

This work was borne out of the preceding frustrating experiences, spawned by authors who came to the realization that there must be a better way. And there is. Why not an atlas that depicts both extremities and does away with "mirror-image" thinking? And while we're at it, let's illustrate the anatomy between the joints, as well. Anyone who interprets cross sectional images would immediately recognize the value of such a work.

Well, here it is. You hold it in your hands. Feast your eyes on its content. Peruse the illustrations. Yes, left and right, both sides at the joints and all points in between are there. All in all, a practical, useful, and instructive contribution.

If you do musculoskeletal imaging, if you interpret musculoskeletal images, or if you are an orthopaedist, rheumatologist, or physiatrist, I am certain this work will be of value to you in your practice. This is the atlas we've been waiting for. The authors are to be commended for their fine efforts. Drs. Pope and Loehr have produced an easy-to-use, comprehensive, and informative atlas that should prove to be of immeasurable value to all who have the need for precise knowledge of musculoskeletal anatomy as displayed by all forms of musculoskeletal imaging.

Lee F. Rogers, M.D.
Winston-Salem, North Carolina

Preface

This atlas was conceived at the view box while reading clinical MR images. While interpreting these images, we would invariably need to consult the standard anatomy books. However, these texts were often insufficient: The image to be interpreted showed the right extremity, but the anatomy book demonstrated the left, or vice versa. This mismatch resulted in some interesting and challenging translations from the reference book to our clinical images. Furthermore, the middle regions of the extremities usually were not included in the standard anatomy texts. Therefore, only by extrapolation from the highest or lowest images of the joint exhibited in the textbook could we estimate the anatomy in the midportion of the extremities of our images. Finally, many textbooks of anatomy do not include the origin and insertion of muscles or any discussion of the joints that are exhibited. These shortfalls prompted us to consider how we could design a text to overcome most of these problems.

The solution, in our opinion, was to create an atlas that not only demonstrated both right- and left-sided images as they are usually interpreted at the view box, but that also included the middle regions of the extremities. Such an atlas would also need to include the origin and insertion of the major muscles of each anatomic region and a brief introduction to the joint at the beginning of each chapter. *Atlas of Musculoskeletal Imaging* is the result of our ideas. The major joints, the pelvis, and selected images of the spine are included. Detailed, yet practical labeling of each anatomic image is provided. The atlas is not intended to be all-inclusive, and we have selected only the most clinically practical images.

Each chapter is organized as follows: A brief "introduction" to the anatomic area precedes the "practical protocol suggestions" section that outlines general hints about obtaining optimal images. Next is the "menu of protocols" that includes the more common technical parameters used in each anatomic area. An outline of "major osteochondral structures/landmarks" is next and lists the important structures with which to be familiar in each organ system. Finally, the "origin/insertion/innervation of major muscles" section provides a practical body of information often needed when interpreting clinical images. These sections were created because they seem to be most practical in the day-to-day clinical situations.

Our intention is for this text to serve as a practical and user-friendly guide that can be used in the day-to-day interpretation of MR images. We hope that it will find a home on the shelves beside the reading room rollerscopes or workstations, in the libraries, or in the offices of radiologists who interpret musculoskeletal MR images, and on the shelves of the offices of orthopaedic surgeons and rheumatologists who request these studies.

We solicit the suggestions of anyone who has an opportunity to use the book and look forward to hearing your comments. No book is without flaws, and this one may contain some errors that were missed. If so, please let us know, and we will ensure that they are addressed in the next edition.

Thomas Lee Pope, Jr., M.D., F.A.C.R.
Stephen Loehr, M.D.

Acknowledgments

No textbook is a single-handed endeavor, and this book is no exception. We greatly appreciate the frustration expressed by many musculoskeletal fellows and residents because they could not find a simple-to-use atlas. Without their difficulty, the idea for this book would not have been developed.

We thank Ms. Sharon Meister for her tireless dedication to excellence in transcribing the text for the book, and for coordinating and collating text. We also thank Dr. Donna Garrison and Mr. Terry Poovey, the medical editors of our department, who made sure that we all sound good on paper. Finally, we thank our Chair, Dr. C. Douglas Maynard, for creating a professional atmosphere conducive to academic productivity and cooperative interpersonal relationships, both requirements for completing projects like this one.

Thomas Lee Pope, Jr., M.D., F.A.C.R.
Stephen Loehr, M.D.

1

INTRODUCTION: GENERAL TECHNICAL CONSIDERATIONS

Patients undergoing musculoskeletal magnetic resonance (MR) imaging should be examined with the smallest coil that covers the body part, thereby achieving the highest signal-to-noise ratio and the best spatial resolution. For imaging of the joints and extremities, surface coils are mandatory as they improve the signal-to-noise ratio by four to six times compared to the head or body coils. The smallest field of view possible should be used. Individual variations are present among the wide range of scanners now available, and each location should determine for itself which sequences are best. The protocols described in each section were developed primarily on General Electric 1.5-T magnets. Obviously, images of diagnostic quality can be obtained with a variety of scanners, and the recommended protocols may require modification to suit the scanner at the institution and the personal preferences of the imager. The general principles regarding selection of pulse sequence and planes are most important. Furthermore, the major indicator of success is the satisfaction of the imager and the referring physician with their diagnostic results when these results are confirmed by arthroscopy, surgery, or patient outcome.

Positioning the patient properly in the MR imaging scanner is critical to obtaining diagnostic images. Technologists should pay particular attention to the placement of an extremity within the coil for an optimal selection of the slices. For best results, images should be obtained in axial, coronal, and sagittal planes. Axial MR images are probably most critical in the evaluation of a soft-tissue mass thought to be a tumor, so that the relationship of the mass to the neurovascular bundles and other important structures can be ascertained.

KEY TO ACRONYMS

Acronym	Explanation/Meaning
EPI	Echoplanar imaging
ETL	Echo-train length
FA	Flip angle (90° unless otherwise specified)
FMPIR	Fast multiplanar inversion recovery
FOV	Field of view (cm)
FS	Fat saturation
FSE	Fast spin echo
GAD	Gadolinium
GRASS	Gradient-recalled acquisition in the steady state
GRE	Gradient echo, gradient-recalled echo
IR	Inversion recovery
MPGR	Multiplanar GRASS
NEX	Number of excitations
PS	Pulse sequence
RL	Right to left
SE	Spin echo
SI	Superior to inferior
SPGR	Spoiled GRASS
ST/G	Slice thickness and gap (mm)
TE	Time to echo (msec)
TI	Inversion time
TR	Time to repetition (msec)
VAR	Variable (dependent upon size of abnormality or patient)

SUMMARY OF FAST MR TERMS

Term	Abbreviation	Explanation	Example of Manufacturer	Characteristic Feature
General				
	EPI	Echoplanar imaging		
	ETL	Echo train length		
	FOV	Field of view		
	GRE	Gradient-recalled echo		
	IR	Inversion recovery		
	MR	Magnetic resonance		
	NEX	Number of excitations		
	NSA	Number of signals averaged		
	SE	Spin echo		
	SNR	Signal-to-noise ratio		
	TE	Echo time		
	TI	Inversion time		
	TR	Repetition time		
T1-weighted sequence				
	FLASH	Fast low-angle shot	Siemens, Bruker	GRE sequence with spoiling gradient
	FFE	Fast field echo	Philips	GRE sequence with spoiling gradient
	PSR	Partial saturation recovery	Picker	GRE sequence with spoiling gradient
	FE	Field echo	Elscint	GRE sequence with spoiling gradient
	MP-RAGE	Magnetization-prepared rapid gradient echo		180° IR pulse GRE sequence with spoiling gradient
	SPGR	Spoiled gradient-recalled imaging	General Electric	GRE sequence with spoiling gradient
T2-weighted sequence				
	SSFP	Steady-state free precession	Siemens	GRE sequence with TE > TR
	PSIF	Reversed fast imaging with steady state precession, collection of the refocused echo	Siemens	GRE sequence with TE > TR
	CE-FAST	Contrast-enhanced Fourier-acquired steady-state technique	Picker	GRE sequence with TE > TR
	FSE	Fast spin echo		More than one echo per excitation with multiple 180° pulses
	FAIST	Fast-acquisition interleaved spin echo		More than one echo per excitation with multiple 180° pulses
	GRASE	Gradient and spin echo		Multiple 180° pulses and gradient-recalled echoes

(continued)

SUMMARY OF FAST MR TERMS (*CONTINUED*)

Term	Abbreviation	Explanation	Example of Manufacturer	Characteristic Feature
	GREASE	Gradient echo and spin echo		GRE with multiple 180° pulses
	RARE	Rapid acquisition with relaxation enhancement		More than one phase-encoding step per excitation
	RASE	Rapid acquisition spin echo	Siemens	Half Fourier imaging
	TGSE	Turbo gradient spin echo, identical to GRASE	Siemens	FRE with multiple 180° pulses
	turboFLASH	Turbo fast low-angle shot	Siemens, Bruker	180° inversion recovery pulse plus GRE sequence
	turboSE	Turbo spin echo, identical to FSE	Siemens	More than one echo per excitation with multiple 180° pulses
T1- + T2-weighted sequence and variable weighting				
	GRASS	Gradient-recalled acquisition in the steady state	General Electric	GRE without spoiling gradient
	FISP	Fast imaging with steady-state precession	Siemens	GRE without spoiling gradient
	FAST	Fourier-acquired steady-state technique	Picker	GRE without spoiling gradient
Echoplanar sequence	ABEST	Asymmetric blipped echoplanar single-pulse technique		One 90° pulse, rectangular scanning of K-space
	BEST	Blipped echoplanar signal-pulse technique		One 90° pulse, rectangular scanning of K-space
	EPISTAR	Echoplanar imaging with signal targeting and alternating radiofrequency		One 90° pulse, rectangular scanning of K-space
	Instascan	Brand name for EPI sequence	Advanced NMR Systems	One 90° pulse, rectangular scanning of K-space
	MBEST	Modulus-blipped echoplanar single-pulse technique		One 90° pulse, rectangular scanning of K-space
	mesh	Interleaved K-space scan		Meshed scanning of K-space

(*continued*)

SUMMARY OF FAST MR TERMS (*CONTINUED*)

Term	Abbreviation	Explanation	Example of Manufacturer	Characteristic Feature
Motion suppression technique				
	COPE	Cardiac-ordered phase encoding		Phase-encoding steps triggered by ECG
	FAT SAT	Fat saturation pulse		Presaturation pulse suppresses signal from fat
	FRODO	Flow and respiratory artifact obliteration with directed orthogonal pulses		Presaturation pulse suppresses signal from vessels and from tissue outside the area of interest
	MAST	Motion artifact suppression technique		
	ROPE	Respiratory-ordered phase encoding		Phase-encoding steps triggered by respiration
	STIR	Short inversion time inversion recovery		IR sequence with short T1

From Dr. Saini, with permission. Petersein J, Saini S. Appendix: Summary of fast MR terms. Fast MR Imaging: Technical Strategies. *AJR* 1995;165:1105–1109.

2

THE SHOULDER AND THE UPPER EXTREMITY

A. THE SHOULDER

The glenohumeral joint is commonly evaluated by magnetic resonance (MR) imaging. The major indications for MR imaging are suspected rotator cuff abnormality, glenohumeral instability, and chronic and unexplained shoulder pain. The most common pathologic processes are tendinosis, partial or complete tears of the rotator cuff tendons (injuries to the supraspinatus are by far the most frequent), glenoid labral abnormalities, biceps tendon displacement or injury, and spinoglenoid ganglia.

PRACTICAL PROTOCOL CONSIDERATIONS

The patient is routinely imaged in the supine position, with either a surface coil or paired flat coils placed above and below the shoulder in a Helmholtz configuration. The advantage of the Helmholtz configuration is the additive signal-to-noise ratio created by the two coils. Flexible quadrature and phased-array coils have also been used recently to improve the signal-to-noise ratio and increase the anatomic area covered by the study.

The patient's arm is at his or her side and is either in the neutral position or slightly externally rotated position to decrease overlapping of the infraspinatus and supraspinatus tendons. Abduction and external rotation have also been used to facilitate evaluation of partial rotator cuff tears, but this positioning is not in common use today.

Menu of Protocols: Glenohumeral Joint

Plane	Pulse Sequence	FA (degrees)	TR (msec)	TE (msec)	TI (msec)	FOV (cm)	Matrix (256X-)	ST/G (mm)	NEX	Comments
Localizer (coronal)	FMPIR		2,500	30	150	36	128	5/1.5	1	Either is acceptable
Localizer (coronal)	FSE		600	17		35	128	5/1.5	2	
Localizer (axial)	2D SPGR		30	min		20	128	5/0	2	
Coronal (oblique)	SE, double echo		2,000	20/80		14	192	4/1	1	Either is acceptable
Coronal (oblique)	FSE, double echo, (+/−1-FS)		3,000	17/102		16	192	5/1	2	
Sagittal (oblique)	SE, double echo		2,000	17/70		16	192	3/1	1	Either is acceptable
Sagittal (oblique)	FSE (+/−1-FS)		3,000	20		14	192	4/1	2	
Sagittal (oblique)	FSE (+/−1-FS)		5,500	85		16	192	4/.5	2	
Transaxial	SE, double echo		2,000	20/80		14	192	4/1	1	Either is acceptable
Transaxial	MPGR	30	450	15		14	192	4/1	1	
Transaxial	3D GRE	20	30	15		15	128	1.2/0	2	
Transaxial	FSE (+/−1-FS)		3,000	85		16	192	4/.5	2	

MAJOR OSTEOCHONDRAL STRUCTURES/LANDMARKS

- Scapula
  - Acromion
  - Spine of scapula
  - Glenoid cavity of scapula (with its articular cartilage)
  - Body of scapula
  - Coracoid process
- Infraglenoid tubercle (origin of long head of biceps tendon)
  - Proximal humerus
  - Humeral articular cartilage
  - Greater tuberosity of humerus
  - Lesser tuberosity of humerus
  - Intertubercular sulcus (for biceps tendon)
  - Clavicle
  - Acromioclavicular joint
  - Anterior glenoid labrum
  - Posterior glenoid labrum
  - Superior glenoid labrum
  - Inferior glenoid labrum

MAJOR LIGAMENTS/TENDONS/BURSAE

Tendons
- "SITS" tendons
  - Supraspinatus
  - Infraspinatus
  - Teres minor
- Subscapularis
- Long head of biceps
- Coracobrachialis

Ligaments
- Coracoclavicular (conoid and trapezoid components)
- Acromioclavicular
- Coracoacromial
- Sternoclavicular
- Coracohumeral
- Glenohumeral ligaments (focal thickenings of the anterior joint capsule)
  - Superior
  - Middle
  - Inferior

Bursae
- Subacromial/subdeltoid (most important)
- Subscapularis (normally communicates with glenohumeral joint)
- Infraspinatus
- Subcoracoid
- Coracobrachialis (not identified often on MR images)
- Latissimus dorsi
- Teres major
- Pectoralis major

ORIGIN/INSERTION/INNERVATION OF MAJOR MUSCLES

Muscle	Origin	Insertion	Innervation
Dorsal Group			
–Supraspinatus (SS)	Supraspinatus fossa of scapula	Greater tuberosity of humerus	Suprascapular nerve (N.) (C5, C6)
–Infraspinatus (IS)	Infraspinatus fossa of scapula	Greater tuberosity of humerus (below SS insertion)	Suprascapular N. (C5, C6)
–Teres minor (TM)	Lateral margin of scapula	Posterior facet of greater tuberosity	Axillary N. (C5, C6)
–Deltoid	Lateral third of clavicle, acromion, scapular spine	Deltoid tuberosity of humerus	Axillary N. (C5, C6)
–Subscapularis	Suprascapular fossa	Lesser tuberosity	Subscapular N. (C5, C6)
–Latissimus dorsi	Spinous processes (T6–T12), thoracolumbar fascia of L spine and sacrum	Medial aspect of intertubercular groove	Thoracodorsal N. (C6–C8)
Ventral Group			
–Pectoralis major	Sternal half of clavicle, sternum, costochondral junctions	Lateral aspect of intertubercular groove	Medial/lateral anterior thoracic N. (C5–T1)
–Pectoralis minor	Anterior ribs 2–5	Coracoid process of scapula	Medial pectoral N. (C8–T1)
–Corabrachialis	Coracoid process of scapula	Inner surface of humerus	Musculocutaneous N.

(*continued*)

ORIGIN/INSERTION/INNERVATION OF MAJOR MUSCLES (*CONTINUED*)

Muscle	*Origin*	*Insertion*	*Innervation*
Other Muscles			
–Teres major	Inferior and lateral aspect of scapula	Medial aspect, intertubercular groove	Subscapular N. (C5, C6)
–Trapezius	Ligamentum nuchae, spinous processes of thoracic vertebrae	Distal clavicle, acromion, spine of scapula	Spinal accessory and C2, C3
–Levator scapulae	Posterior tubercles, transverse processes of C1–C4	Upper and medial scapula	Cervical plexus (C3–C4)
–Rhomboids			
–Major	Spinous processes of C2–T5	Posterior and medial scapula	Dorsal scapular N. (C5)
–Minor	Ligamentum nuchae, spinous processes of C7/T1	Posterior and medial scapula	Dorsal scapular N. (C5)
–Serratus anterior	Ribs 1–9	Anterior and medial scapula	Long thoracic N. (C5–C7)
–Subclavius	Anterior and medial first rib	Middle and inferior clavicle	Subclavian N.

THE SHOULDER: AXIAL ANATOMY

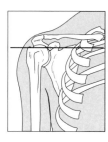

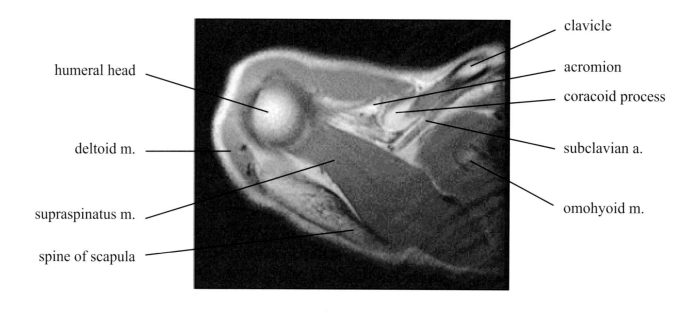

clavicle

humeral head

acromion

coracoid process

deltoid m.

subclavian a.

supraspinatus m.

omohyoid m.

spine of scapula

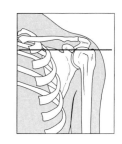

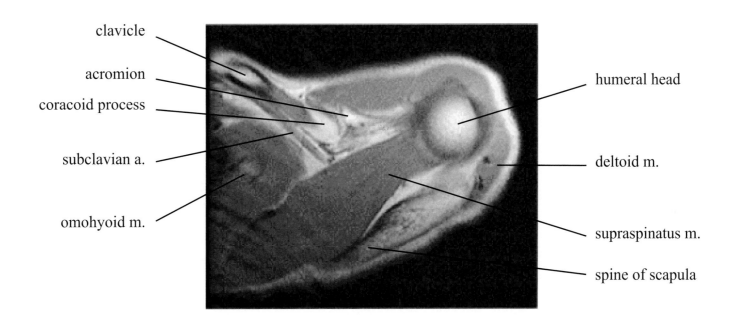

clavicle

acromion

coracoid process

subclavian a.

omohyoid m.

humeral head

deltoid m.

supraspinatus m.

spine of scapula

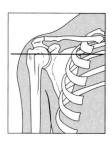

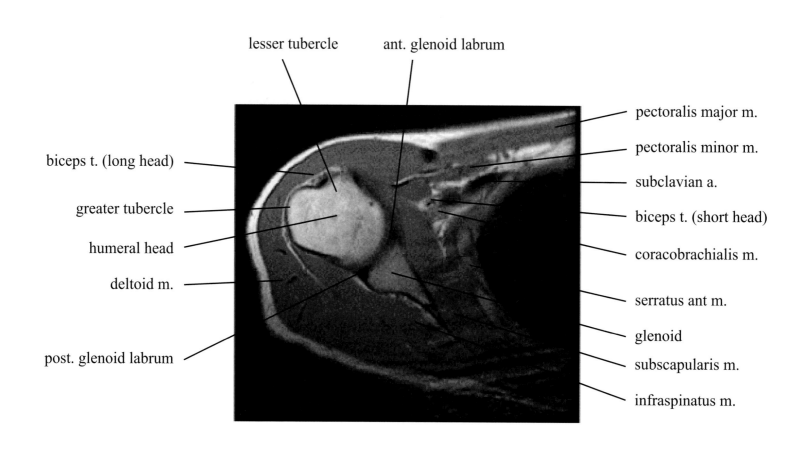

lesser tubercle

ant. glenoid labrum

pectoralis major m.

pectoralis minor m.

biceps t. (long head)

subclavian a.

greater tubercle

biceps t. (short head)

humeral head

coracobrachialis m.

deltoid m.

serratus ant m.

glenoid

subscapularis m.

post. glenoid labrum

infraspinatus m.

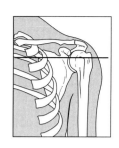

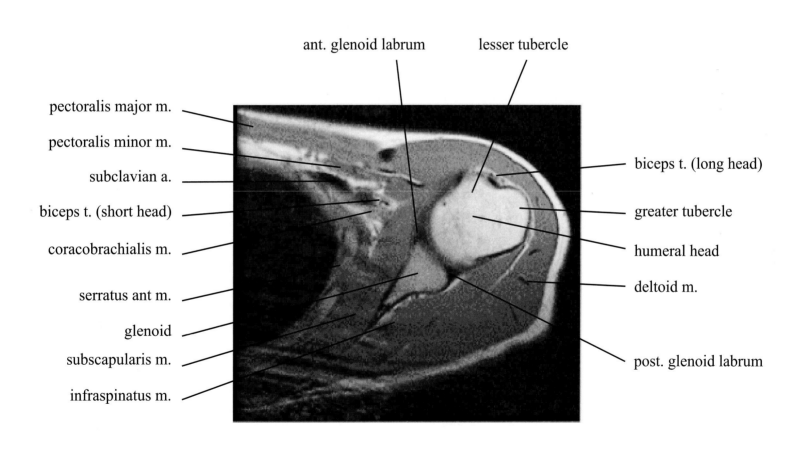

ant. glenoid labrum

lesser tubercle

pectoralis major m.

pectoralis minor m.

subclavian a.

biceps t. (short head)

coracobrachialis m.

serratus ant m.

glenoid

subscapularis m.

infraspinatus m.

biceps t. (long head)

greater tubercle

humeral head

deltoid m.

post. glenoid labrum

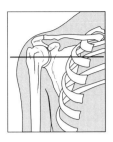

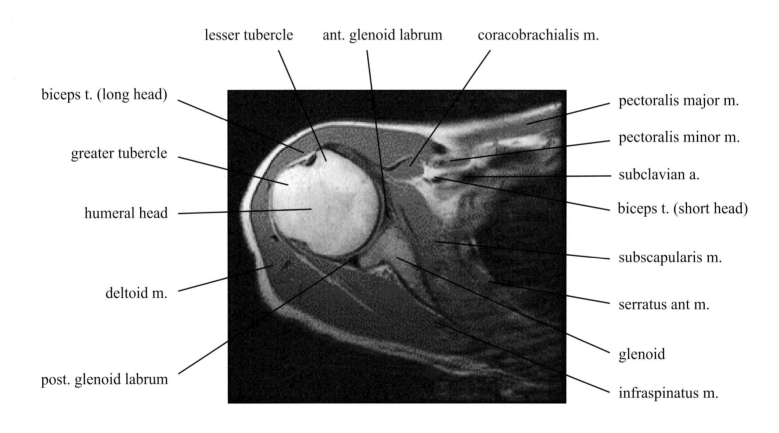

lesser tubercle   ant. glenoid labrum   coracobrachialis m.

biceps t. (long head)

greater tubercle

humeral head

deltoid m.

post. glenoid labrum

pectoralis major m.

pectoralis minor m.

subclavian a.

biceps t. (short head)

subscapularis m.

serratus ant m.

glenoid

infraspinatus m.

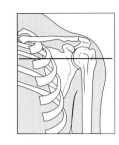

coracobrachialis m.   ant. glenoid labrum   lesser tubercle

pectoralis major m.

pectoralis minor m.

subclavian a.

biceps t. (short head)

subscapularis m.

serratus ant m.

glenoid

infraspinatus m.

biceps t. (long head)

greater tubercle

humeral head

deltoid m.

post. glenoid labrum

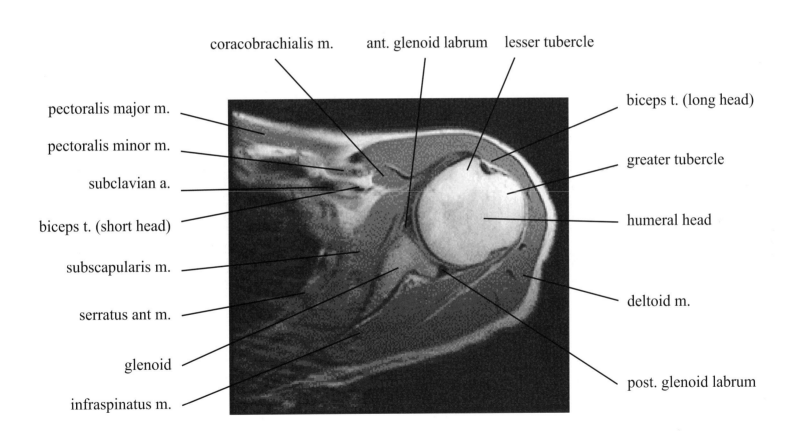

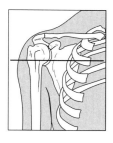

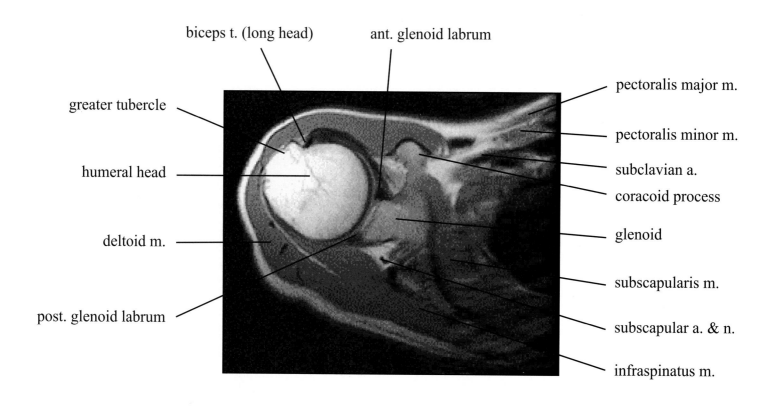

biceps t. (long head)

ant. glenoid labrum

pectoralis major m.

greater tubercle

pectoralis minor m.

humeral head

subclavian a.

coracoid process

deltoid m.

glenoid

subscapularis m.

post. glenoid labrum

subscapular a. & n.

infraspinatus m.

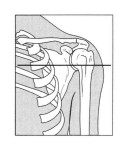

ant. glenoid labrum   biceps t. (long head)

pectoralis major m.

pectoralis minor m.

subclavian a.

coracoid process

glenoid

subscapularis m.

subscapular a. & n.

infraspinatus m.

greater tubercle

humeral head

deltoid m.

post. glenoid labrum

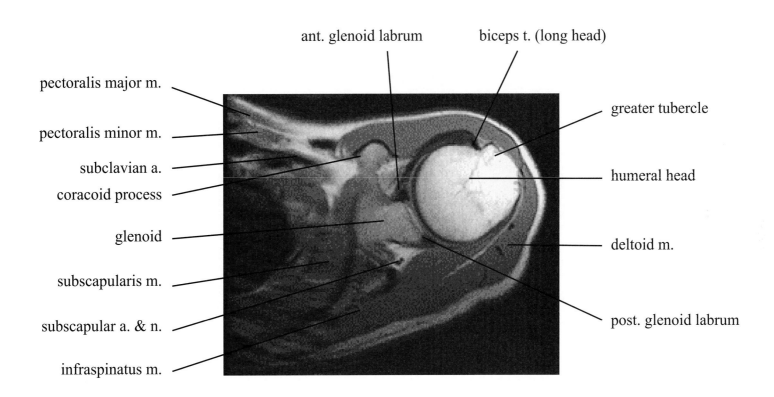

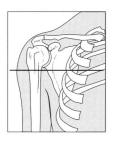

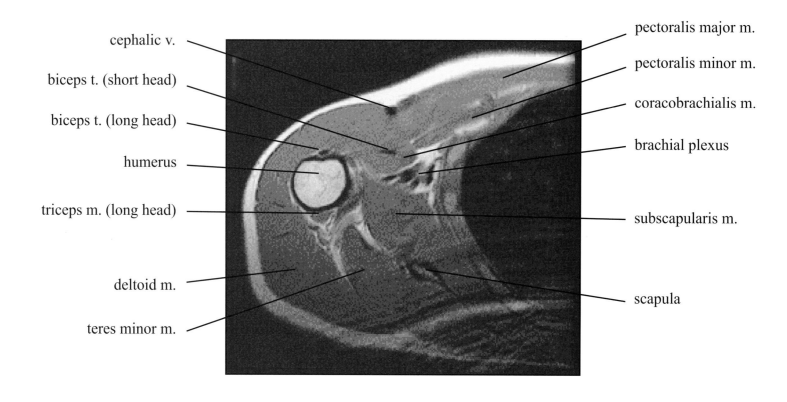

cephalic v.

biceps t. (short head)

biceps t. (long head)

humerus

triceps m. (long head)

deltoid m.

teres minor m.

pectoralis major m.

pectoralis minor m.

coracobrachialis m.

brachial plexus

subscapularis m.

scapula

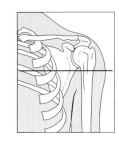

pectoralis major m.

pectoralis minor m.

coracobrachialis m.

brachial plexus

subscapularis m.

scapula

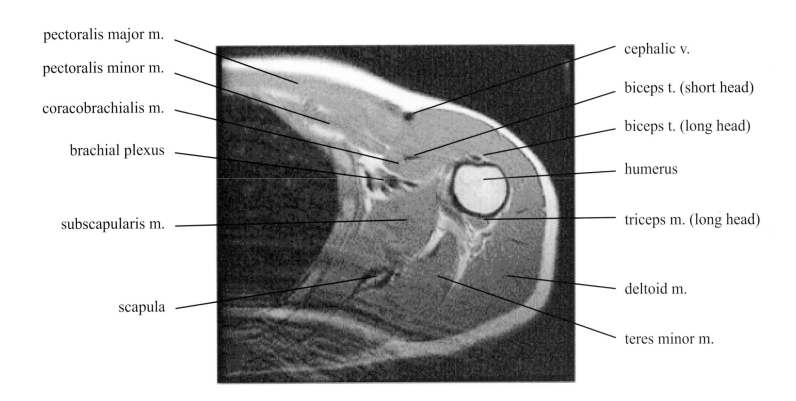

cephalic v.

biceps t. (short head)

biceps t. (long head)

humerus

triceps m. (long head)

deltoid m.

teres minor m.

THE SHOULDER:
OBLIQUE SAGITTAL ANATOMY

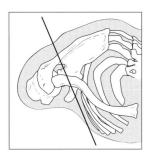

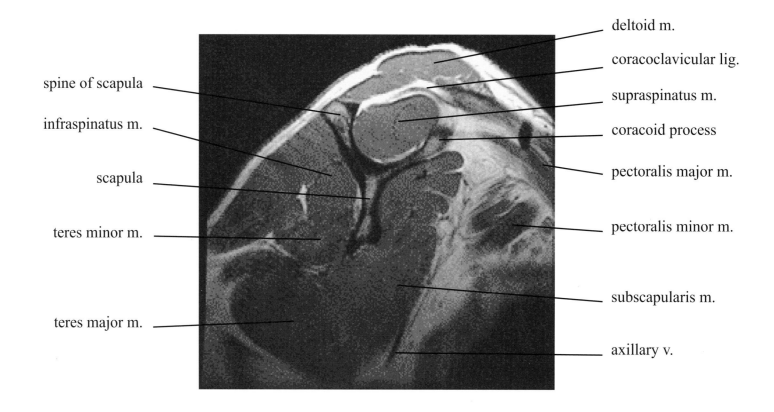

spine of scapula

infraspinatus m.

scapula

teres minor m.

teres major m.

deltoid m.

coracoclavicular lig.

supraspinatus m.

coracoid process

pectoralis major m.

pectoralis minor m.

subscapularis m.

axillary v.

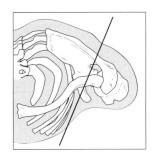

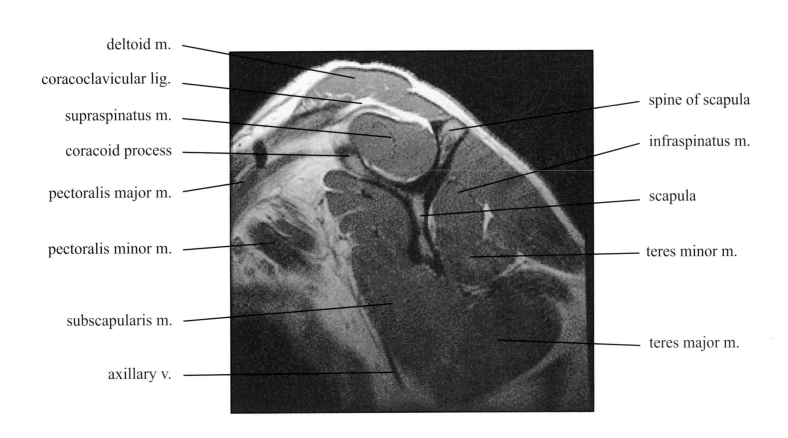

deltoid m.

coracoclavicular lig.

supraspinatus m.

coracoid process

pectoralis major m.

pectoralis minor m.

subscapularis m.

axillary v.

spine of scapula

infraspinatus m.

scapula

teres minor m.

teres major m.

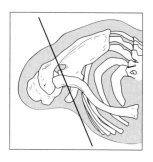

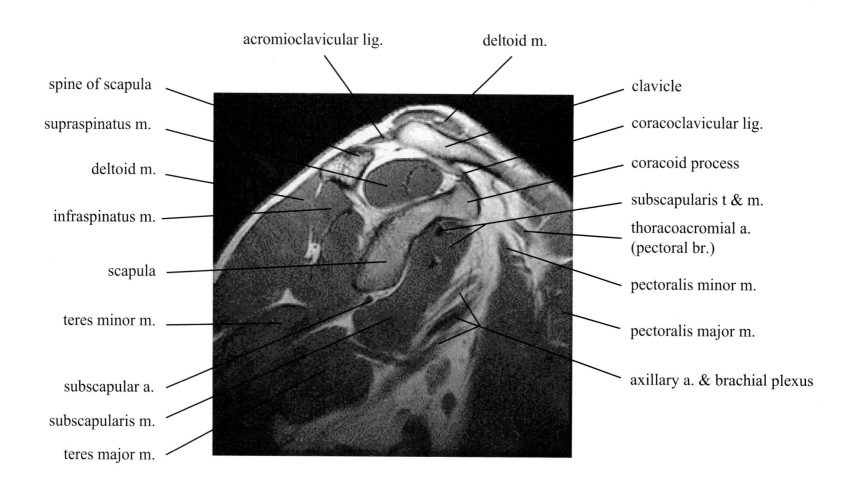

acromioclavicular lig.

deltoid m.

spine of scapula

clavicle

supraspinatus m.

coracoclavicular lig.

deltoid m.

coracoid process

infraspinatus m.

subscapularis t & m.

thoracoacromial a.
(pectoral br.)

scapula

pectoralis minor m.

teres minor m.

pectoralis major m.

subscapular a.

axillary a. & brachial plexus

subscapularis m.

teres major m.

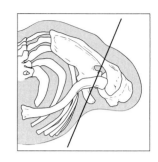

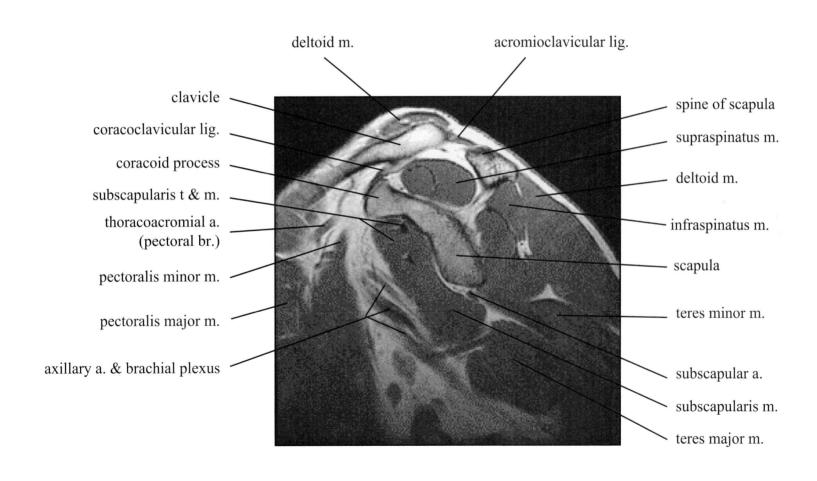

deltoid m.

acromioclavicular lig.

clavicle

coracoclavicular lig.

coracoid process

subscapularis t & m.

thoracoacromial a.
(pectoral br.)

pectoralis minor m.

pectoralis major m.

axillary a. & brachial plexus

spine of scapula

supraspinatus m.

deltoid m.

infraspinatus m.

scapula

teres minor m.

subscapular a.

subscapularis m.

teres major m.

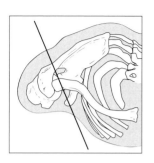

acromioclavicular lig.   clavicle   coracoclavicular lig.

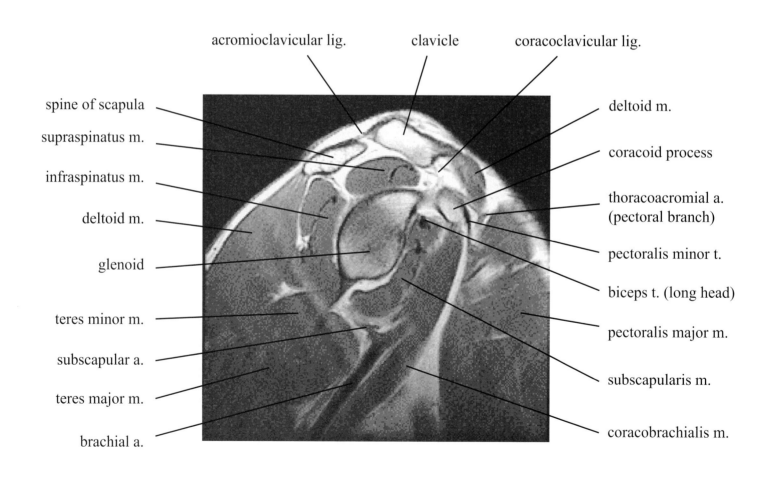

spine of scapula

supraspinatus m.

infraspinatus m.

deltoid m.

glenoid

teres minor m.

subscapular a.

teres major m.

brachial a.

deltoid m.

coracoid process

thoracoacromial a.
(pectoral branch)

pectoralis minor t.

biceps t. (long head)

pectoralis major m.

subscapularis m.

coracobrachialis m.

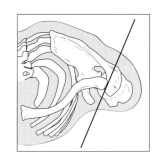

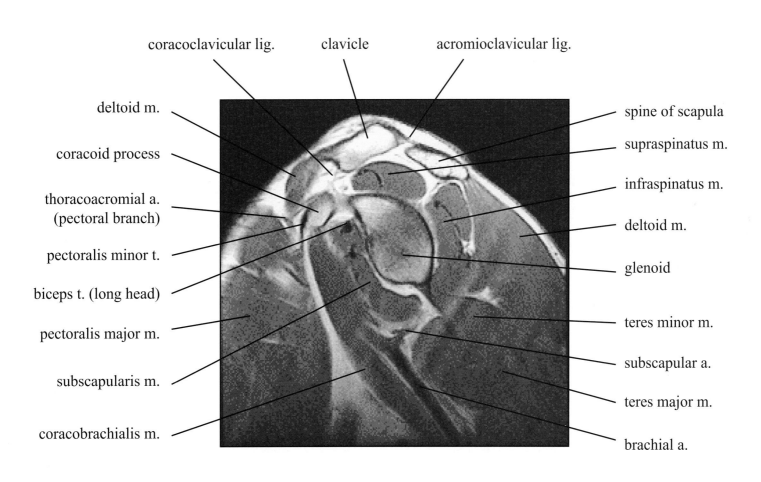

coracoclavicular lig.   clavicle   acromioclavicular lig.

deltoid m.

coracoid process

thoracoacromial a.
(pectoral branch)

pectoralis minor t.

biceps t. (long head)

pectoralis major m.

subscapularis m.

coracobrachialis m.

spine of scapula

supraspinatus m.

infraspinatus m.

deltoid m.

glenoid

teres minor m.

subscapular a.

teres major m.

brachial a.

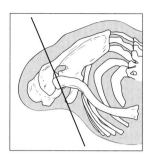

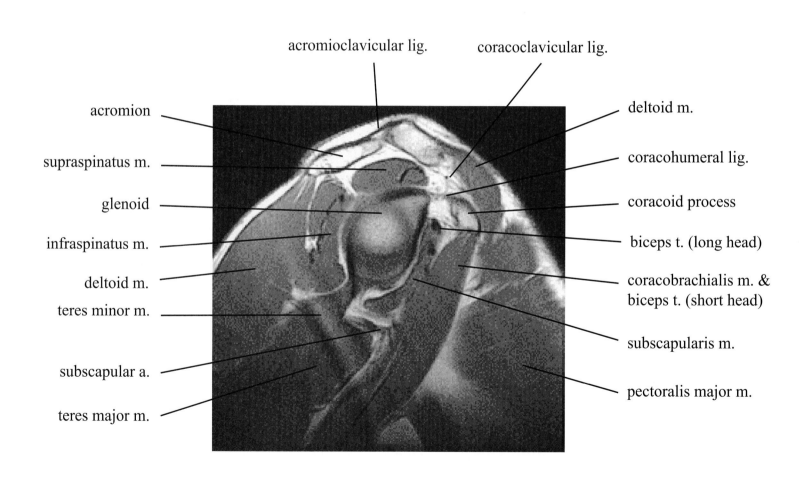

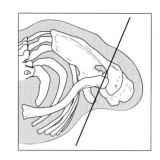

coracoclavicular lig.   acromioclavicular lig.

deltoid m.

coracohumeral lig.

coracoid process

biceps t. (long head)

coracobrachialis m. &
biceps t. (short head)

subscapularis m.

pectoralis major m.

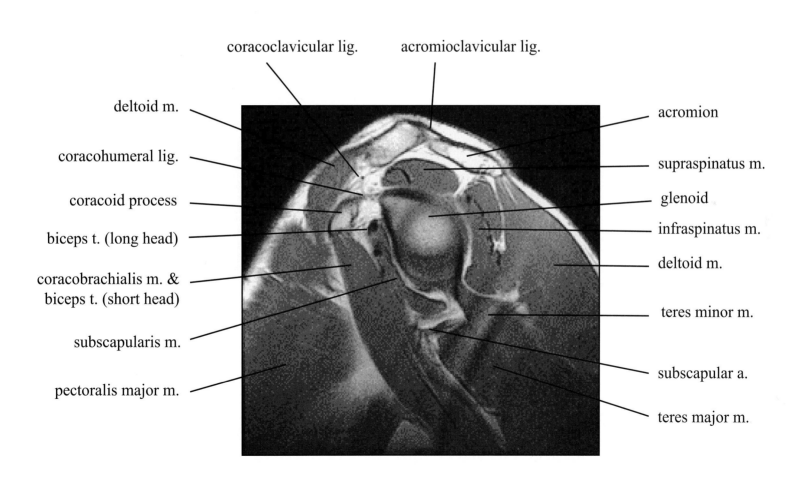

acromion

supraspinatus m.

glenoid

infraspinatus m.

deltoid m.

teres minor m.

subscapular a.

teres major m.

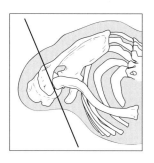

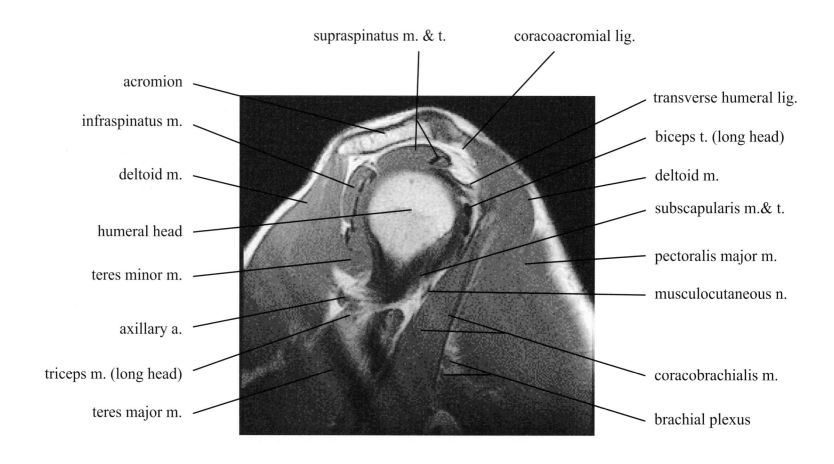

supraspinatus m. & t.

coracoacromial lig.

acromion

infraspinatus m.

deltoid m.

humeral head

teres minor m.

axillary a.

triceps m. (long head)

teres major m.

transverse humeral lig.

biceps t. (long head)

deltoid m.

subscapularis m.& t.

pectoralis major m.

musculocutaneous n.

coracobrachialis m.

brachial plexus

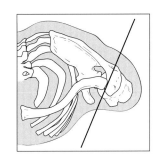

coracoacromial lig.

supraspinatus m. & t.

transverse humeral lig.

acromion

biceps t. (long head)

infraspinatus m.

deltoid m.

deltoid m.

subscapularis m.& t.

humeral head

pectoralis major m.

teres minor m.

musculocutaneous n.

axillary a.

coracobrachialis m.

triceps m. (long head)

brachial plexus

teres major m.

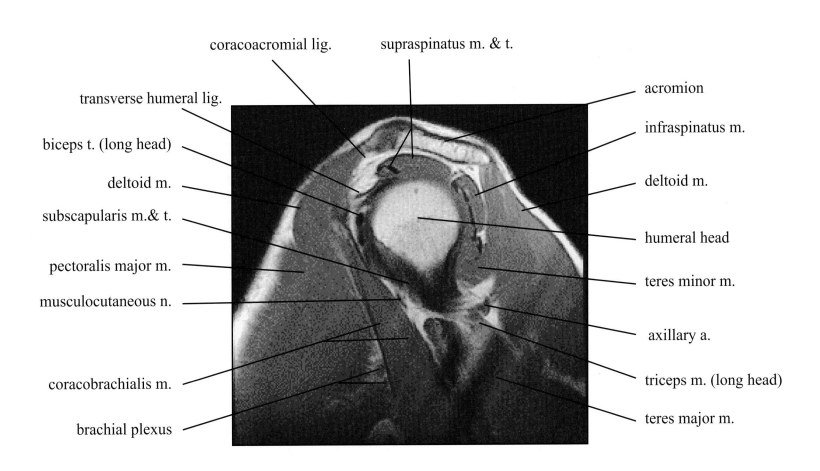

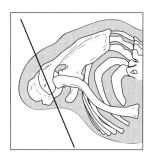

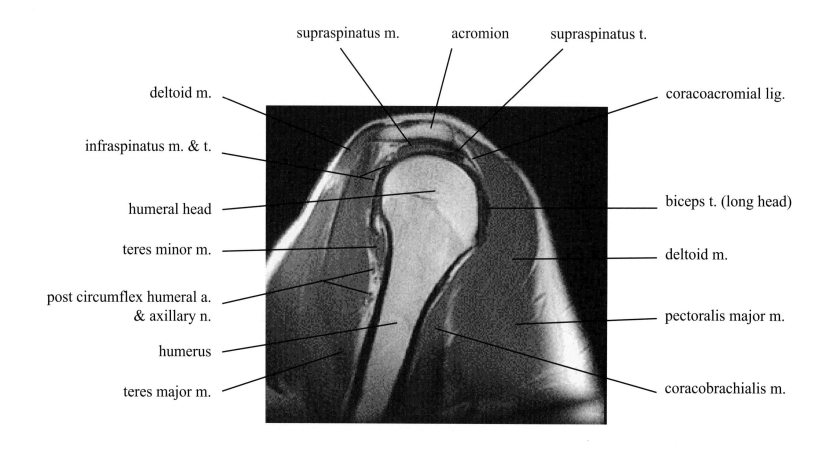

supraspinatus m.   acromion   supraspinatus t.

deltoid m.

coracoacromial lig.

infraspinatus m. & t.

humeral head

biceps t. (long head)

teres minor m.

deltoid m.

post circumflex humeral a.
& axillary n.

pectoralis major m.

humerus

teres major m.

coracobrachialis m.

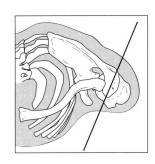

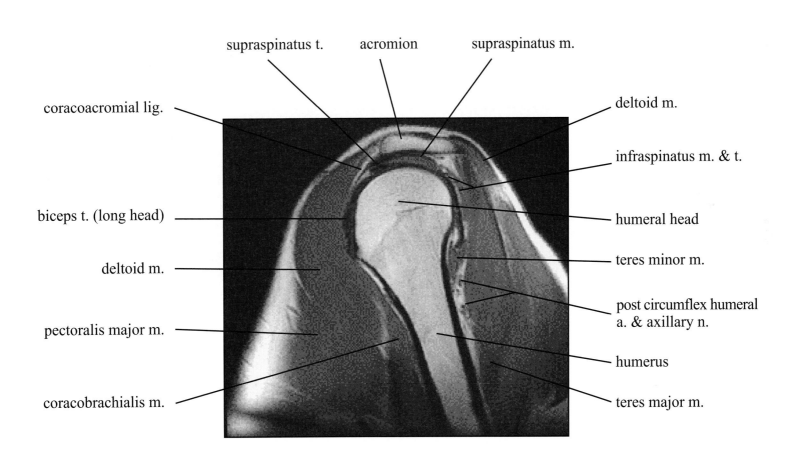

supraspinatus t.

acromion

supraspinatus m.

coracoacromial lig.

deltoid m.

infraspinatus m. & t.

biceps t. (long head)

humeral head

deltoid m.

teres minor m.

post circumflex humeral a. & axillary n.

pectoralis major m.

humerus

coracobrachialis m.

teres major m.

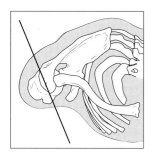

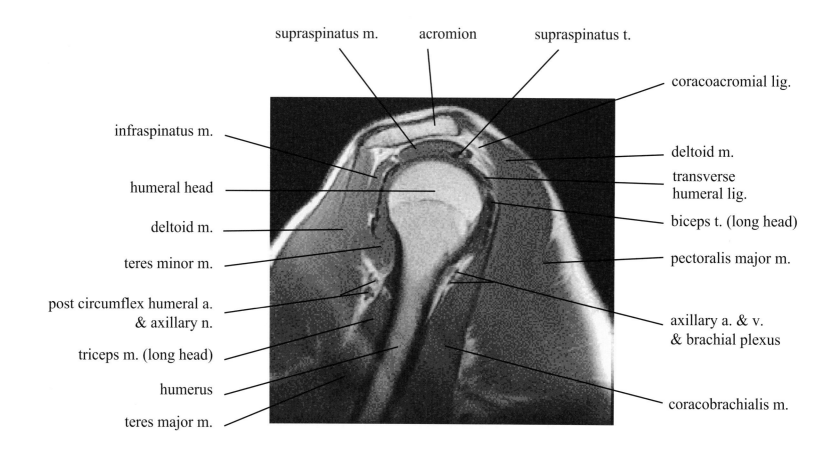

supraspinatus m.   acromion   supraspinatus t.

coracoacromial lig.

infraspinatus m.

deltoid m.

transverse
humeral lig.

humeral head

biceps t. (long head)

deltoid m.

pectoralis major m.

teres minor m.

post circumflex humeral a.
& axillary n.

axillary a. & v.
& brachial plexus

triceps m. (long head)

humerus

coracobrachialis m.

teres major m.

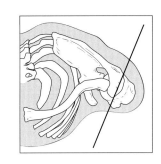

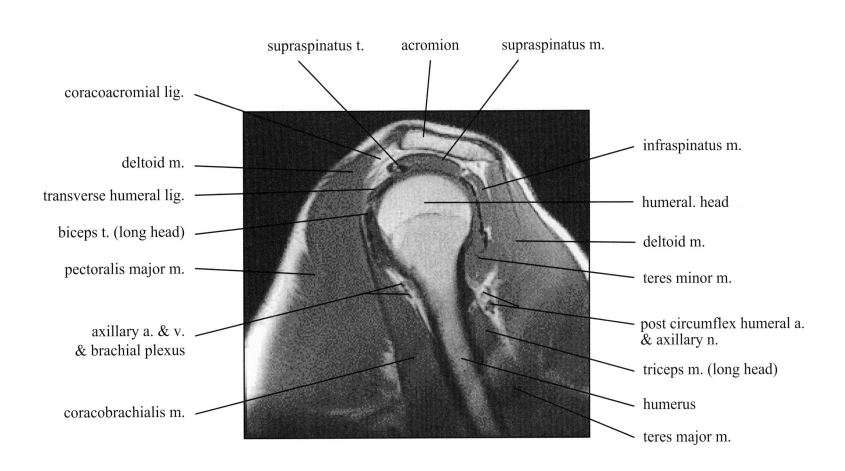

supraspinatus t.   acromion   supraspinatus m.

coracoacromial lig.

infraspinatus m.

deltoid m.

transverse humeral lig.

humeral. head

biceps t. (long head)

deltoid m.

pectoralis major m.

teres minor m.

axillary a. & v.
& brachial plexus

post circumflex humeral a.
& axillary n.

triceps m. (long head)

humerus

coracobrachialis m.

teres major m.

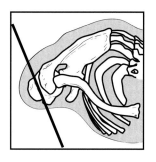

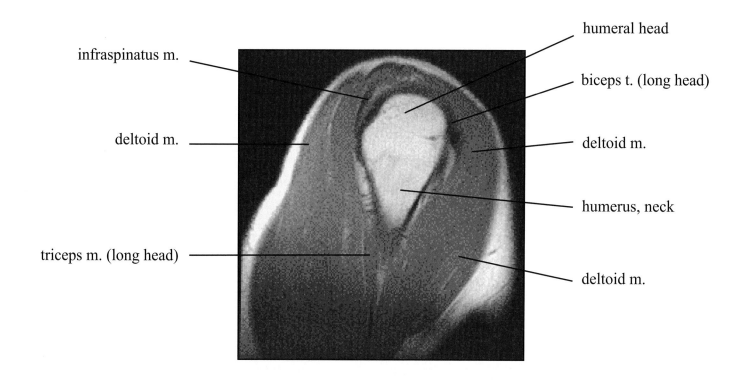

infraspinatus m.

humeral head

biceps t. (long head)

deltoid m.

deltoid m.

humerus, neck

triceps m. (long head)

deltoid m.

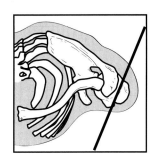

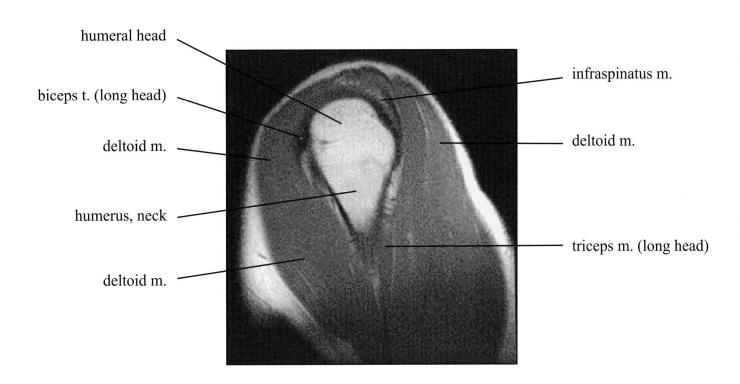

humeral head

biceps t. (long head)

deltoid m.

humerus, neck

deltoid m.

infraspinatus m.

deltoid m.

triceps m. (long head)

THE SHOULDER:
OBLIQUE CORONAL ANATOMY

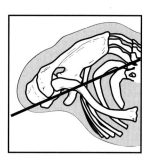

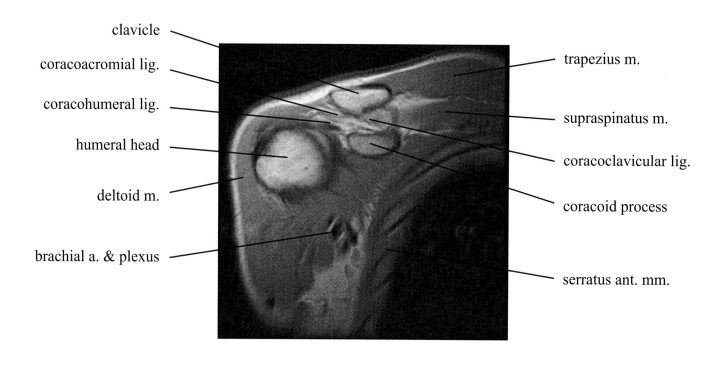

clavicle

coracoacromial lig.

coracohumeral lig.

humeral head

deltoid m.

brachial a. & plexus

trapezius m.

supraspinatus m.

coracoclavicular lig.

coracoid process

serratus ant. mm.

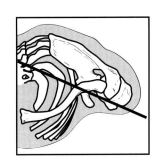

trapezius m.

clavicle

coracoacromial lig.

supraspinatus m.

coracohumeral lig.

coracoclavicular lig.

humeral head

coracoid process

deltoid m.

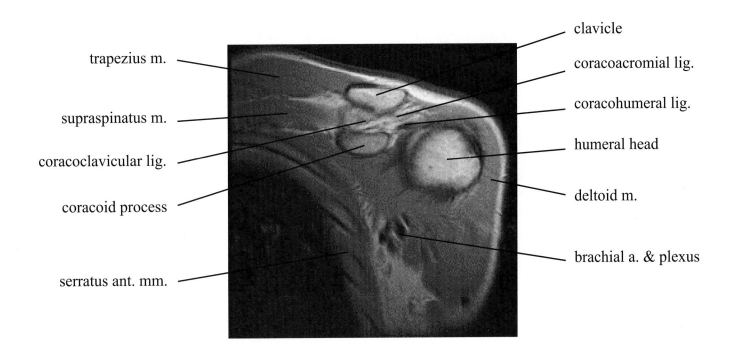

brachial a. & plexus

serratus ant. mm.

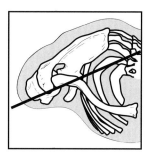

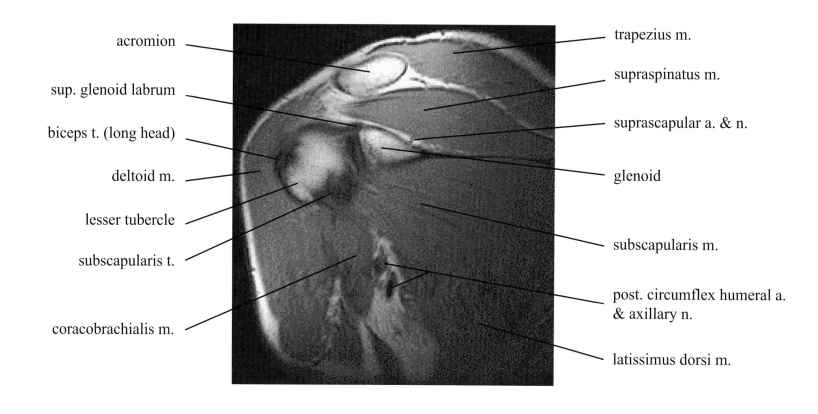

acromion

sup. glenoid labrum

biceps t. (long head)

deltoid m.

lesser tubercle

subscapularis t.

coracobrachialis m.

trapezius m.

supraspinatus m.

suprascapular a. & n.

glenoid

subscapularis m.

post. circumflex humeral a.
& axillary n.

latissimus dorsi m.

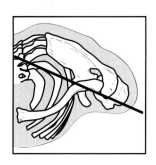

trapezius m.

supraspinatus m.

suprascapular a. & n.

glenoid

subscapularis m.

post. circumflex humeral a.
& axillary n.

latissimus dorsi m.

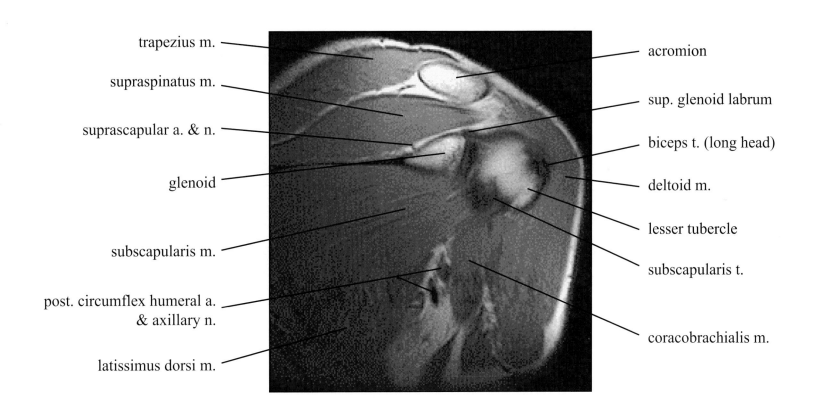

acromion

sup. glenoid labrum

biceps t. (long head)

deltoid m.

lesser tubercle

subscapularis t.

coracobrachialis m.

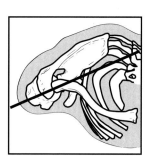

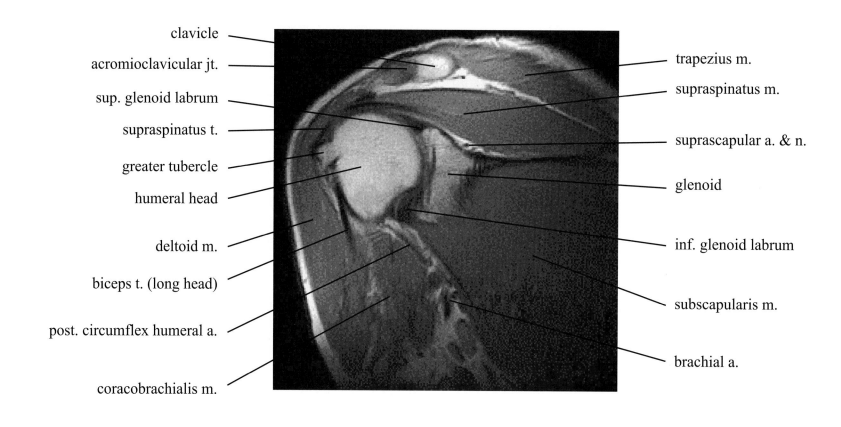

clavicle

acromioclavicular jt.

sup. glenoid labrum

supraspinatus t.

greater tubercle

humeral head

deltoid m.

biceps t. (long head)

post. circumflex humeral a.

coracobrachialis m.

trapezius m.

supraspinatus m.

suprascapular a. & n.

glenoid

inf. glenoid labrum

subscapularis m.

brachial a.

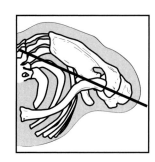

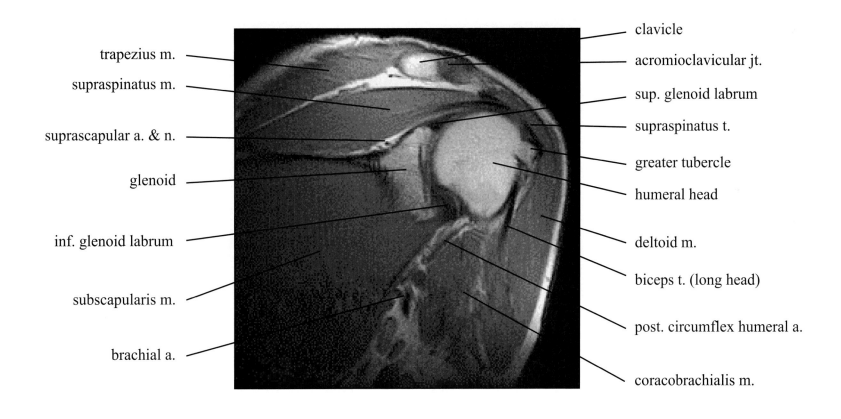

trapezius m.

supraspinatus m.

suprascapular a. & n.

glenoid

inf. glenoid labrum

subscapularis m.

brachial a.

clavicle

acromioclavicular jt.

sup. glenoid labrum

supraspinatus t.

greater tubercle

humeral head

deltoid m.

biceps t. (long head)

post. circumflex humeral a.

coracobrachialis m.

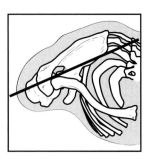

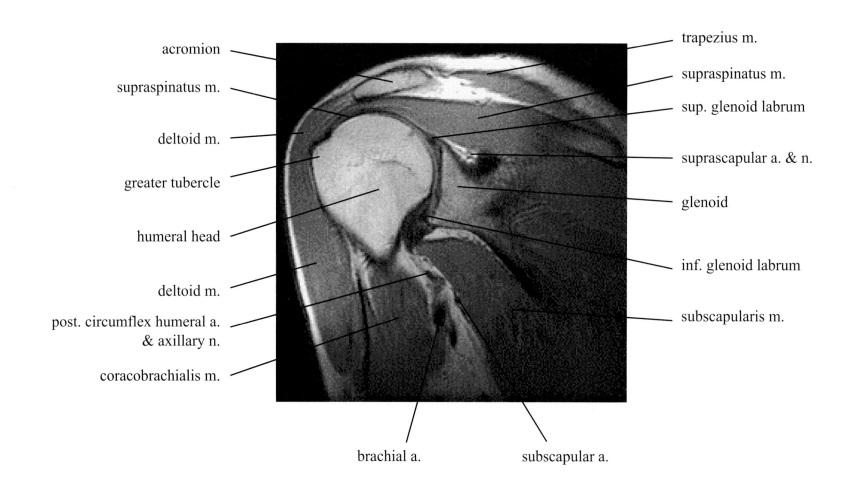

acromion

supraspinatus m.

deltoid m.

greater tubercle

humeral head

deltoid m.

post. circumflex humeral a.
& axillary n.

coracobrachialis m.

trapezius m.

supraspinatus m.

sup. glenoid labrum

suprascapular a. & n.

glenoid

inf. glenoid labrum

subscapularis m.

brachial a.   subscapular a.

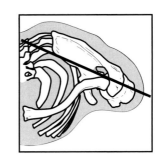

trapezius m.

supraspinatus m.

sup. glenoid labrum

suprascapular a. & n.

glenoid

inf. glenoid labrum

subscapularis m.

acromion

supraspinatus m.

deltoid m.

greater tubercle

humeral head

deltoid m.

post. circumflex humeral a. & axillary n.

coracobrachialis m.

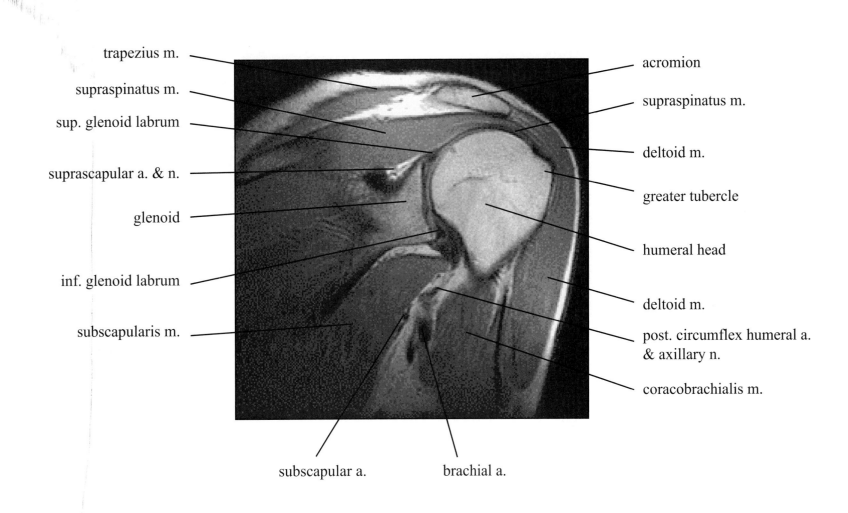

subscapular a.   brachial a.

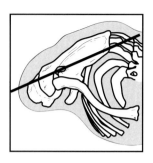

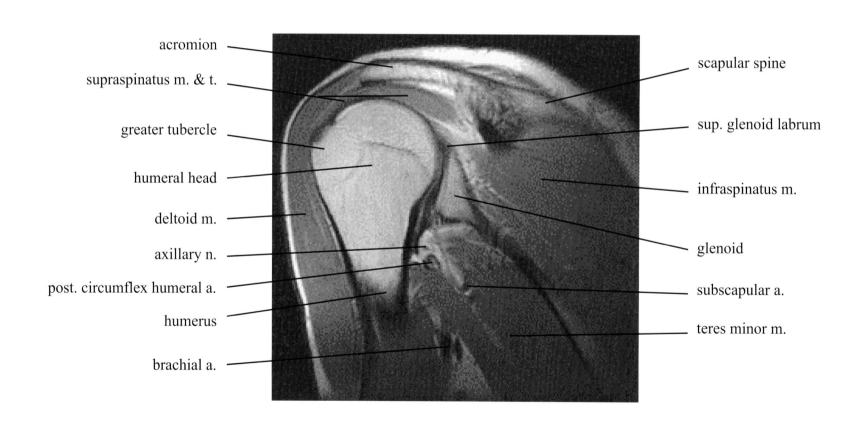

acromion

supraspinatus m. & t.

greater tubercle

humeral head

deltoid m.

axillary n.

post. circumflex humeral a.

humerus

brachial a.

scapular spine

sup. glenoid labrum

infraspinatus m.

glenoid

subscapular a.

teres minor m.

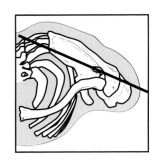

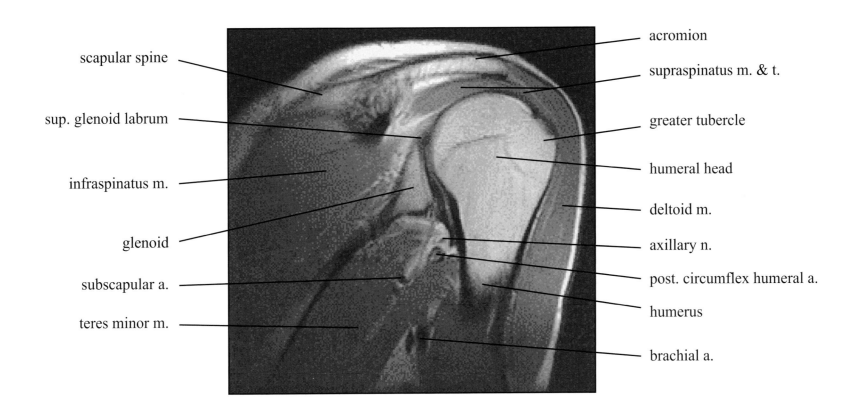

scapular spine

sup. glenoid labrum

infraspinatus m.

glenoid

subscapular a.

teres minor m.

acromion

supraspinatus m. & t.

greater tubercle

humeral head

deltoid m.

axillary n.

post. circumflex humeral a.

humerus

brachial a.

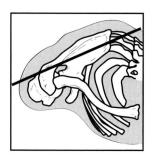

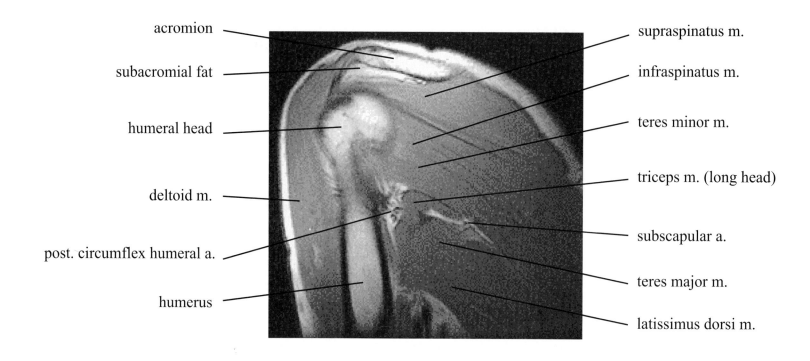

acromion

subacromial fat

humeral head

deltoid m.

post. circumflex humeral a.

humerus

supraspinatus m.

infraspinatus m.

teres minor m.

triceps m. (long head)

subscapular a.

teres major m.

latissimus dorsi m.

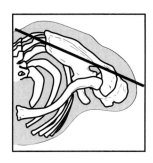

supraspinatus m.

infraspinatus m.

teres minor m.

triceps m. (long head)

subscapular a.

teres major m.

latissimus dorsi m.

acromion

subacromial fat

humeral head

deltoid m.

post. circumflex humeral a.

humerus

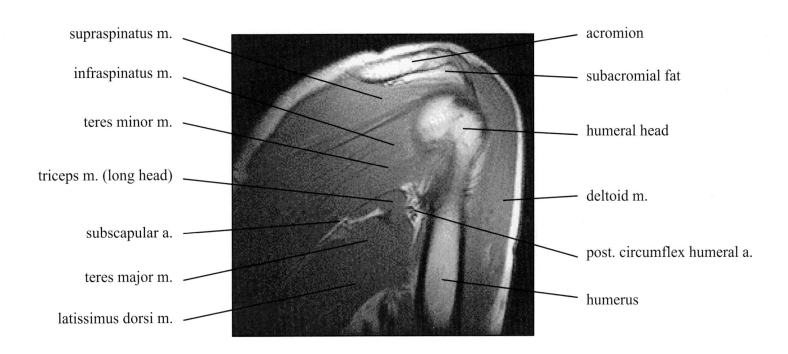

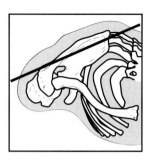

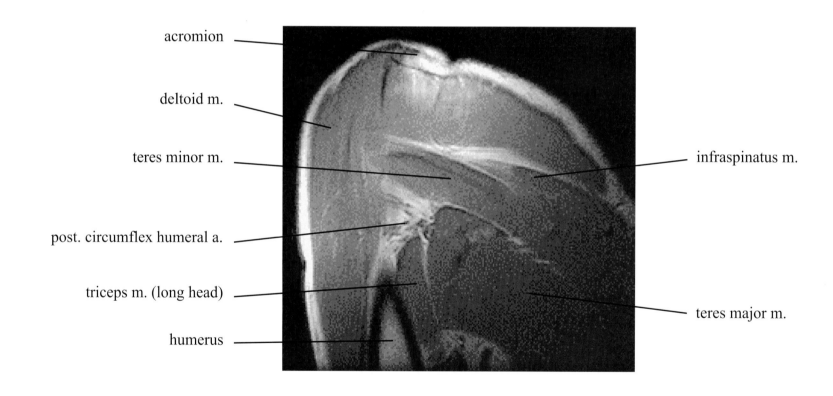

acromion

deltoid m.

teres minor m.

infraspinatus m.

post. circumflex humeral a.

triceps m. (long head)

teres major m.

humerus

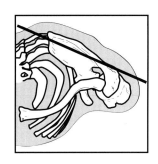

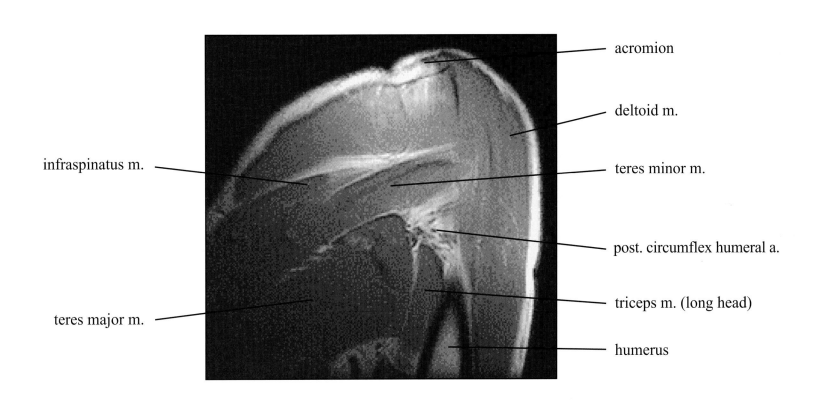

acromion

deltoid m.

infraspinatus m.

teres minor m.

post. circumflex humeral a.

teres major m.

triceps m. (long head)

humerus

B. THE UPPER EXTREMITY

The major indications for MR imaging of the upper arm include suspected metastatic disease, avascular necrosis, infection, and primary soft-tissue tumors. Generally, these studies are monitored while the patient is in the scanner, and the images are approved before the patient leaves the MR imaging suite.

PRACTICAL PROTOCOL CONSIDERATIONS

For an MR imaging examination of the upper arm, the patient is placed in a comfortable supine position. If there is a palpable abnormality or surgical scar, or if a suspicious area is identified during physical examination, a bath oil bead or vitamin E tablet is placed at the site. For a surgical site, both the proximal and distal ends of the scar should be marked with the bead or tablet.

Whether a body or surface coil is used depends on the clinical indication for the study. In general, sagittal, coronal, and axial planes are used. The axial plane is the most important of these because it shows the relationship of any abnormality to the neurovascular bundle and other vital structures best.

Menu of Protocols: Upper Arm

Plane	Pulse Sequence	FA (degrees)	TR (msec)	TE (msec)	TI (msec)	FOV (cm)	Matrix (256X-)	ST/G (mm)	NEX	Comments
Localizer (transaxial)	SE		500	min		VAR	128	4/	1	Mark area of concern
Coronal, sagittal	SE		500	min		VAR	192	5/1.5	2	
Coronal	SE		1,000	min		VAR	192	5/1.5	2	
Coronal	FMPIR		2,500	30	150	VAR	128	5/1.5	2	
Sagittal	SE		1,000	min		VAR	192	5/1.5	2	
Sagittal	FMPIR		2,500	30	150	VAR	128	5/1.5	2	
Axial	SE, double echo, FS		3,000	19/90		VAR	192	4/1	2	
Axial, pre-GAD	SE		600	20		VAR	192	4/1	2	Repeat after GAD
Axial, pre-GAD	SE, FS		600	20		VAR	192	4/1	2	Repeat after GAD

MAJOR OSTEOCHONDRAL STRUCTURES/LANDMARKS

(See Glenohumeral Joint and Elbow)

MAJOR LIGAMENTS/TENDONS/BURSAE

(See Glenohumeral Joint and Elbow)

MAJOR MUSCLES

Compartments

The muscles of the upper arm are divided into an anterior group and a posterior group.
- Anterior compartment
  - Coracobrachialis
  - Biceps brachii
    - Long head
    - Short head
  - Brachialis
- Posterior compartment
  - Triceps brachii
    - Long head
    - Medial head
    - Lateral head
  - Anconeus

ORIGIN/INSERTION/INNERVATION OF MAJOR MUSCLES

Muscle	Origin	Insertion	Innervation
Anterior Compartment			
–Coracobrachialis	Tip of coracoid process in common with short head of biceps brachii muscle	Medial surface of humerus just proximal to its mid-portion	Musculocutaneous N.
–Biceps brachii, long head	Supraglenoid tubercle of scapula	After union with short head, into radial tuberosity	Median N.

(continued)

ORIGIN/INSERTION/INNERVATION OF MAJOR MUSCLES (*CONTINUED*)

Muscle	Origin	Insertion	Innervation
–Biceps brachii, short head	Tip of coracoid process in common with coracobrachialis muscle	After union with long head, into radial tuberosity	Median N.
–Brachialis	Lower half of anterior humeral surface and two intermuscular septae	Tuberosity of ulna and anterior surface of coronoid process	Median N.
Posterior compartment			
–Triceps brachii, long head	Infraglenoid tubercle of humerus	Joins lateral and medial heads in a common insertion on posterior aspect of olecranon and deep fascia of upper arm	Radial N.
–Triceps brachii, lateral head	Posterior surface and lateral border of humerus above and lateral to radial groove, lateral intermuscular septum	Joins long and medial heads in a common insertion	Radial N.

(continued)

ORIGIN/INSERTION/INNERVATION OF MAJOR MUSCLES (*CONTINUED*)

Muscle	Origin	Insertion	Innervation
–Triceps brachii, medial head	Humerus medial and below radial groove and as high as insertion of teres major muscle to as low as humeral olecranon fascia, entire aspect of medial intermuscular septum	Joins lateral and long heads in a common insertion	Radial N. (Branches of ulnar N.)
–Anconeus	Lateral epicondyle of humerus	The side of olecranon and one-fourth of posterior surface of ulna	Radial N.

THE UPPER EXTREMITY: AXIAL ANATOMY

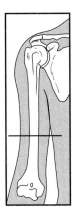

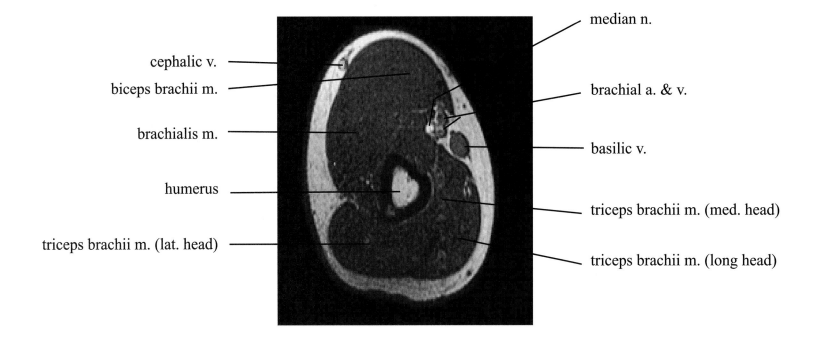

cephalic v.

biceps brachii m.

brachialis m.

humerus

triceps brachii m. (lat. head)

median n.

brachial a. & v.

basilic v.

triceps brachii m. (med. head)

triceps brachii m. (long head)

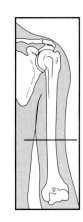

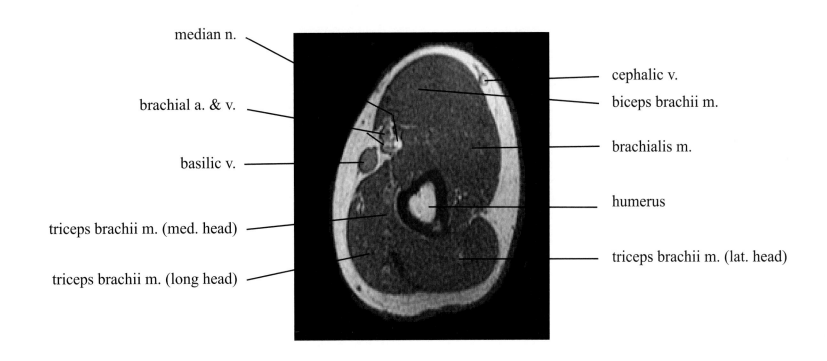

median n.

cephalic v.

biceps brachii m.

brachial a. & v.

brachialis m.

basilic v.

humerus

triceps brachii m. (med. head)

triceps brachii m. (lat. head)

triceps brachii m. (long head)

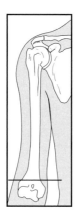

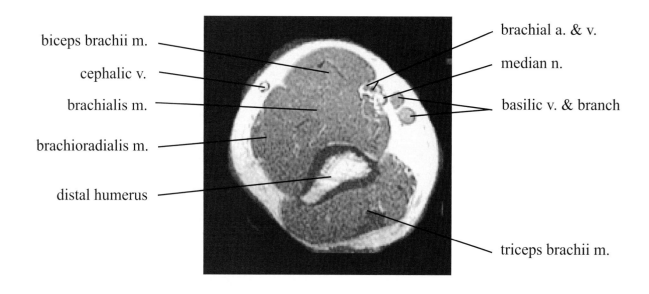

biceps brachii m.

cephalic v.

brachialis m.

brachioradialis m.

distal humerus

brachial a. & v.

median n.

basilic v. & branch

triceps brachii m.

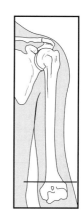

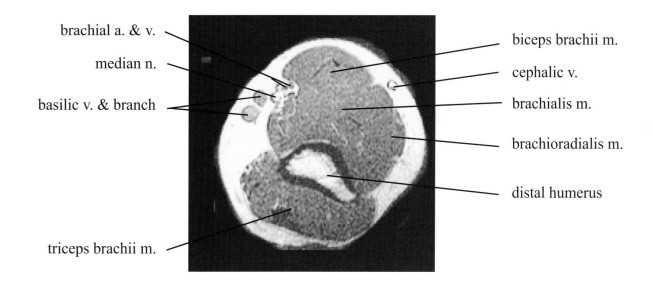

brachial a. & v.

median n.

basilic v. & branch

biceps brachii m.

cephalic v.

brachialis m.

brachioradialis m.

distal humerus

triceps brachii m.

THE UPPER EXTREMITY: SAGITTAL ANATOMY

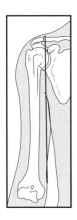

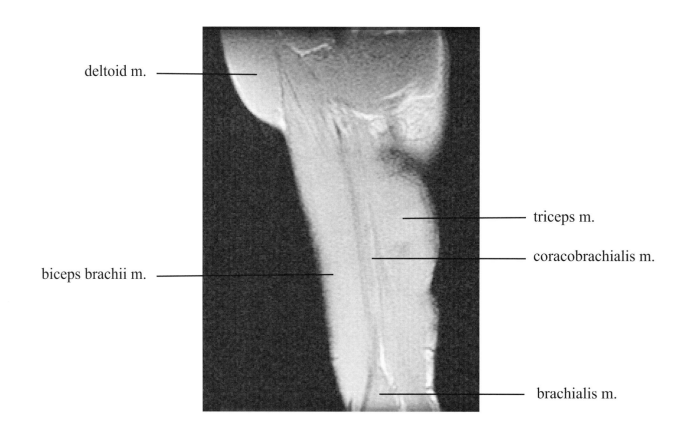

deltoid m. ————

triceps m.

coracobrachialis m.

biceps brachii m. ————

brachialis m.

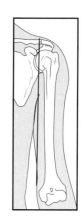

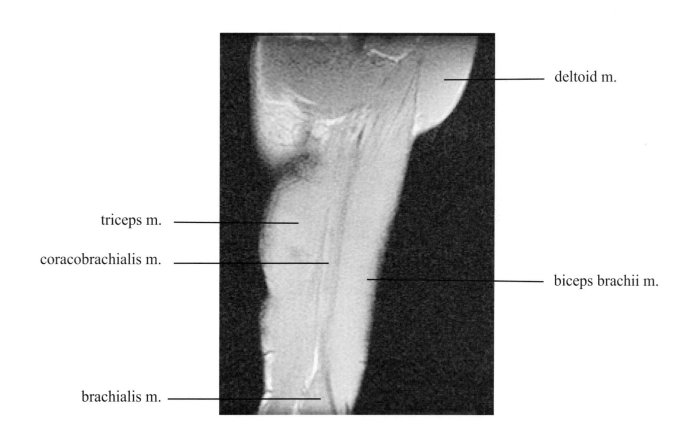

deltoid m.

triceps m.

coracobrachialis m.

biceps brachii m.

brachialis m.

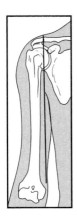

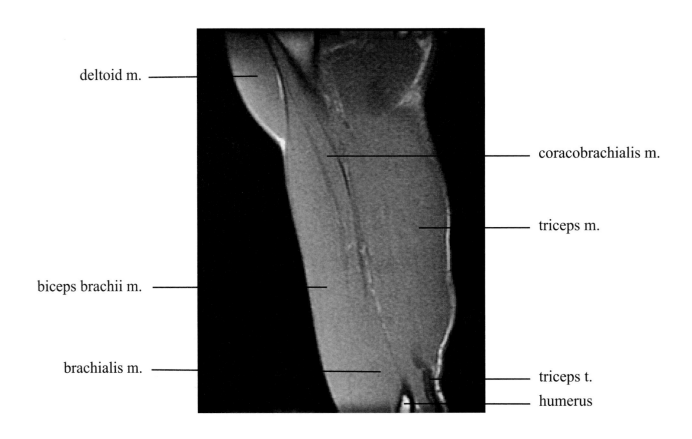

deltoid m. ——

—— coracobrachialis m.

—— triceps m.

biceps brachii m. ——

brachialis m. ——

—— triceps t.

—— humerus

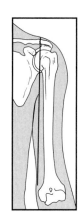

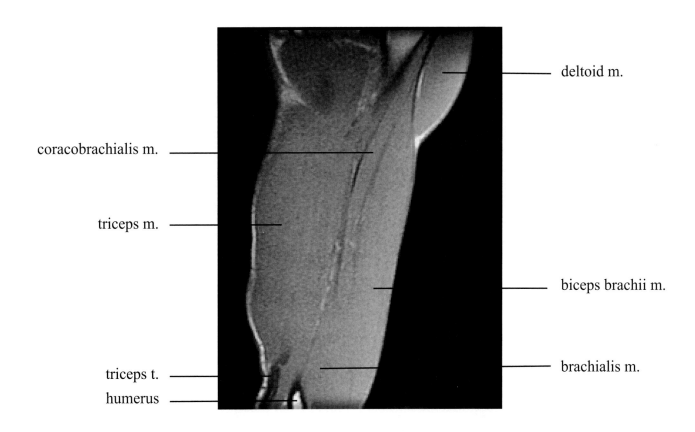

deltoid m.

coracobrachialis m.

triceps m.

biceps brachii m.

brachialis m.

triceps t.

humerus

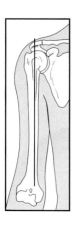

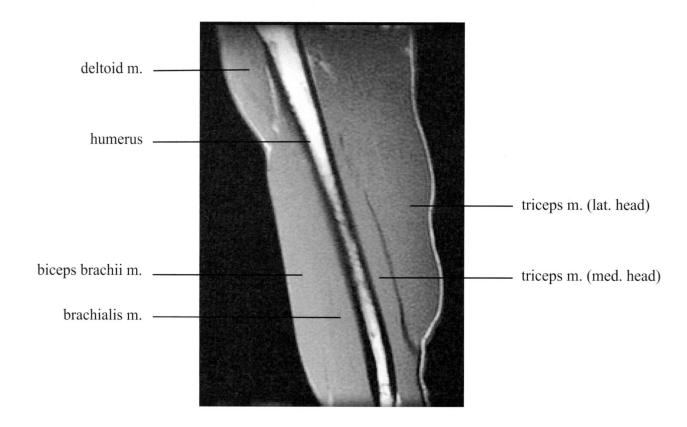

deltoid m.

humerus

biceps brachii m.

brachialis m.

triceps m. (lat. head)

triceps m. (med. head)

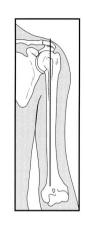

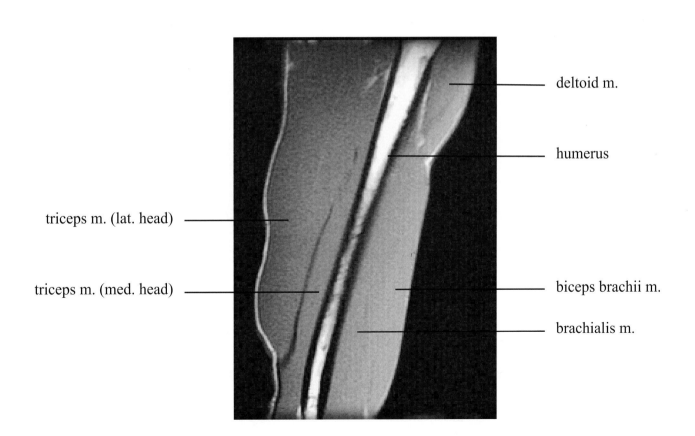

deltoid m.

humerus

triceps m. (lat. head)

triceps m. (med. head)

biceps brachii m.

brachialis m.

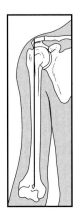

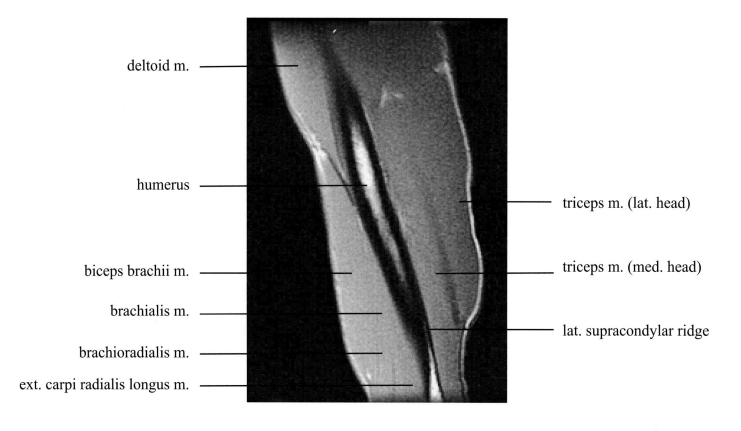

deltoid m. —

humerus —

biceps brachii m. —

brachialis m. —

brachioradialis m. —

ext. carpi radialis longus m. —

— triceps m. (lat. head)

— triceps m. (med. head)

— lat. supracondylar ridge

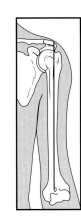

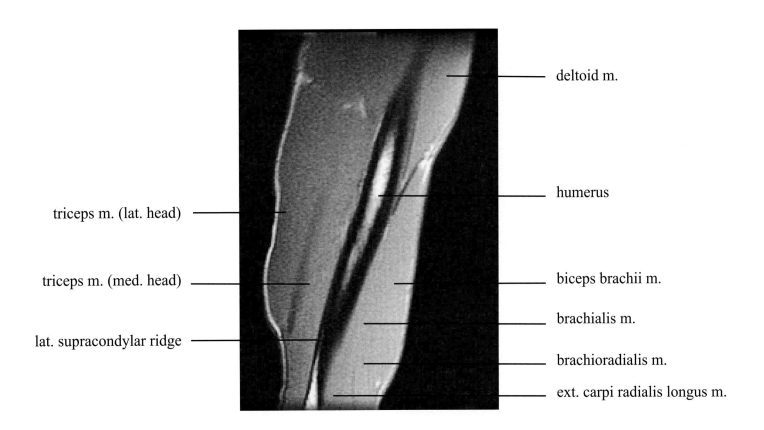

deltoid m.

humerus

triceps m. (lat. head)

triceps m. (med. head) — biceps brachii m.

brachialis m.

lat. supracondylar ridge — brachioradialis m.

ext. carpi radialis longus m.

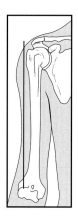

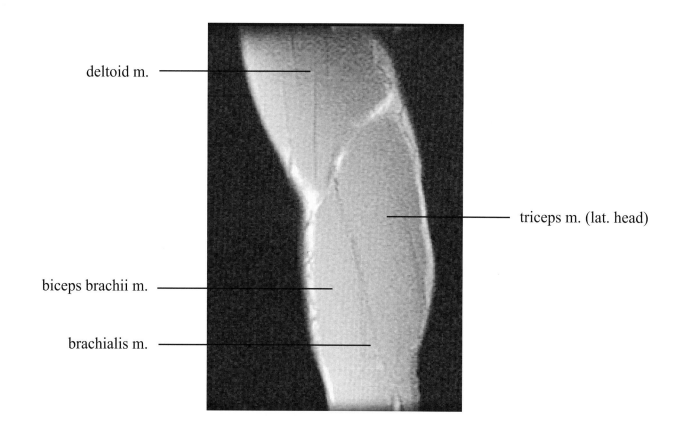

deltoid m. ———————————

triceps m. (lat. head)

biceps brachii m. ———————

brachialis m. ————————

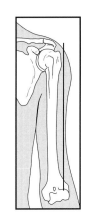

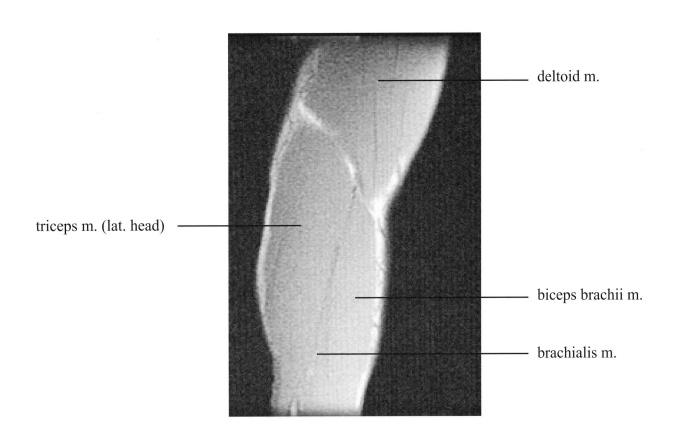

deltoid m.

triceps m. (lat. head)

biceps brachii m.

brachialis m.

THE UPPER EXTREMITY: CORONAL ANATOMY

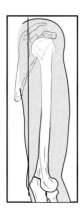

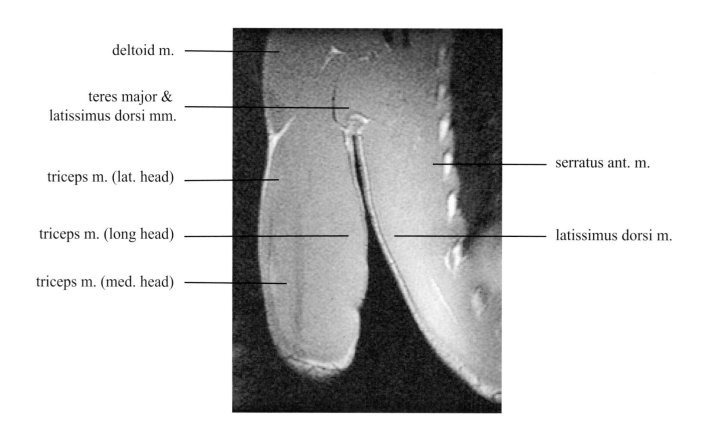

deltoid m.

teres major &
latissimus dorsi mm.

serratus ant. m.

triceps m. (lat. head)

triceps m. (long head)

latissimus dorsi m.

triceps m. (med. head)

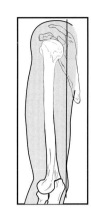

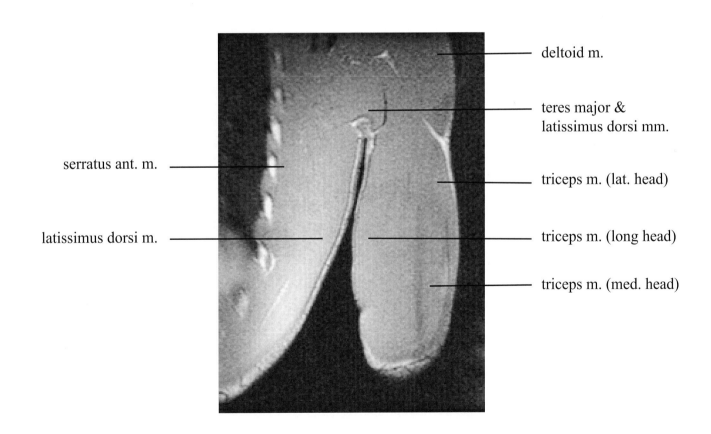

deltoid m.

teres major &
latissimus dorsi mm.

serratus ant. m.

triceps m. (lat. head)

latissimus dorsi m.

triceps m. (long head)

triceps m. (med. head)

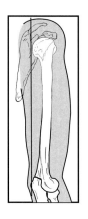

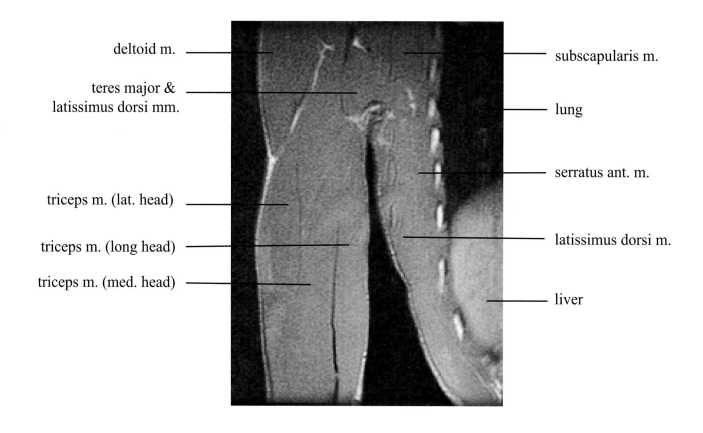

deltoid m. —————

teres major &
latissimus dorsi mm. —————

triceps m. (lat. head) —————

triceps m. (long head) —————

triceps m. (med. head) —————

————— subscapularis m.

————— lung

————— serratus ant. m.

————— latissimus dorsi m.

————— liver

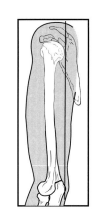

subscapularis m. ———

lung ———

serratus ant. m. ———

latissimus dorsi m. ———

liver ———

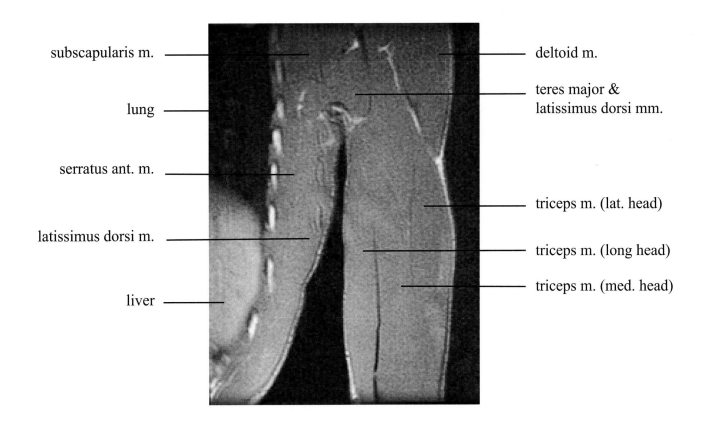

——— deltoid m.

——— teres major &
latissimus dorsi mm.

——— triceps m. (lat. head)

——— triceps m. (long head)

——— triceps m. (med. head)

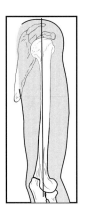

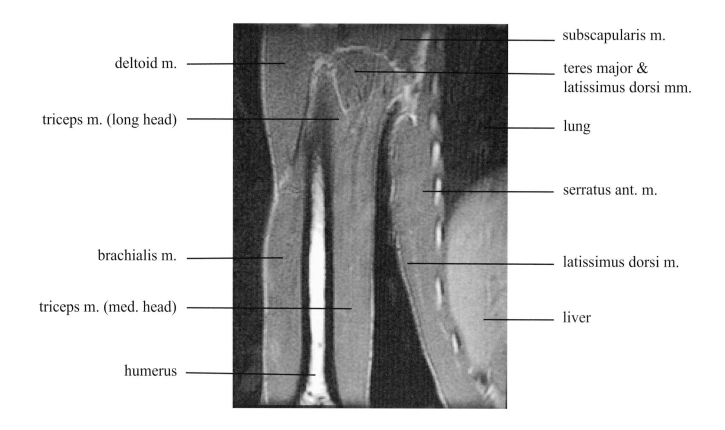

deltoid m.

triceps m. (long head)

brachialis m.

triceps m. (med. head)

humerus

subscapularis m.

teres major &
latissimus dorsi mm.

lung

serratus ant. m.

latissimus dorsi m.

liver

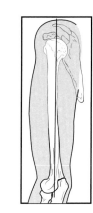

subscapularis m. —————————

teres major &
latissimus dorsi mm. —————

lung —————

serratus ant. m. —————

latissimus dorsi m. —————

liver —————

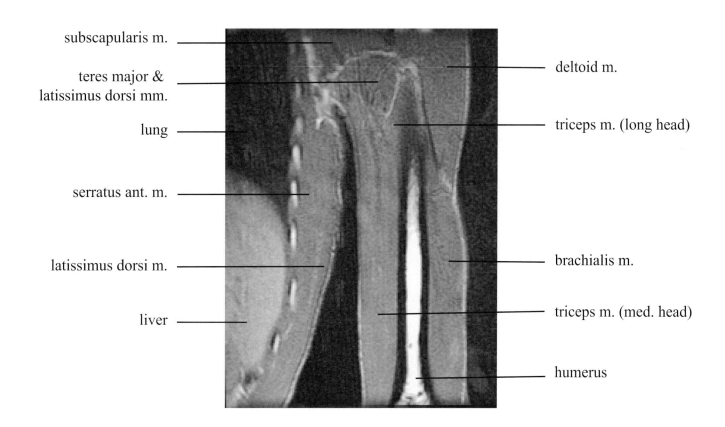

————— deltoid m.

————— triceps m. (long head)

————— brachialis m.

————— triceps m. (med. head)

————— humerus

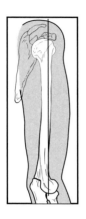

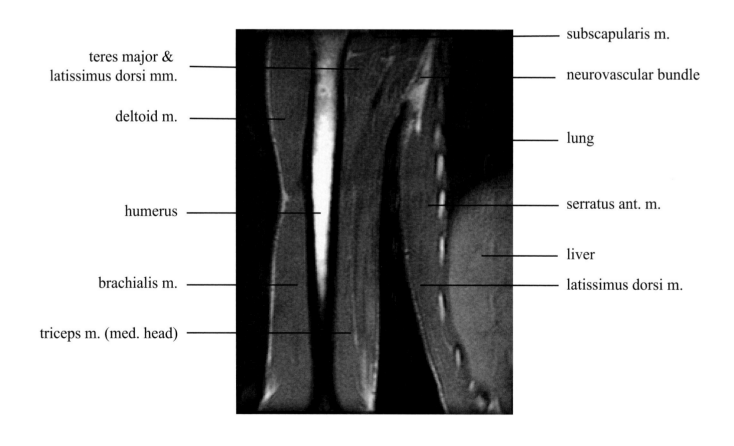

teres major &
latissimus dorsi mm.

deltoid m.

humerus

brachialis m.

triceps m. (med. head)

subscapularis m.

neurovascular bundle

lung

serratus ant. m.

liver

latissimus dorsi m.

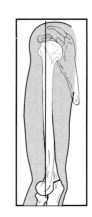

subscapularis m. ————

teres major &
latissimus dorsi mm.

neurovascular bundle ————

deltoid m.

lung ————

serratus ant. m. ————

humerus

liver ————

latissimus dorsi m. ————

brachialis m.

triceps m. (med. head)

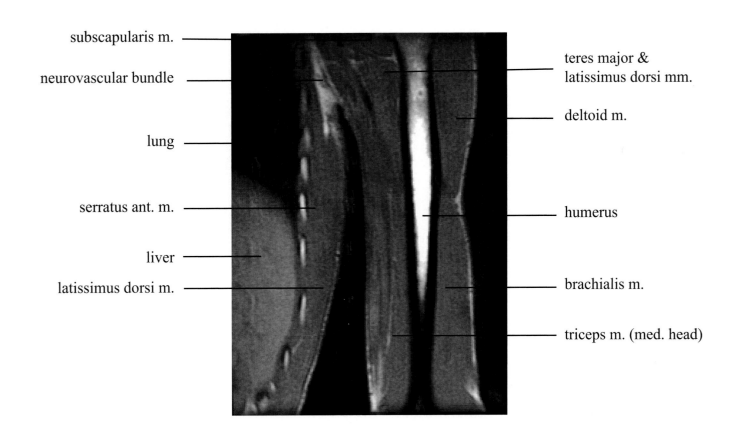

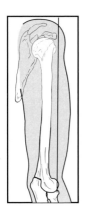

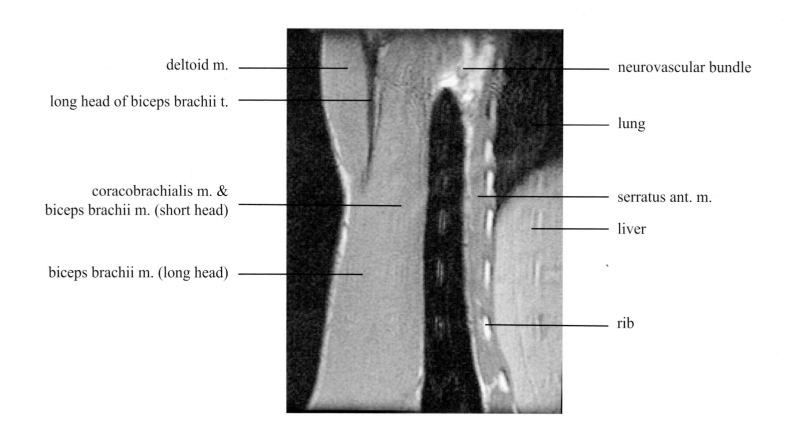

deltoid m.

long head of biceps brachii t.

coracobrachialis m. &
biceps brachii m. (short head)

biceps brachii m. (long head)

neurovascular bundle

lung

serratus ant. m.

liver

rib

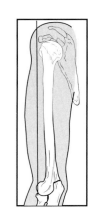

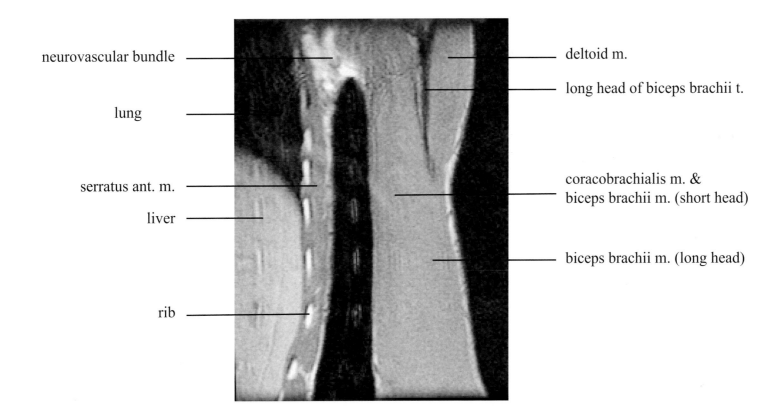

neurovascular bundle —————————— deltoid m.

————— long head of biceps brachii t.

lung ——————————

serratus ant. m. ————————— coracobrachialis m. &
                            biceps brachii m. (short head)

liver —————

————— biceps brachii m. (long head)

rib ——————

3

THE ELBOW AND FOREARM

Imaging of the elbow is not performed as commonly as that of other anatomic sites such as the shoulder or knee. MR imaging can evaluate all of the osseous and soft-tissue structures of the elbow. The major indications for MR imaging of the elbow are fractures when evaluation of the nonossified cartilage is necessary, fractures with suspected injury to tendons and ligaments, acute or chronic repetitive injury to the ligaments or tendons, evaluation of osteochondritis dissecans, suspected entrapment neuropathies, and, rarely, evaluation of arthritides such as rheumatoid or infectious arthritis.

PRACTICAL PROTOCOL CONSIDERATIONS

The elbow can be imaged in a variety of ways. Typically, the patient is placed in the supine position with the arm resting comfortably at his or her side. Alternatively, the patient may be semiprone with the arm extended overhead; however, this position is not as well tolerated by the patient because of the placement of the shoulder, and images may be degraded as a result of motion.

Dedicated or surface coils are mandatory to obtain diagnostic-quality images of the elbow. As in every anatomic area, if there is a suspicion of a soft-tissue mass or significant pain, a vitamin E capsule or other marker should be taped to the skin at the superior and inferior margins or the medial and lateral margins of the suspected abnormality for best results. A combination of imaging sequences can be used, and these are demonstrated in the table that follows.

Menu of Protocols

Elbow

Plane	Pulse Sequence	FA (degrees)	TR (msec)	TE (msec)	TI (msec)	FOV (cm)	Matrix (256X-)	ST/G (mm)	NEX	Comments
Localizer (transaxial)	FMPIR		2,500	25	150	22–24	128	5/2.5	2	Excellent for edema
Localizer (transaxial)	SE		300	20		40	128	4/1	1	Either is acceptable
Sagittal, transaxial	SE		200	15		30	128	10/5	1	
Transaxial	FSE, double echo		3,000	17/102		12	192	4/1	2	Either is acceptable
Transaxial	FSE, FS		2,500	40		12–13	256	5/1	2	
Transaxial	SE		300	20		12–16	128	3/1	2	
Sagittal	FMPIR		8,000	20	150	16–18	256	5/1	2	Either is acceptable
Sagittal	SE, double echo		2,000	20/80		14–16	128	3/1	2	
Sagittal	SE		600	20		12	128	3/1	2	

Forearm

Plane	Pulse Sequence	FA (degrees)	TR (msec)	TE (msec)	TI (msec)	FOV (cm)	Matrix (256X-)	ST/G (mm)	NEX	Comments
Localizer (transaxial)	SE		300	20		VAR	128	4/1	1	Mark area of concern
Coronal, sagittal	SE		500	min		VAR	192	5/1.5	1	
Coronal	SE		1,000	min		VAR	192	5/1.5	2	
Coronal	FMPIR		2,500	30	150	VAR	128	5/1.5	1	
Sagittal	SE		1,000	min		VAR	192	5/1.5	2	
Sagittal	FMPIR		2,500	30	150	VAR	128	5/1.5	2	
Axial	SE		600	20		VAR	192	4/1	2	
Axial, pre-GAD	SE		600	20		VAR	192	4/1	2	Repeat after GAD
Axial, pre-GAD	SE, FS		600	20		VAR	192	4/1	2	Repeat after GAD

MAJOR OSTEOCARTILAGINOUS STRUCTURES/LANDMARKS

- Distal humerus
  - Medial condyle
  - Lateral condyle
  - Articular surface of trochlea
  - Articular surface of capitellum
  - Olecranon fascia
  - Coronoid fascia
  - Radial fascia
  - Medial and lateral supracondylar crests
- Proximal ulna
  - Coronoid process
  - Olecranon
  - Radial notch of ulna
- Proximal radius
  - Radial head
  - Radial neck
  - Radial tuberosity

MAJOR LIGAMENTS/TENDONS

Ligaments

- Medial collateral ligamentous complex
  - Anterior band (bundle)—from inferior aspect of the medial epicondyle to the medial aspect of the coronoid process, seen best on coronal images. The anterior bundle is the primary constraint to valgus stress and is commonly injured in athletes whose sport involves throwing
  - Posterior bundle
  - Oblique band (transverse ligament)
    - The posterior bundle and transverse ligament are deep to the ulnar nerve and make up the floor of the cubital tunnel

- Lateral collateral ligamentous complex
  - Radial collateral ligament (RCL)
    - Arises from the anterior portion of the lateral epicondyle, blending with the fibers of the annular ligament and surrounding the radial head
  - Annular ligament
    - Primary stabilizer of the proximal radial ulnar joint
    - Best evaluated on axial images
    - Lateral ulnar collateral ligament (LUCL)—variably seen

Tendons

- Anterior compartment
  - Biceps tendon
  - Brachialis tendon
- Posterior compartment
  - Triceps tendon
  - Anconeus tendon
- Medial compartment
  - Pronator teres tendon
  - Hand and wrist flexors (common flexor tendon)
- Lateral compartment
  - Supinator tendon
  - Brachioradialis tendon
  - Extensor carpi radialis longus tendon
  - Hand and wrist extensors (common extensor tendon)

Bursae

- Olecranon

MAJOR MUSCLES

The 19 muscles in the forearm are arranged in anterior (flexor) and posterior (extensor) compartments. They can be divided into groups by either their actions or layers as superficial and deep flexors or extensors, as demonstrated in the following categories.

Compartments

Grouped by Muscle Action

- Anterior compartment
  - Rotation (Radius on ulna)
    - Pronator teres
    - Pronator quadratus
    - Supinator
  - Flexion (Hand at wrist)
    - Flexor carpi radialis
    - Flexor carpi ulnaris
    - Palmaris longus
  - Flexion (Digits)
    - Flexor digitorum superficialis
    - Flexor digitorum profundus
    - Flexor pollicis longus
- Posterior compartment
  - Extension (Hand at wrist)
    - Extensor carpi radialis longus
    - Extensor carpi radialis brevis
    - Extensor carpi ulnaris
  - Extension (Digits except thumb)
    - Extensor digitorum
    - Extensor indicis
    - Extensor digiti minimi
  - Extension (Thumb)
    - Abductor pollicis longus
    - Extensor pollicis brevis
    - Extensor pollicis longus

Grouped by Layers

- Flexor muscles
  - Superficial layer
    - Pronator teres
    - Flexor carpi radialis
    - Palmaris longus
    - Flexor carpi ulnaris
    - Flexor digitorum superficialis
  - Deep layer
    - Flexor digitorum profundus
    - Flexor pollicis longus
    - Pronator quadratus
- Extensor muscles
  - Superficial layer
    - Brachioradialis
    - Extensor carpi radialis longus
    - Extensor carpi radialis brevis
    - Extensor digitorum
    - Extensor digiti minimi
    - Extensor carpi ulnaris
  - Deep layer
    - Supinator
    - Abductor pollicis longus
    - Extensor pollicis brevis
    - Extensor pollicis longus

ORIGIN/INSERTION/INNERVATION OF MAJOR MUSCLES

Muscle	Origin	Insertion	Innervation
Anterior Compartment			
Flexor Muscles—Superficial Layer			
– Pronator teres	Two heads: (1) humeral head—medial epicondyle of humerus and (2) ulnar head—medial side of coronoid process of ulna	Middle third of lateral surface of radius	Median N. (C6, C7)
– Flexor carpi radialis	Medial epicondyle of humerus	Base of second metacarpal and, frequently, a slip to base of third metacarpal	Median N. (C6, C7)
– Palmaris longus (absent in 13% of patients)	Medial epicondyle of humerus	Forms chief portion of palmar aponeurosis	Median N. (C7, C8)
– Flexor carpi ulnaris	Two heads: (1) humeral head—medial epicondyle of humerus and (2) ulnar head—medial side of olecranon, upper two-thirds of posterior ulnar border	Primarily pisiform, hamulus of hamate, and base of fifth metacarpal	Ulnar N. (C7, C8)

(continued)

ORIGIN/INSERTION/INNERVATION OF MAJOR MUSCLES (*CONTINUED*)

Muscle	Origin	Insertion	Innervation
– Flexor digitorum superficialis	Two heads: (1) humeroulnar head—medial epicondyle, anterior epicondylar surface, ulnar collateral ligament, ulnar tuberosity, medial border of coronoid process and (2) radial head—upper two-thirds of anterior border of radius	Palmar aspect of shafts of middle phalanges of digits II–V	Median N. (C7, C8, T1)

Flexor Muscles—Deep Layer

Muscle	Origin	Insertion	Innervation
– Flexor digitorum profundus	Proximal two-thirds of medial surface face of ulna, posterior border of ulna, interosseus membrane	Bases of distal phalanges of digits II–V	Median N., anterior interosseous branch (C8, T1)
– Flexor pollicis longus	Anterior surface of radius and adjacent interosseus membrane	Base of distal phalanx of thumb	Median N., anterior interosseus branch (C8, T1)
– Pronator quadratus	Anterior surface of distal one-fourth of ulna	Anterior surface of radius	Median, anterior interosseous N. (C8, T1)

(continued)

ORIGIN/INSERTION/INNERVATION OF MAJOR MUSCLES (*CONTINUED*)

Muscle	*Origin*	*Insertion*	*Innervation*
Extensor Muscles—Superficial Layer			
– Brachioradialis	Upper two-thirds of lateral epicondylar ridge of humerus	Lateral side of base of styloid process of radius	Radial N. (C5, C6, C7)
– Extensor carpi radialis longus	Common extensor tendon of lateral epicondyle of humerus, lower one-third of lateral epicondylar ridge, lateral intermuscular septum	Dorsum of second metacarpal	Radial N. (C5, C6, C7)
– Extensor carpi radialis brevis	Common extensor tendon of lateral epicondyle of humerus, intermuscular septa, and radial collateral ligament of elbow	Dorsum of base of third metacarpal	Radial or deep radial (posterior interosseus) N. (C7, C8)
– Extensor digitorum	Common extensor tendon of lateral epicondyle of humerus	By four tendons on bases of middle and distal phalanges of digits II–V	Deep radial (posterior interosseus) N. (C7, C8)
– Extensor digiti minimi	Common extensor tendon of lateral epicondyle of humerus, intermuscular septa, overlying fascia	Base of proximal phalanx of fifth digit	Deep radial (posterior interosseus) N. (C7, C8)

(*continued*)

ORIGIN/INSERTION/INNERVATION OF MAJOR MUSCLES (*CONTINUED*)

Muscle	*Origin*	*Insertion*	*Innervation*
– Extensor carpi ulnaris	Two heads: (1) common extensor tendon lateral to epicondyle of humerus and (2) middle one-half of posterior border of ulna	Ulnar side of base of fifth metacarpal	Deep radial (posterior interosseus) N. (C7, C8)

Extensor Muscles—Deep Layer

– Supinator	Lateral epicondyle of humerus, radial collateral ligament, annular ligament, and fossa of ulna	Lateral surface of upper one-third of radius between anterior and posterior oblique lines	Deep radial (posterior interosseous) N. (C5, C6)
– Abductor pollicis longus	Middle third of posterior surface of ulna, posterior (dorsal) surface of radius, interosseus membrane	Radial side of base of first metacarpal	Deep radial (posterior interosseus) N. (C7, C8)
– Extensor pollicis brevis	Distal end and dorsal surface of middle third of radius, interosseus membrane, and ulna (sometimes)	Base of proximal phalanx of thumb	Deep radial (posterior interosseus) N. (C7, C8)

(*continued*)

ORIGIN/INSERTION/INNERVATION OF MAJOR MUSCLES (*CONTINUED*)

Muscle	Origin	Insertion	Innervation
– Extensor pollicis longus	Middle third and dorsal surface of ulna, interosseus membrane distal to abductor pollicis longus muscle	Base of distal phalanx of thumb	Deep radial (posterior interosseus) N. (C7, C8)
– Extensor indicis	Posterior surface of distal third of ulna, interosseus membrane	Joins ulnar side of digital extensor muscle to insert on base of proximal phalanx of second digit	Deep radial (posterior interosseus) N. (C7, C8)

THE ELBOW: AXIAL ANATOMY

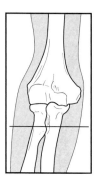

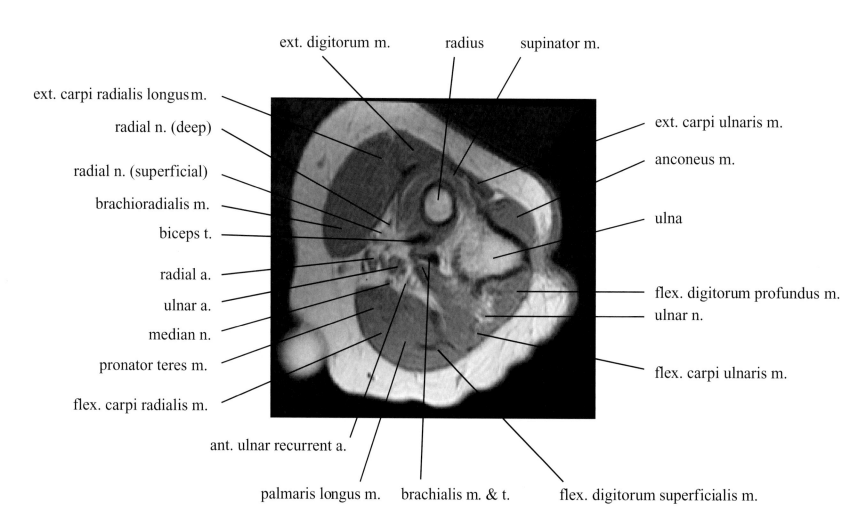

ext. digitorum m.   radius   supinator m.

ext. carpi radialis longus m.

radial n. (deep)

radial n. (superficial)

brachioradialis m.

biceps t.

radial a.

ulnar a.

median n.

pronator teres m.

flex. carpi radialis m.

ext. carpi ulnaris m.

anconeus m.

ulna

flex. digitorum profundus m.

ulnar n.

flex. carpi ulnaris m.

ant. ulnar recurrent a.

palmaris longus m.   brachialis m. & t.   flex. digitorum superficialis m.

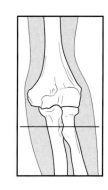

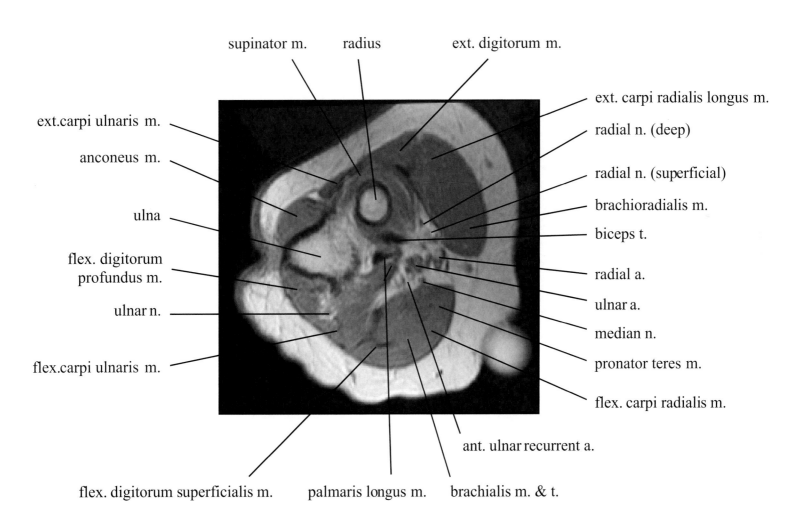

supinator m.   radius   ext. digitorum m.

ext. carpi radialis longus m.

ext.carpi ulnaris m.

radial n. (deep)

anconeus m.

radial n. (superficial)

brachioradialis m.

ulna

biceps t.

flex. digitorum
profundus m.

radial a.

ulnar n.

ulnar a.

median n.

flex.carpi ulnaris m.

pronator teres m.

flex. carpi radialis m.

ant. ulnar recurrent a.

flex. digitorum superficialis m.   palmaris longus m.   brachialis m. & t.

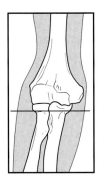

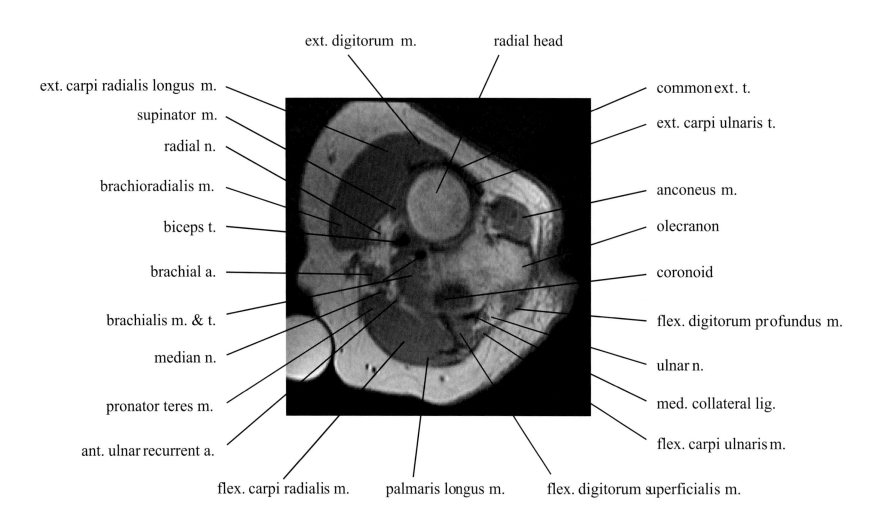

ext. digitorum m.

radial head

ext. carpi radialis longus m.

common ext. t.

supinator m.

ext. carpi ulnaris t.

radial n.

brachioradialis m.

anconeus m.

biceps t.

olecranon

brachial a.

coronoid

brachialis m. & t.

flex. digitorum profundus m.

median n.

ulnar n.

pronator teres m.

med. collateral lig.

ant. ulnar recurrent a.

flex. carpi ulnaris m.

flex. carpi radialis m.

palmaris longus m.

flex. digitorum superficialis m.

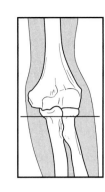

common ext t.   radial head   ext. digitorum m.

ext. carpi radialis longus m.

ext. carpi ulnaris t.

supinator m.

radial n.

anconeus m.

brachioradialis m.

olecranon

biceps t.

coronoid

flex. digitorum profundus m.

brachial a.

ulnar n.

brachialis m & t.

med. collateral lig.

median n.

flex. carpi ulnaris m.

pronator teres m.

ant. ulnar recurrent a.

flex. digitorum superficialis m.   palmaris longus m.   flex. carpi radialis m.

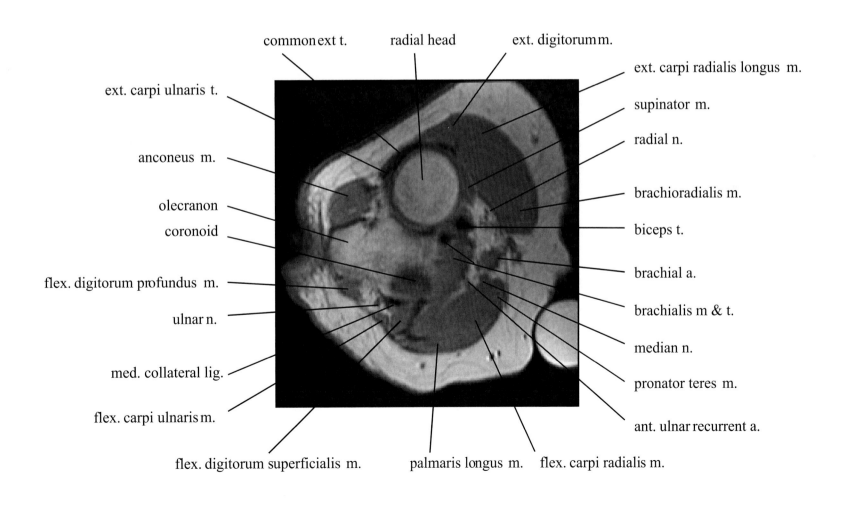

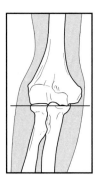

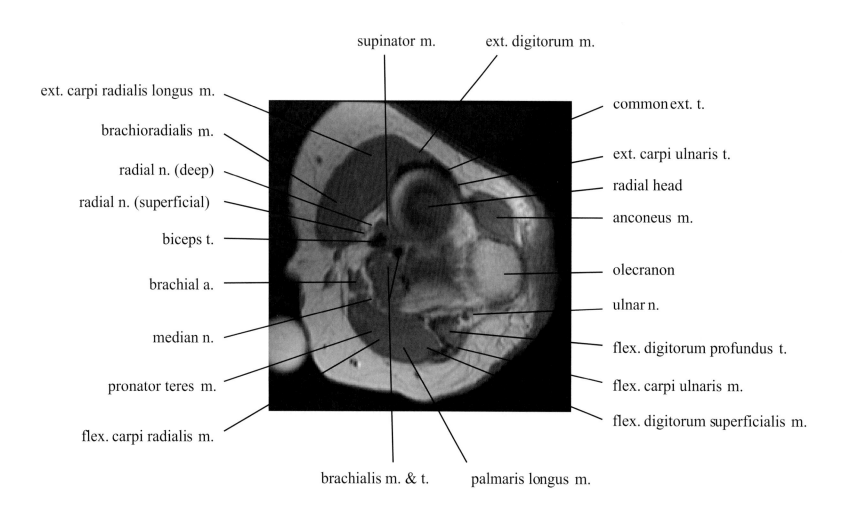

supinator m.

ext. digitorum m.

ext. carpi radialis longus m.

common ext. t.

brachioradialis m.

ext. carpi ulnaris t.

radial n. (deep)

radial head

radial n. (superficial)

anconeus m.

biceps t.

brachial a.

olecranon

median n.

ulnar n.

pronator teres m.

flex. digitorum profundus t.

flex. carpi radialis m.

flex. carpi ulnaris m.

flex. digitorum superficialis m.

brachialis m. & t.

palmaris longus m.

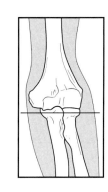

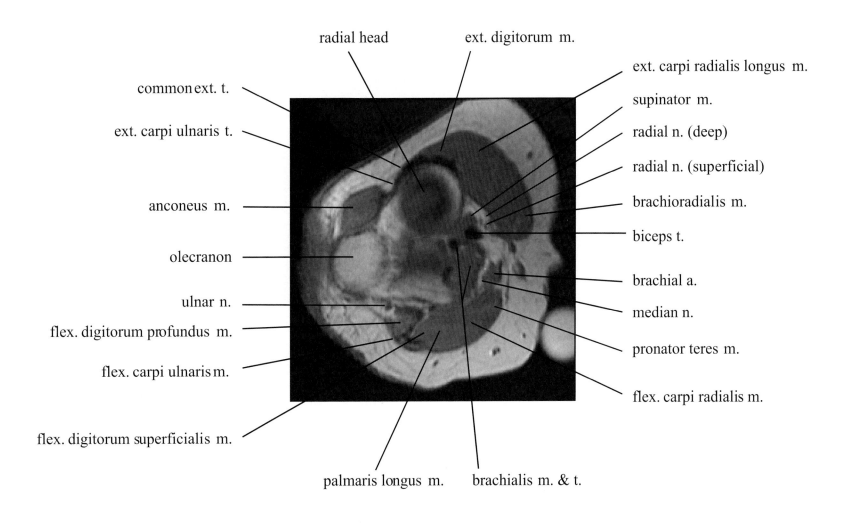

radial head

ext. digitorum m.

ext. carpi radialis longus m.

common ext. t.

supinator m.

ext. carpi ulnaris t.

radial n. (deep)

radial n. (superficial)

anconeus m.

brachioradialis m.

biceps t.

olecranon

brachial a.

ulnar n.

median n.

flex. digitorum profundus m.

pronator teres m.

flex. carpi ulnaris m.

flex. carpi radialis m.

flex. digitorum superficialis m.

palmaris longus m.

brachialis m. & t.

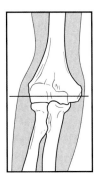

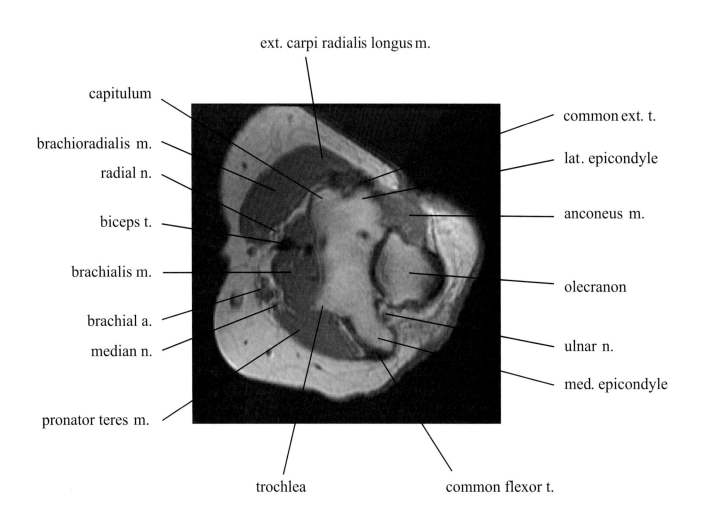

ext. carpi radialis longus m.

capitulum

brachioradialis m.

radial n.

biceps t.

brachialis m.

brachial a.

median n.

pronator teres m.

common ext. t.

lat. epicondyle

anconeus m.

olecranon

ulnar n.

med. epicondyle

trochlea

common flexor t.

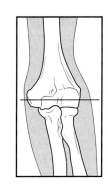

ext. carpi radialis longus m.

common ext. t.

lat. epicondyle

anconeus m.

olecranon

ulnar n.

med. epicondyle

capitulum

brachioradialis m.

radial n.

biceps t.

brachialis m.

brachial a.

median n.

pronator teres m.

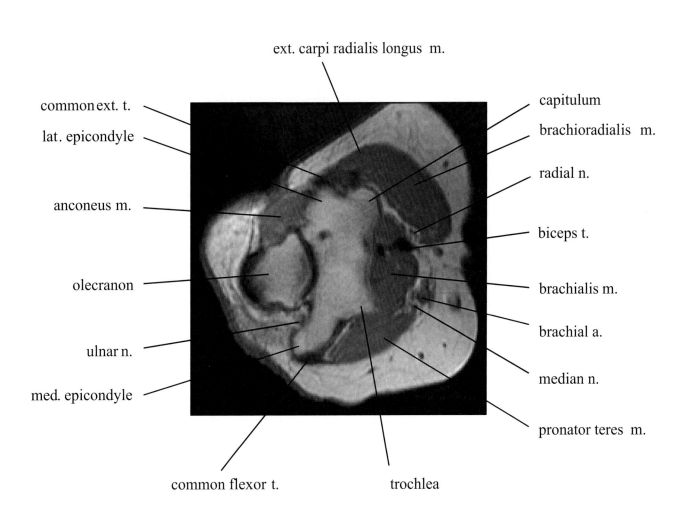

common flexor t.

trochlea

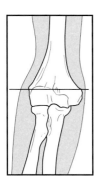

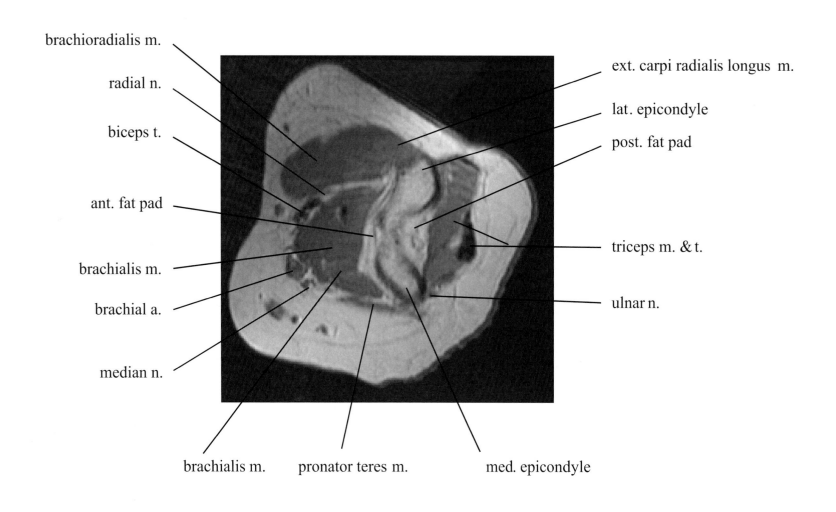

brachioradialis m.

radial n.

biceps t.

ant. fat pad

brachialis m.

brachial a.

median n.

ext. carpi radialis longus m.

lat. epicondyle

post. fat pad

triceps m. & t.

ulnar n.

brachialis m.   pronator teres m.   med. epicondyle

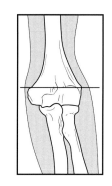

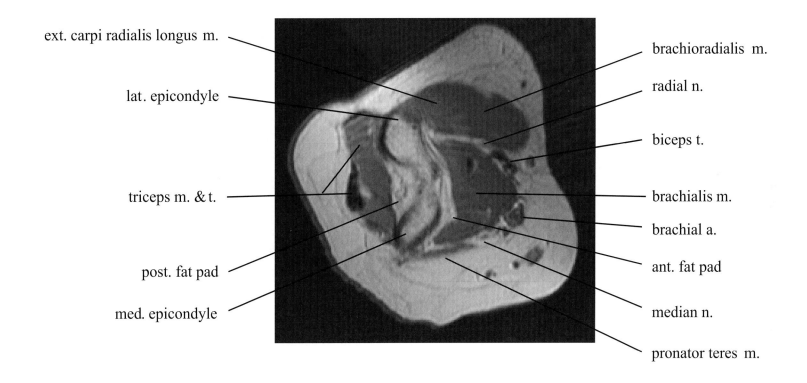

ext. carpi radialis longus m.

lat. epicondyle

triceps m. & t.

post. fat pad

med. epicondyle

brachioradialis m.

radial n.

biceps t.

brachialis m.

brachial a.

ant. fat pad

median n.

pronator teres m.

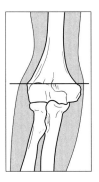

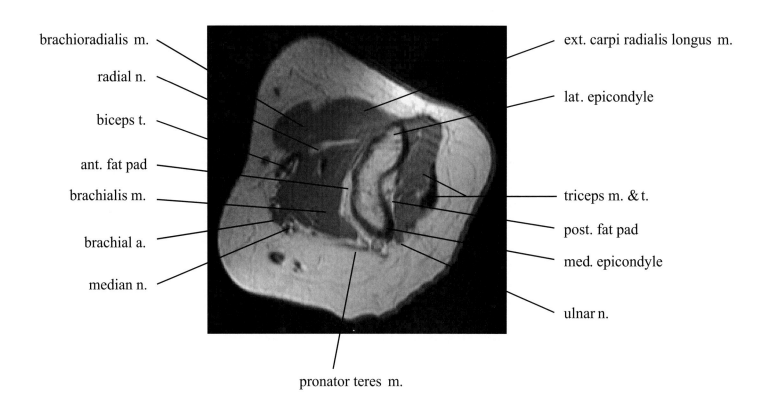

brachioradialis m.

radial n.

biceps t.

ant. fat pad

brachialis m.

brachial a.

median n.

ext. carpi radialis longus m.

lat. epicondyle

triceps m. & t.

post. fat pad

med. epicondyle

ulnar n.

pronator teres m.

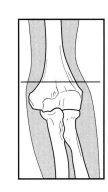

ext. carpi radialis longus m.

brachioradialis m.

lat. epicondyle

radial n.

biceps t.

triceps m. & t.

brachialis m.

ant. fat pad

post. fat pad

brachial a.

med. epicondyle

median n.

pronator teres m.

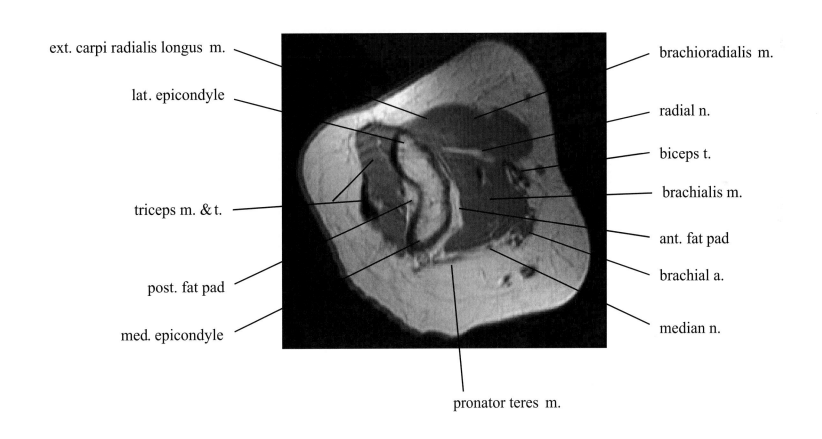

THE ELBOW: SAGITTAL ANATOMY

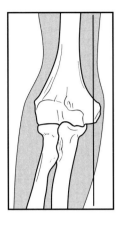

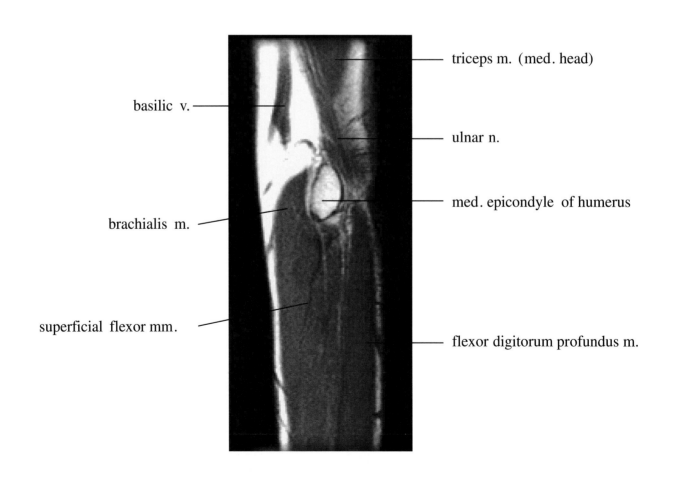

basilic v.

brachialis m.

superficial flexor mm.

triceps m. (med. head)

ulnar n.

med. epicondyle of humerus

flexor digitorum profundus m.

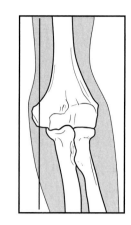

triceps m. (med. head) —————

ulnar n. ——

med. epicondyle of humerus ——

flexor digitorum profundus m. ——

————— basilic v.

————— brachialis m.

————— superficial flexor mm.

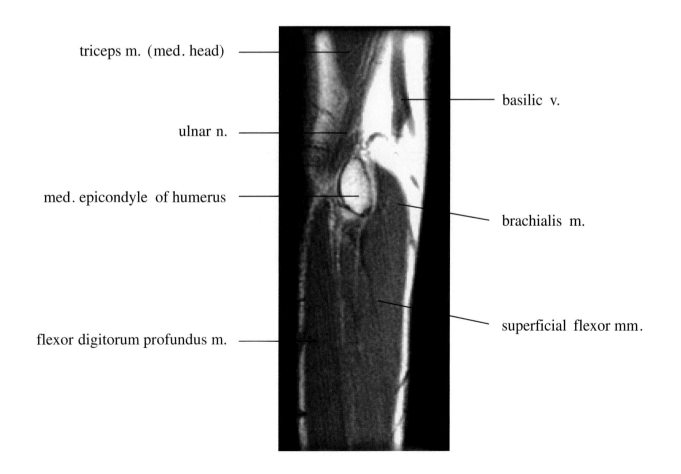

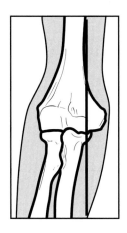

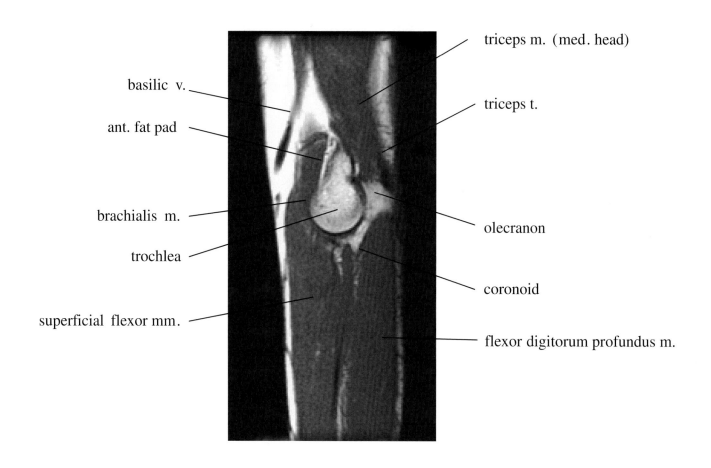

triceps m. (med. head)

basilic v.

triceps t.

ant. fat pad

brachialis m.

olecranon

trochlea

coronoid

superficial flexor mm.

flexor digitorum profundus m.

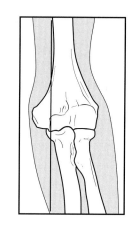

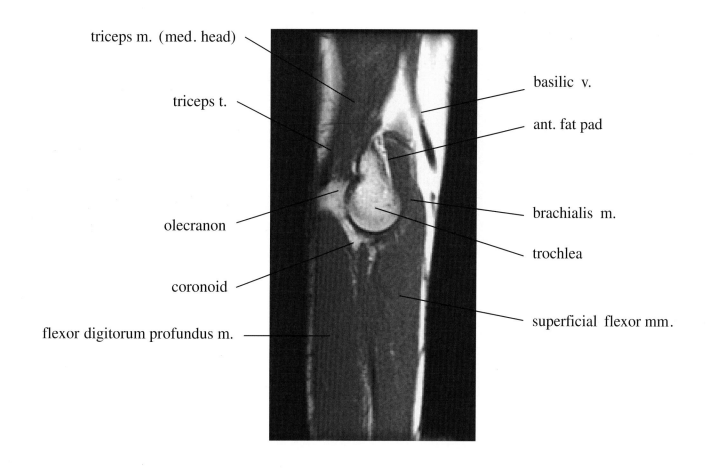

triceps m. (med. head)

triceps t.

olecranon

coronoid

flexor digitorum profundus m.

basilic v.

ant. fat pad

brachialis m.

trochlea

superficial flexor mm.

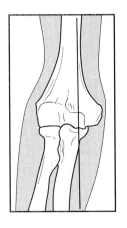

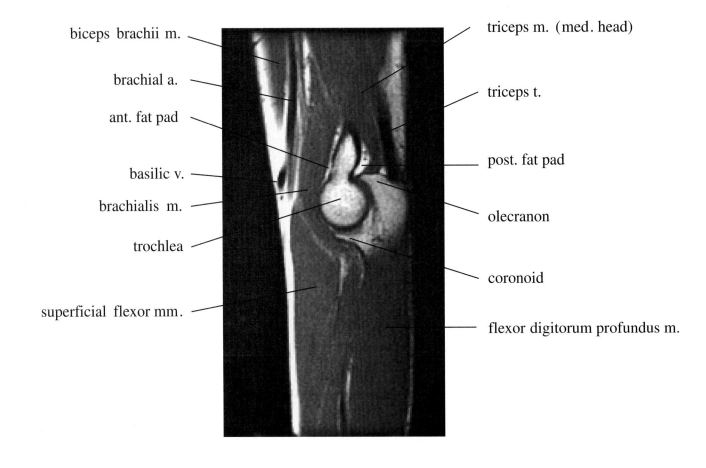

biceps brachii m.

brachial a.

ant. fat pad

basilic v.

brachialis m.

trochlea

superficial flexor mm.

triceps m. (med. head)

triceps t.

post. fat pad

olecranon

coronoid

flexor digitorum profundus m.

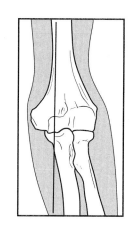

triceps m. (med. head)

triceps t.

post. fat pad

olecranon

coronoid

flexor digitorum profundus m.

biceps brachii m.

brachial a.

ant. fat pad

basilic v.

brachialis m.

trochlea

superficial flexor mm.

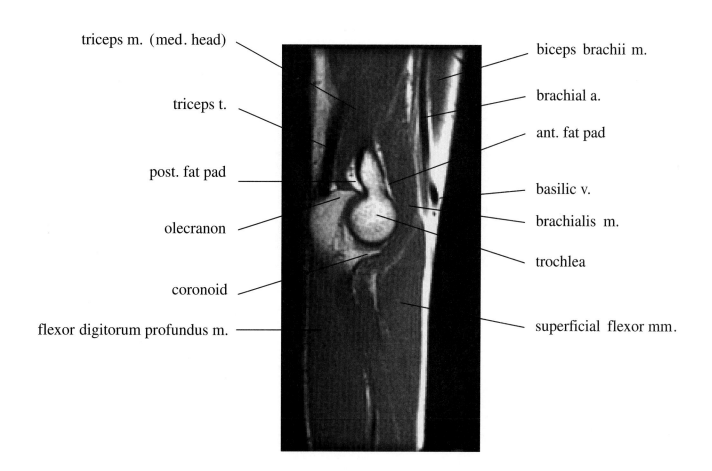

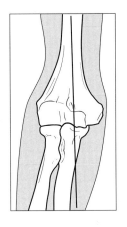

biceps brachii m.

ant. fat pad

brachial a.

basilic v.

brachialis m.

trochlea

superficial flexor mm.

triceps m. (med. head)

triceps t.

post. fat pad

olecranon

coronoid

flexor digitorum profundus m.

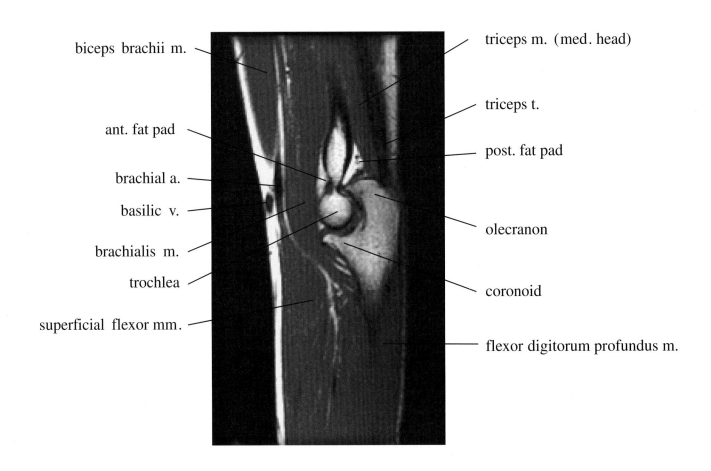

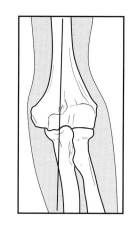

triceps m. (med. head)

biceps brachii m.

triceps t.

ant. fat pad

post. fat pad

brachial a.

olecranon

basilic v.

brachialis m.

coronoid

trochlea

superficial flexor mm.

flexor digitorum profundus m.

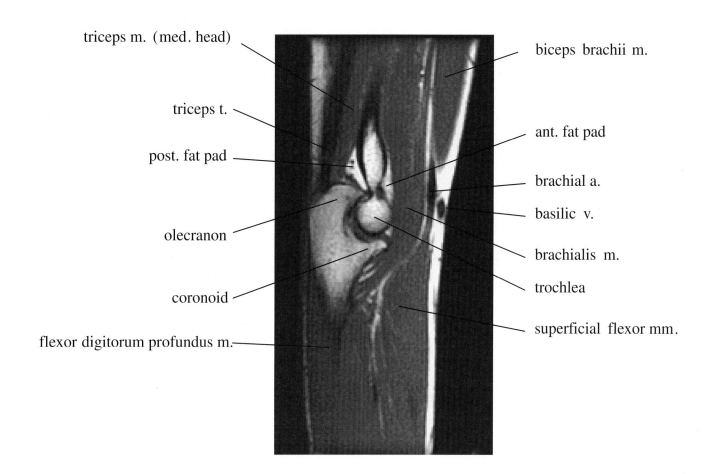

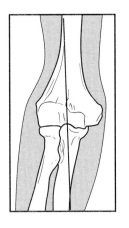

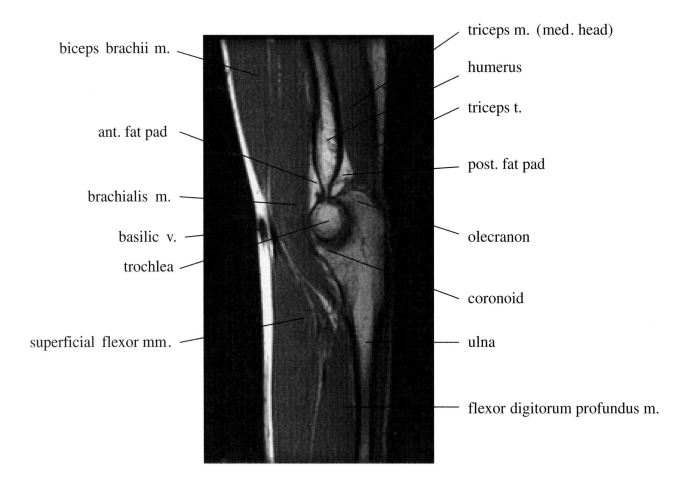

biceps brachii m.

ant. fat pad

brachialis m.

basilic v.

trochlea

superficial flexor mm.

triceps m. (med. head)

humerus

triceps t.

post. fat pad

olecranon

coronoid

ulna

flexor digitorum profundus m.

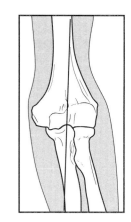

triceps m. (med. head)

humerus

triceps t.

post. fat pad

olecranon

coronoid

ulna

flexor digitorum profundus m.

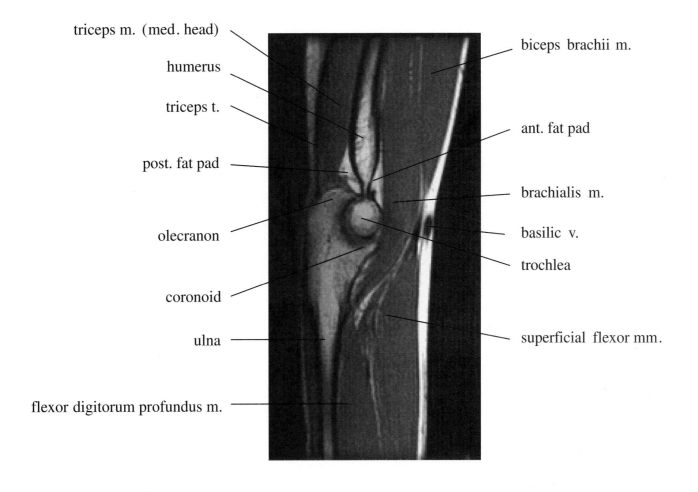

biceps brachii m.

ant. fat pad

brachialis m.

basilic v.

trochlea

superficial flexor mm.

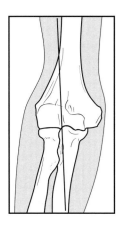

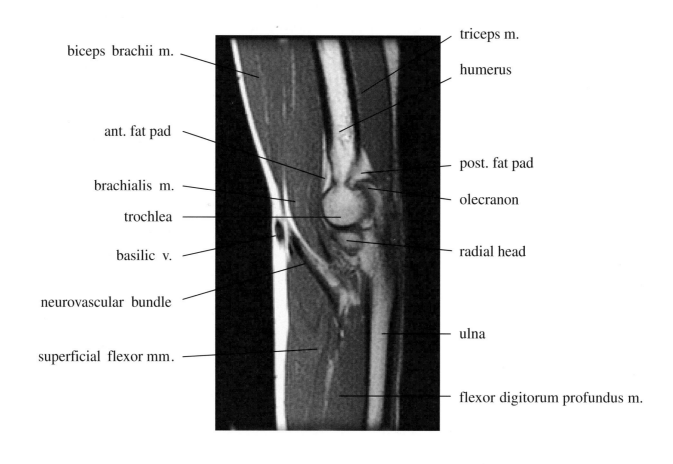

biceps brachii m.

ant. fat pad

brachialis m.

trochlea

basilic v.

neurovascular bundle

superficial flexor mm.

triceps m.

humerus

post. fat pad

olecranon

radial head

ulna

flexor digitorum profundus m.

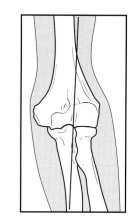

triceps m.

humerus

biceps brachii m.

ant. fat pad

post. fat pad

brachialis m.

olecranon

trochlea

radial head

basilic v.

neurovascular bundle

ulna

superficial flexor mm.

flexor digitorum profundus m.

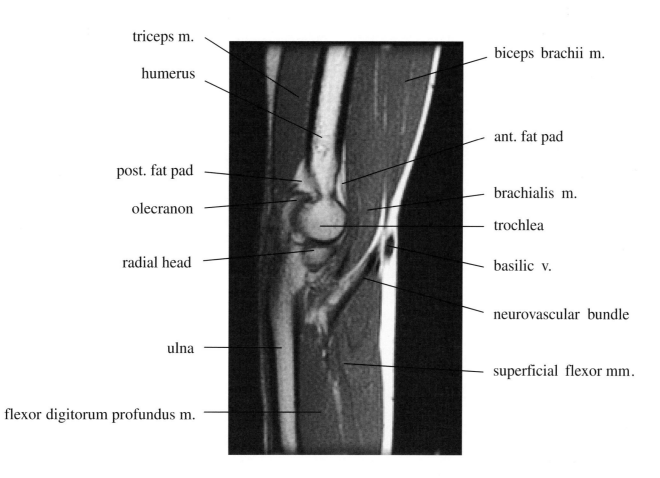

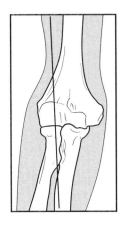

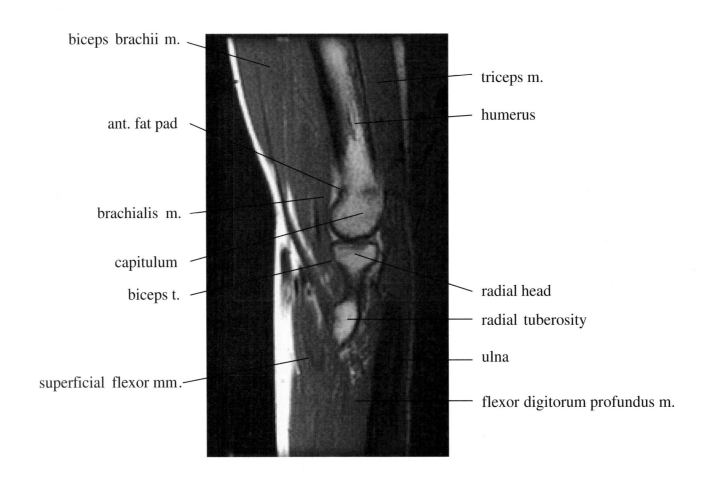

biceps brachii m.

triceps m.

humerus

ant. fat pad

brachialis m.

capitulum

radial head

biceps t.

radial tuberosity

ulna

superficial flexor mm.

flexor digitorum profundus m.

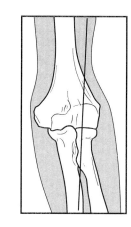

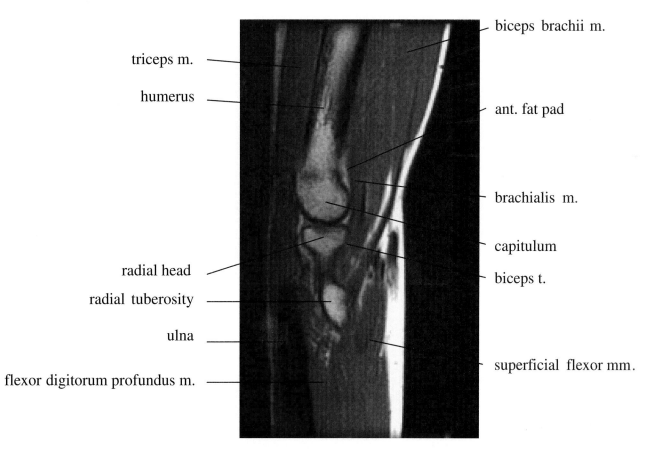

triceps m.

humerus

radial head

radial tuberosity

ulna

flexor digitorum profundus m.

biceps brachii m.

ant. fat pad

brachialis m.

capitulum

biceps t.

superficial flexor mm.

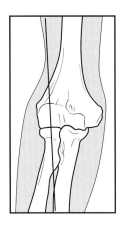

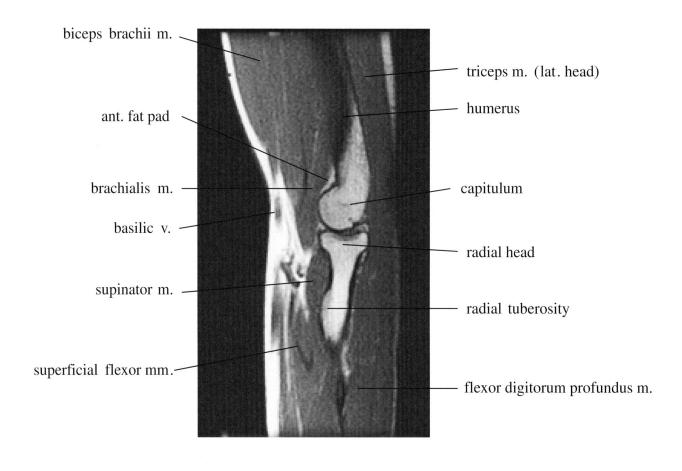

biceps brachii m.

triceps m. (lat. head)

humerus

ant. fat pad

brachialis m.

capitulum

basilic v.

radial head

supinator m.

radial tuberosity

superficial flexor mm.

flexor digitorum profundus m.

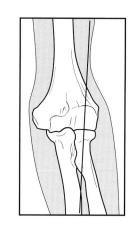

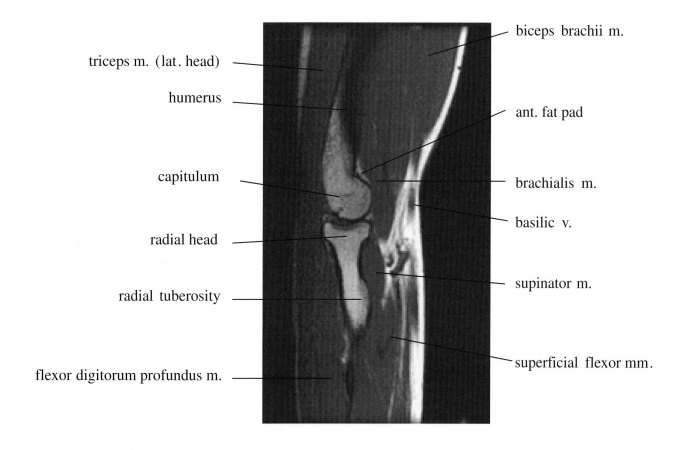

triceps m. (lat. head)

humerus

capitulum

radial head

radial tuberosity

flexor digitorum profundus m.

biceps brachii m.

ant. fat pad

brachialis m.

basilic v.

supinator m.

superficial flexor mm.

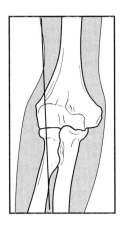

biceps brachii m.

triceps m. (lat. head)

ant. fat pad

brachialis m.

capitulum

radial head

supinator m.

brachioradialis m.

radius

superficial flexor mm.

extensor carpi ulnaris m.

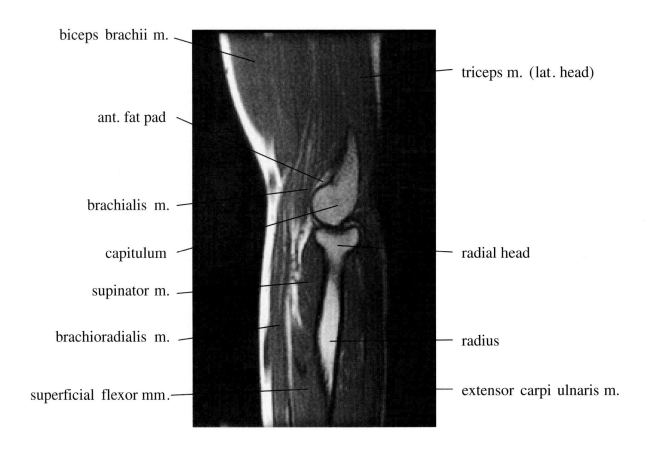

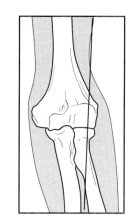

triceps m. (lat. head) —

biceps brachii m.

ant. fat pad

brachialis m.

radial head —

capitulum

supinator m.

radius —

brachioradialis m.

extensor carpi ulnaris m. —

superficial flexor mm.

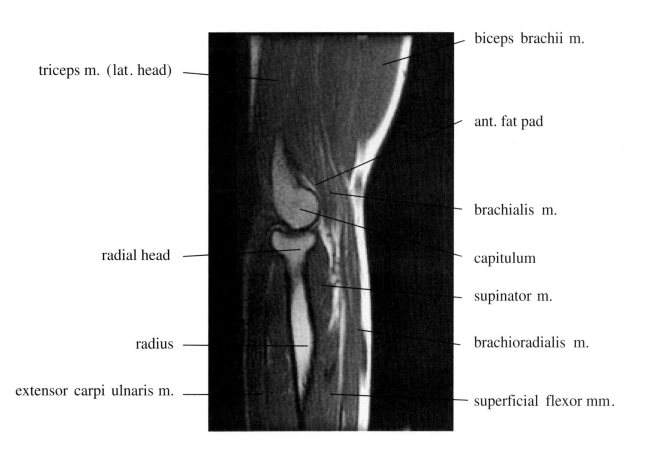

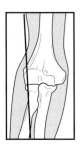

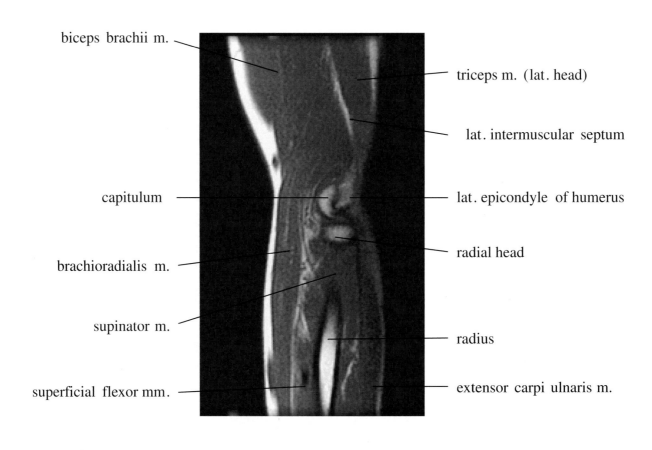

biceps brachii m.

triceps m. (lat. head)

lat. intermuscular septum

capitulum

lat. epicondyle of humerus

radial head

brachioradialis m.

supinator m.

radius

superficial flexor mm.

extensor carpi ulnaris m.

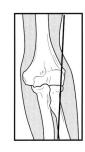

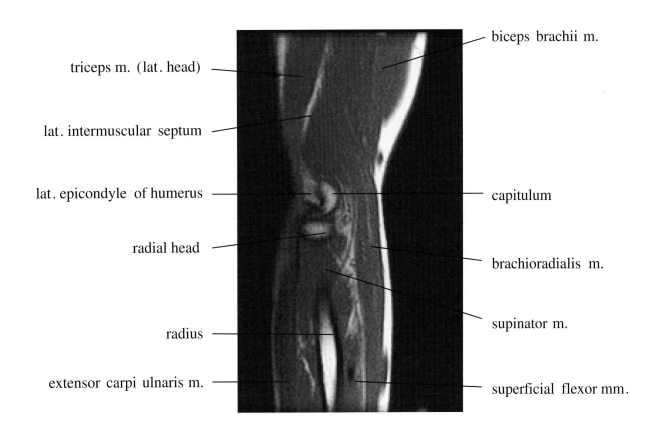

triceps m. (lat. head)

lat. intermuscular septum

lat. epicondyle of humerus

radial head

radius

extensor carpi ulnaris m.

biceps brachii m.

capitulum

brachioradialis m.

supinator m.

superficial flexor mm.

THE ELBOW: CORONAL ANATOMY

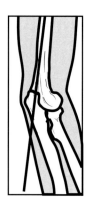

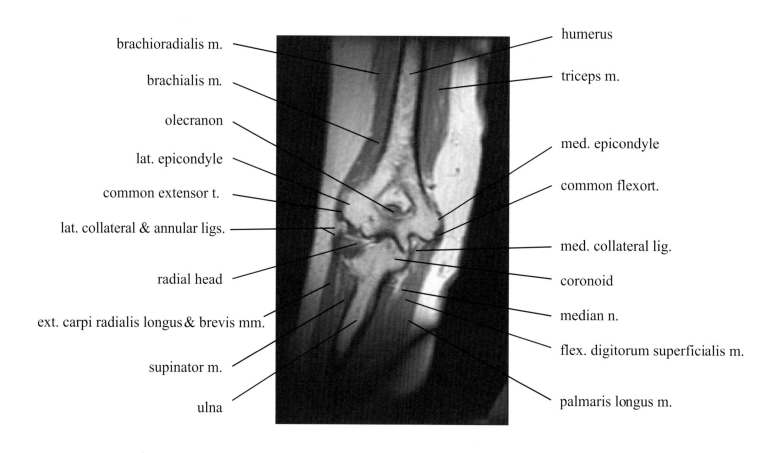

brachioradialis m.

brachialis m.

olecranon

lat. epicondyle

common extensor t.

lat. collateral & annular ligs.

radial head

ext. carpi radialis longus & brevis mm.

supinator m.

ulna

humerus

triceps m.

med. epicondyle

common flexort.

med. collateral lig.

coronoid

median n.

flex. digitorum superficialis m.

palmaris longus m.

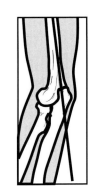

humerus

triceps m.

med. epicondyle

common flexor t.

med. collateral lig.

coronoid

median n.

flex. digitorum superficialis m.

palmaris longus m.

brachioradialis m.

brachialis m.

olecranon

lat. epicondyle

common extensor t.

lat. collateral & annular ligs.

radial head

ext. carpi radialis longus & brevis mm.

supinator m.

ulna

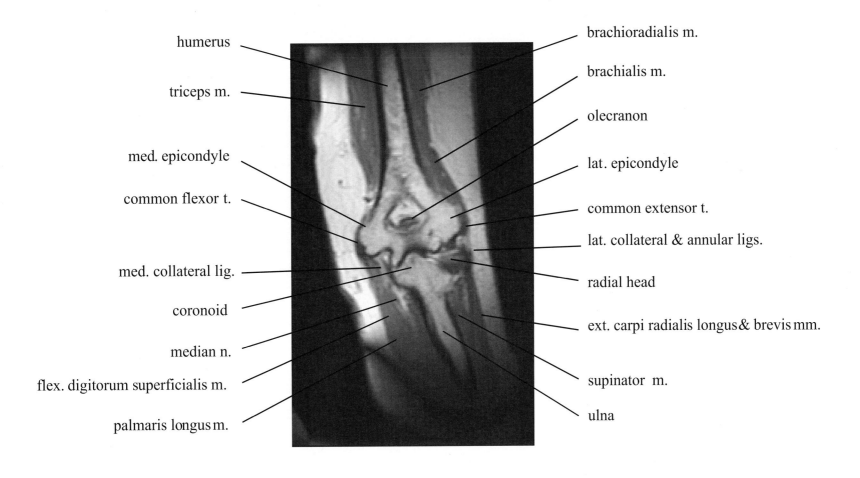

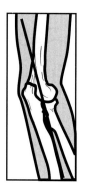

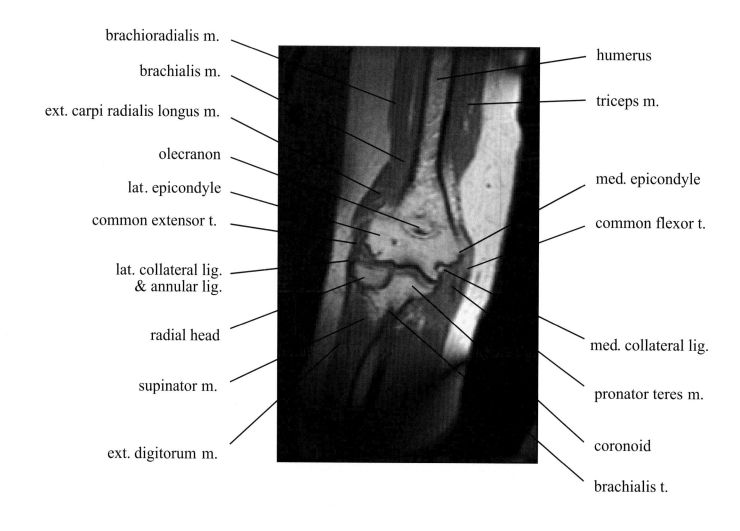

brachioradialis m.

brachialis m.

ext. carpi radialis longus m.

olecranon

lat. epicondyle

common extensor t.

lat. collateral lig.
& annular lig.

radial head

supinator m.

ext. digitorum m.

humerus

triceps m.

med. epicondyle

common flexor t.

med. collateral lig.

pronator teres m.

coronoid

brachialis t.

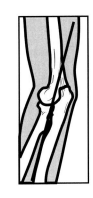

brachioradialis m.

brachialis m.

ext. carpi radialis longus m.

humerus

triceps m.

olecranon

lat. epicondyle

med. epicondyle

common extensor t.

common flexor t.

lat. collateral lig.
& annular lig.

med. collateral lig.

radial head

pronator teres m.

supinator m.

coronoid

brachialis t.

ext. digitorum m.

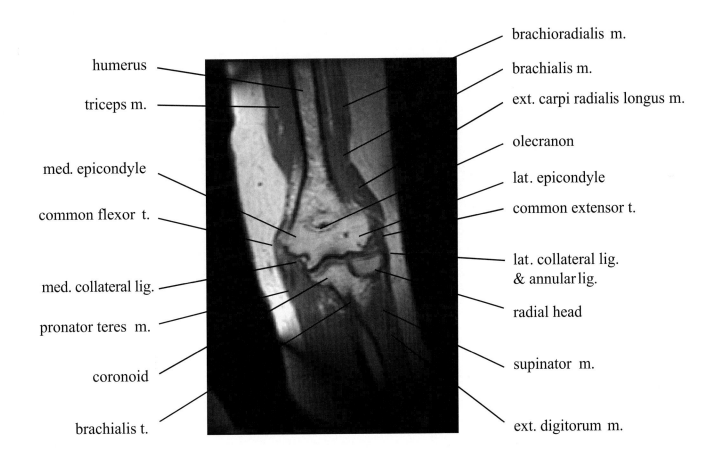

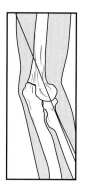

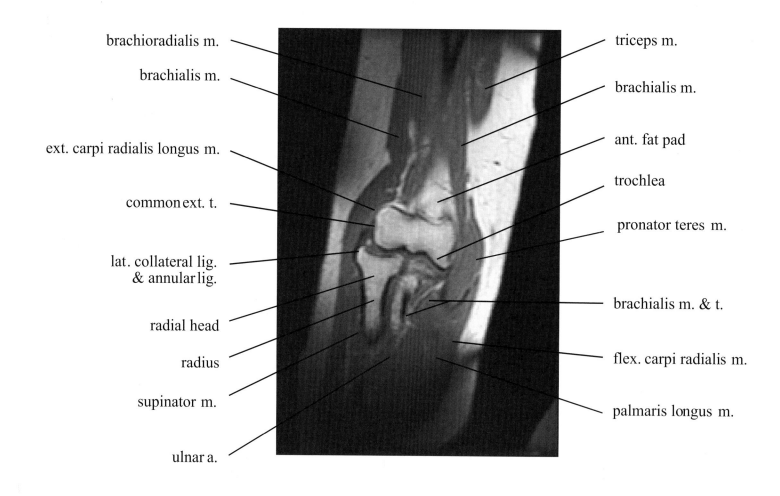

brachioradialis m.

brachialis m.

ext. carpi radialis longus m.

common ext. t.

lat. collateral lig.
& annular lig.

radial head

radius

supinator m.

ulnar a.

triceps m.

brachialis m.

ant. fat pad

trochlea

pronator teres m.

brachialis m. & t.

flex. carpi radialis m.

palmaris longus m.

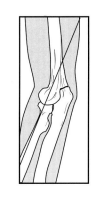

triceps m.

brachialis m.

ant. fat pad

trochlea

pronator teres m.

brachialis m. & t.

flex. carpi radialis m.

palmaris longus m.

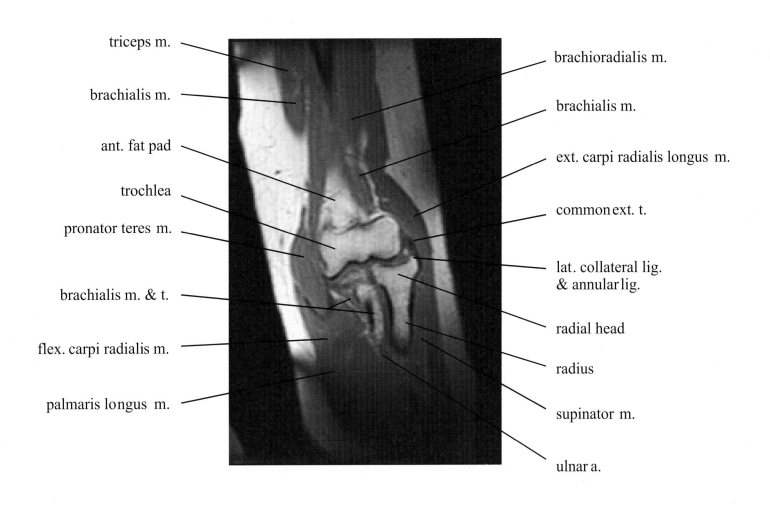

brachioradialis m.

brachialis m.

ext. carpi radialis longus m.

common ext. t.

lat. collateral lig.
& annular lig.

radial head

radius

supinator m.

ulnar a.

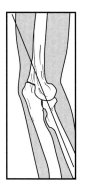

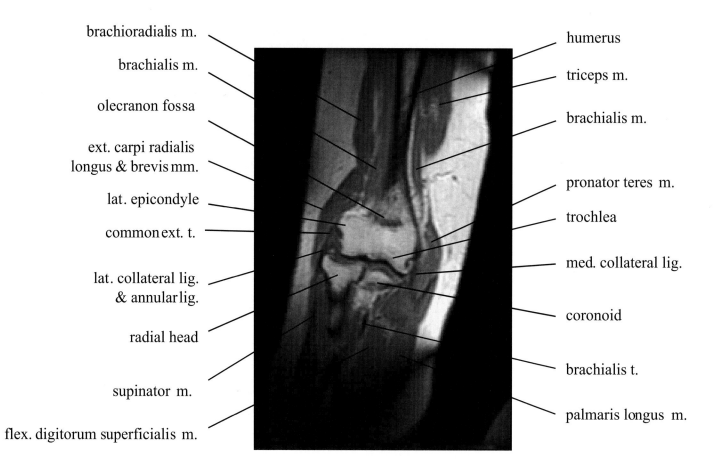

brachioradialis m.

brachialis m.

olecranon fossa

ext. carpi radialis
longus & brevis mm.

lat. epicondyle

common ext. t.

lat. collateral lig.
& annular lig.

radial head

supinator m.

flex. digitorum superficialis m.

humerus

triceps m.

brachialis m.

pronator teres m.

trochlea

med. collateral lig.

coronoid

brachialis t.

palmaris longus m.

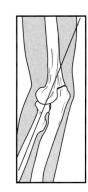

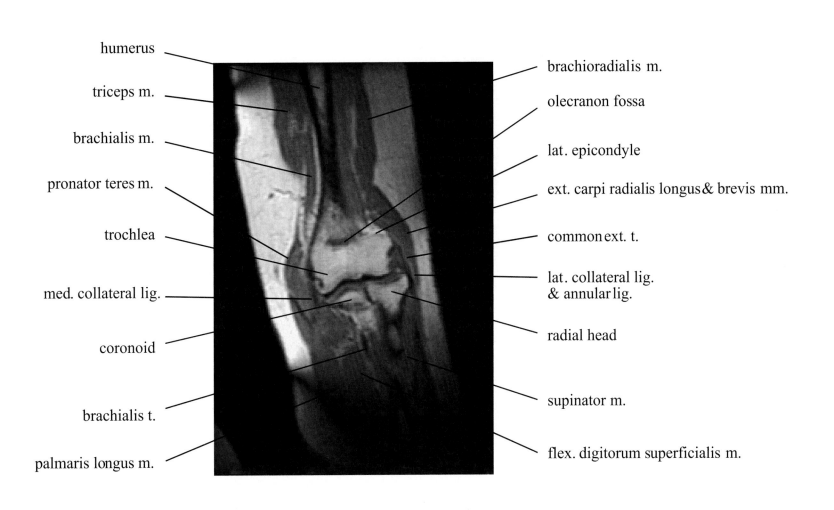

humerus

triceps m.

brachialis m.

pronator teres m.

trochlea

med. collateral lig.

coronoid

brachialis t.

palmaris longus m.

brachioradialis m.

olecranon fossa

lat. epicondyle

ext. carpi radialis longus & brevis mm.

common ext. t.

lat. collateral lig.
& annular lig.

radial head

supinator m.

flex. digitorum superficialis m.

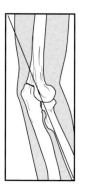

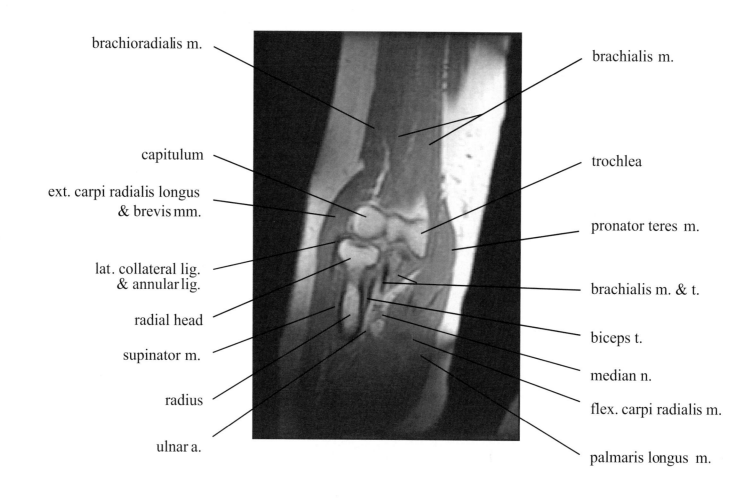

brachioradialis m.

brachialis m.

capitulum

trochlea

ext. carpi radialis longus
& brevis mm.

pronator teres m.

lat. collateral lig.
& annular lig.

brachialis m. & t.

radial head

biceps t.

supinator m.

median n.

radius

flex. carpi radialis m.

ulnar a.

palmaris longus m.

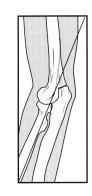

brachialis m.

brachioradialis m.

trochlea

capitulum

pronator teres m.

ext. carpi radialis
longus & brevis mm.

brachialis m. & t.

lat. collateral lig.
& annular lig.

biceps t.

radial head

median n.

supinator m.

flex. carpi radialis m.

radius

palmaris longus m.

ulnar a.

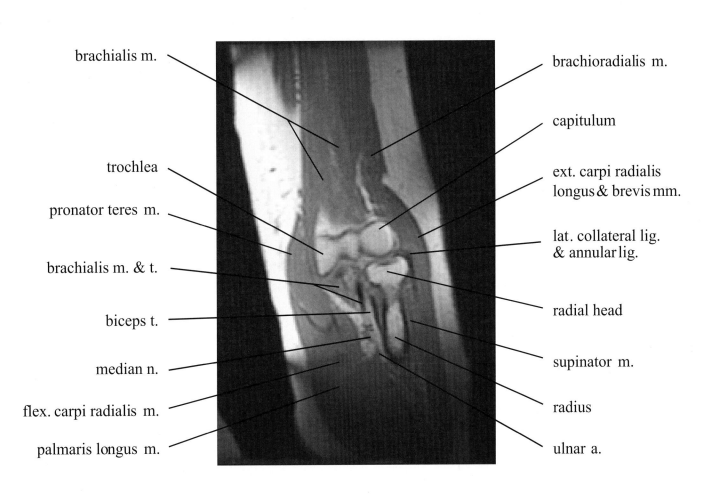

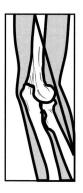

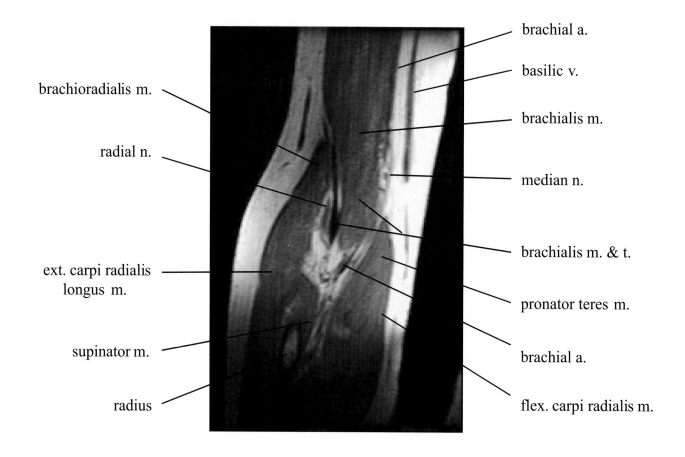

brachioradialis m.

radial n.

ext. carpi radialis
longus m.

supinator m.

radius

brachial a.

basilic v.

brachialis m.

median n.

brachialis m. & t.

pronator teres m.

brachial a.

flex. carpi radialis m.

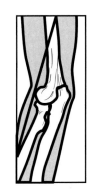

brachial a.

basilic v.

brachialis m.

median n.

brachialis m. & t.

pronator teres m.

brachial a.

flex. carpi radialis m.

brachioradialis m.

radial n.

ext. carpi radialis longus m.

supinator m.

radius

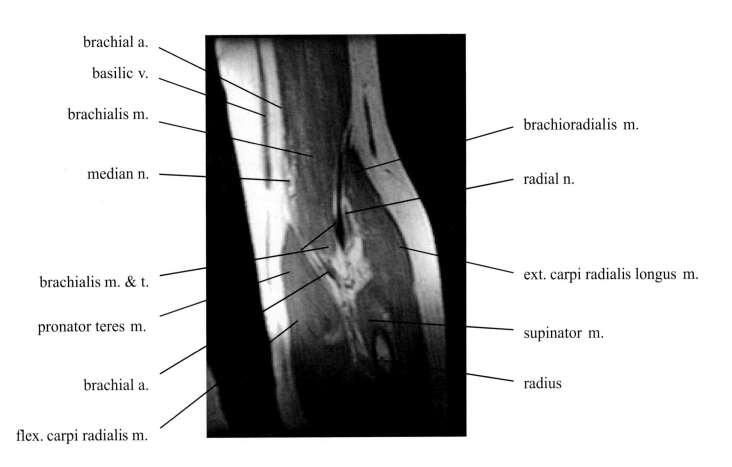

THE FOREARM: AXIAL ANATOMY

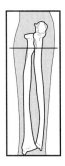

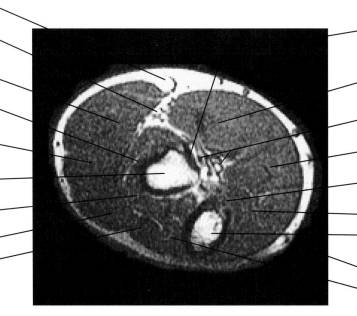

cephalic v.

radial a. & n.

brachioradialis m.

supinator m.

ext. carpi radialis longus m.

radius

ext. carpi radialis brevis m.

ext. digitorum m.

extensor carpi ulnaris m.

biceps t.

flexor digitorum superficialis m.

ulnar a. & median n.

flexor carpi ulnaris m.

brachialis m.

flexor digitorum profundus m.

ulna

basilic v.

anconeus m.

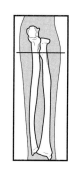

biceps t.

flexor digitorum superficialis m.

ulnar a. & median n.

flexor carpi ulnaris m.

brachialis m.

flexor digitorum profundus m.

ulna

basilic v.

anconeus m.

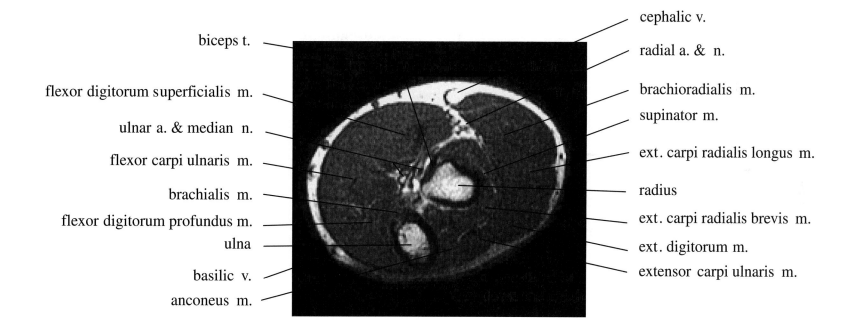

cephalic v.

radial a. & n.

brachioradialis m.

supinator m.

ext. carpi radialis longus m.

radius

ext. carpi radialis brevis m.

ext. digitorum m.

extensor carpi ulnaris m.

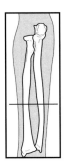

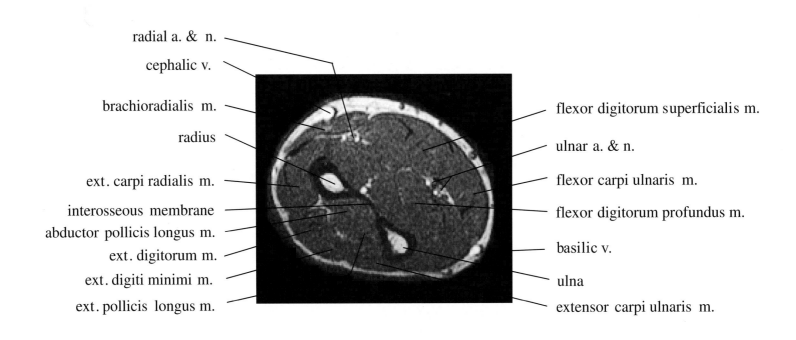

radial a. & n.

cephalic v.

brachioradialis m.

radius

ext. carpi radialis m.

interosseous membrane

abductor pollicis longus m.

ext. digitorum m.

ext. digiti minimi m.

ext. pollicis longus m.

flexor digitorum superficialis m.

ulnar a. & n.

flexor carpi ulnaris m.

flexor digitorum profundus m.

basilic v.

ulna

extensor carpi ulnaris m.

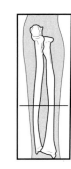

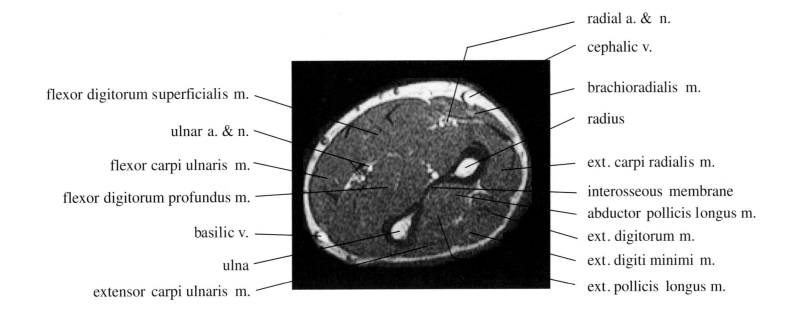

radial a. & n.

cephalic v.

brachioradialis m.

radius

flexor digitorum superficialis m.

ulnar a. & n.

flexor carpi ulnaris m.

flexor digitorum profundus m.

basilic v.

ulna

extensor carpi ulnaris m.

ext. carpi radialis m.

interosseous membrane

abductor pollicis longus m.

ext. digitorum m.

ext. digiti minimi m.

ext. pollicis longus m.

THE FOREARM: SAGITTAL ANATOMY

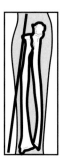

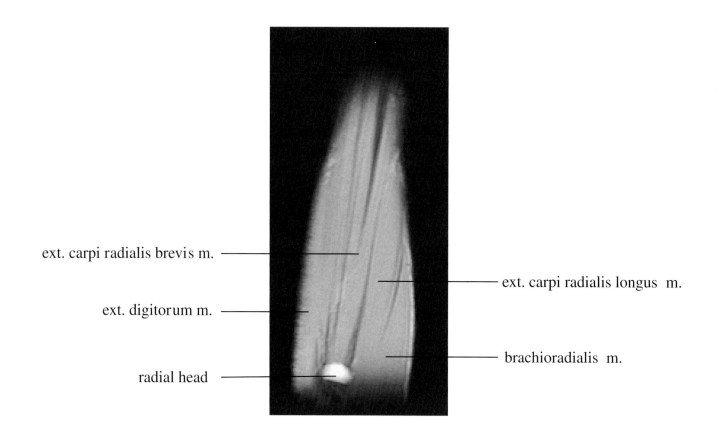

ext. carpi radialis brevis m. ———————

ext. digitorum m. ———————

radial head ———————

——————— ext. carpi radialis longus m.

——————— brachioradialis m.

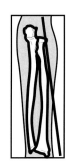

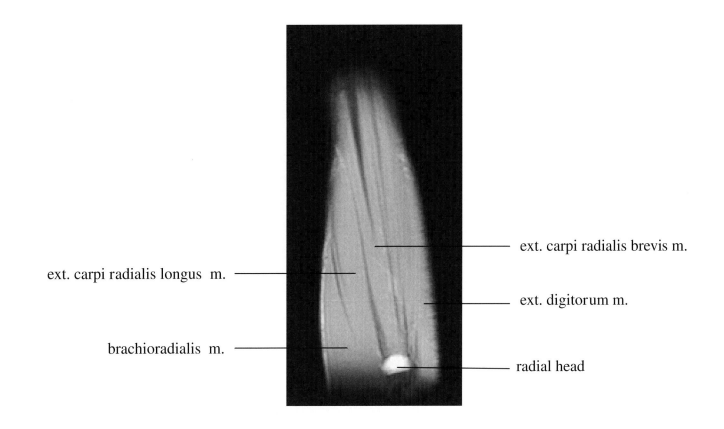

ext. carpi radialis brevis m.

ext. carpi radialis longus m.

ext. digitorum m.

brachioradialis m.

radial head

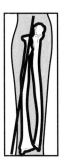

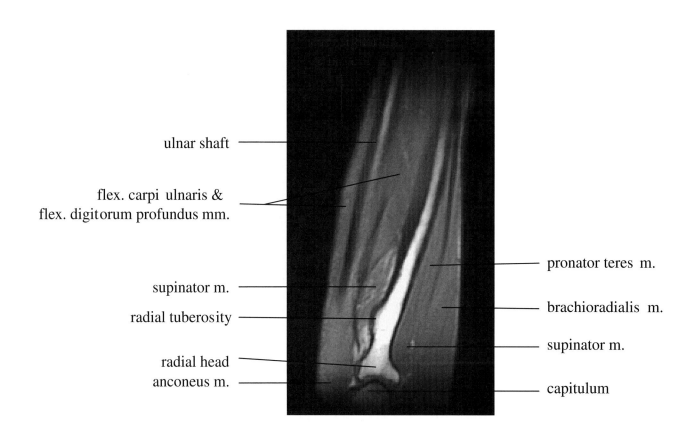

ulnar shaft

flex. carpi ulnaris &
flex. digitorum profundus mm.

pronator teres m.

supinator m.

brachioradialis m.

radial tuberosity

supinator m.

radial head

anconeus m.

capitulum

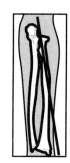

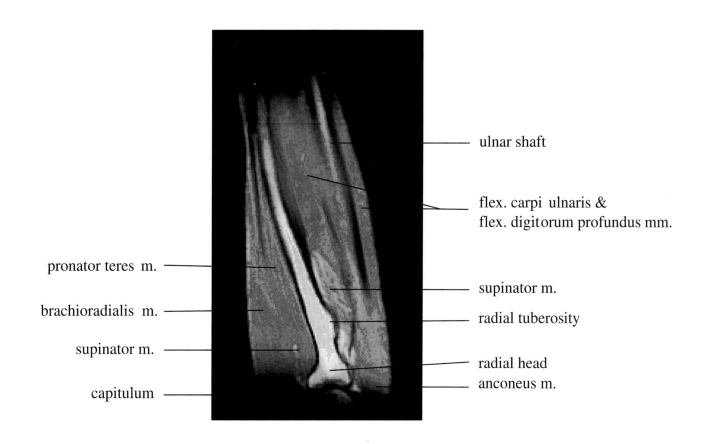

ulnar shaft

flex. carpi ulnaris &
flex. digitorum profundus mm.

pronator teres m.

supinator m.

brachioradialis m.

radial tuberosity

supinator m.

radial head
anconeus m.

capitulum

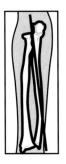

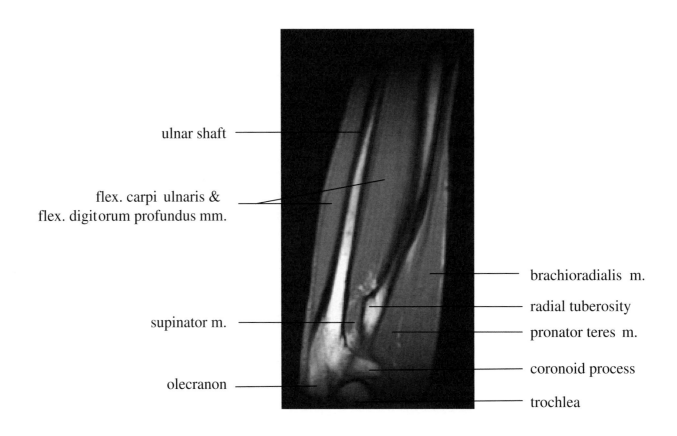

ulnar shaft

flex. carpi ulnaris &
flex. digitorum profundus mm.

brachioradialis m.

radial tuberosity

supinator m.

pronator teres m.

coronoid process

olecranon

trochlea

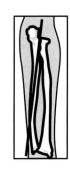

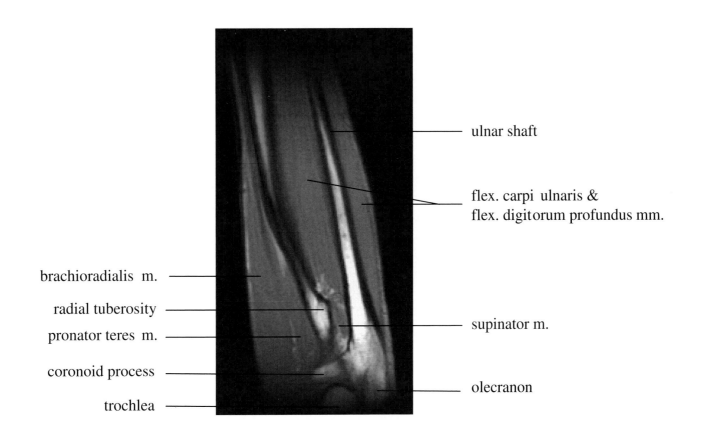

ulnar shaft

flex. carpi ulnaris &
flex. digitorum profundus mm.

brachioradialis m.

radial tuberosity

pronator teres m.

coronoid process

trochlea

supinator m.

olecranon

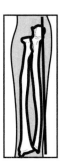

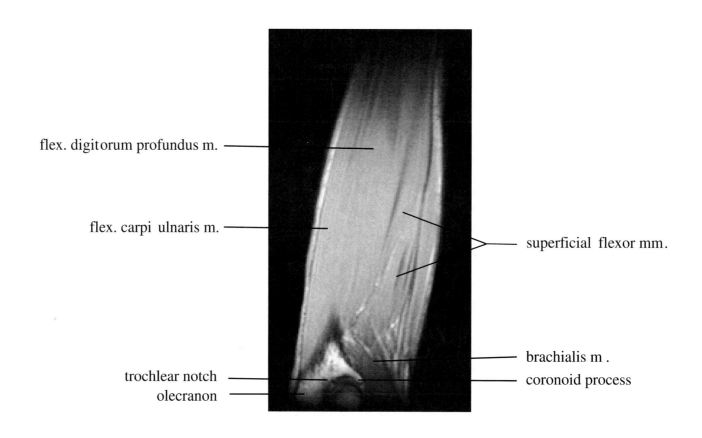

flex. digitorum profundus m. ———

flex. carpi ulnaris m. ———

⟩——— superficial flexor mm.

——— brachialis m .

trochlear notch ———
——— coronoid process

olecranon ———

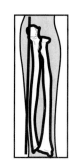

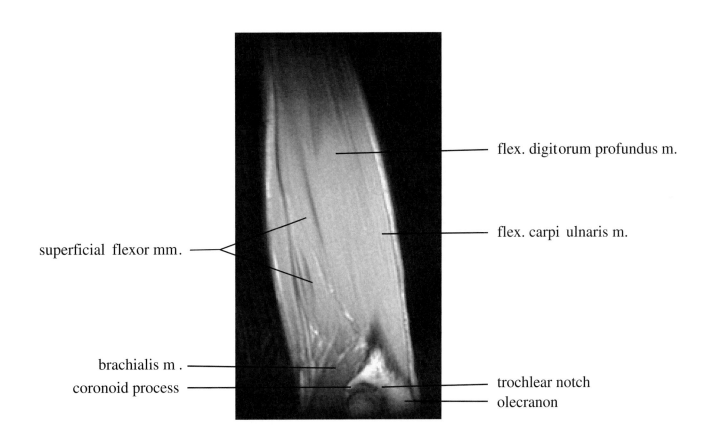

flex. digitorum profundus m.

flex. carpi ulnaris m.

superficial flexor mm.

brachialis m.

coronoid process

trochlear notch

olecranon

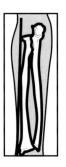

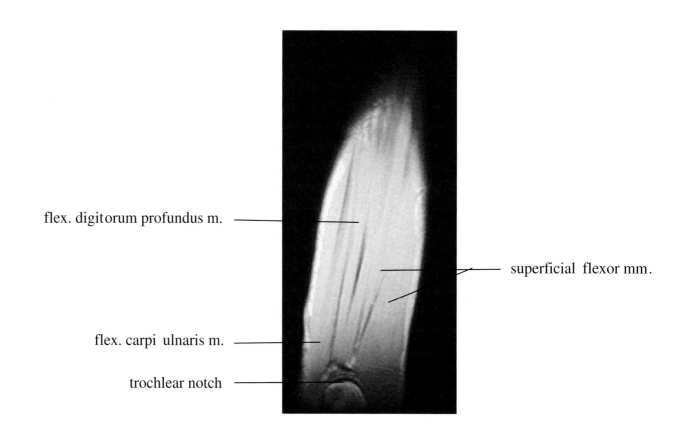

flex. digitorum profundus m. ——————

————— superficial flexor mm.

flex. carpi ulnaris m. ——————

trochlear notch ——————

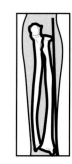

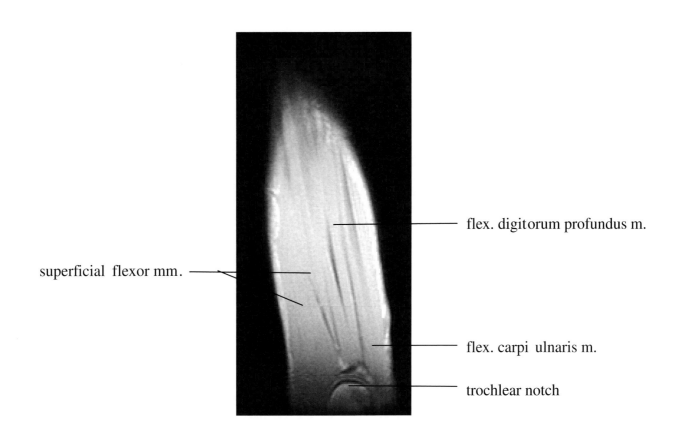

flex. digitorum profundus m.

superficial flexor mm.

flex. carpi ulnaris m.

trochlear notch

THE FOREARM: CORONAL ANATOMY

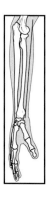

flex. carpi superficialis m. ——————

pronator teres m. ——————   —————— ext. carpi radialis longus m.

flex. carpi radialis m . ——————   —————— radius

—————— brachioradialis m.

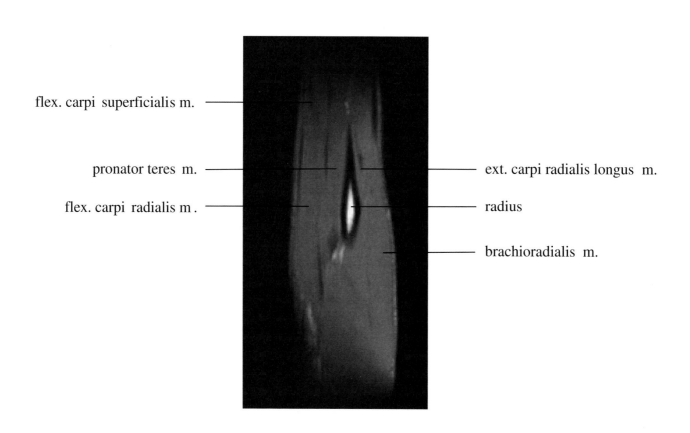

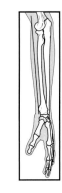

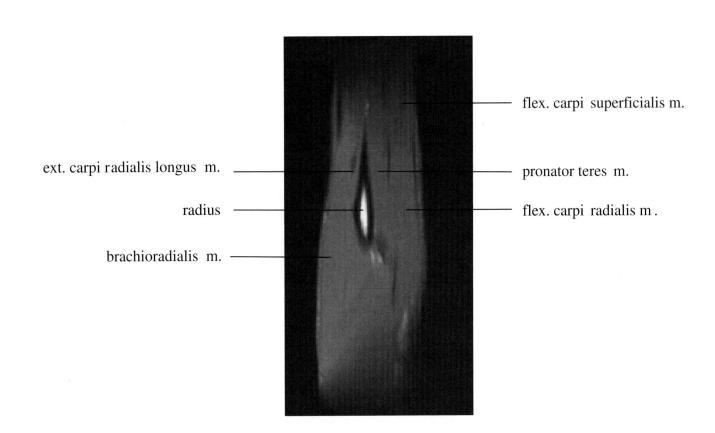

flex. carpi superficialis m.

ext. carpi radialis longus m.

pronator teres m.

radius

flex. carpi radialis m .

brachioradialis m.

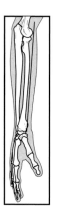

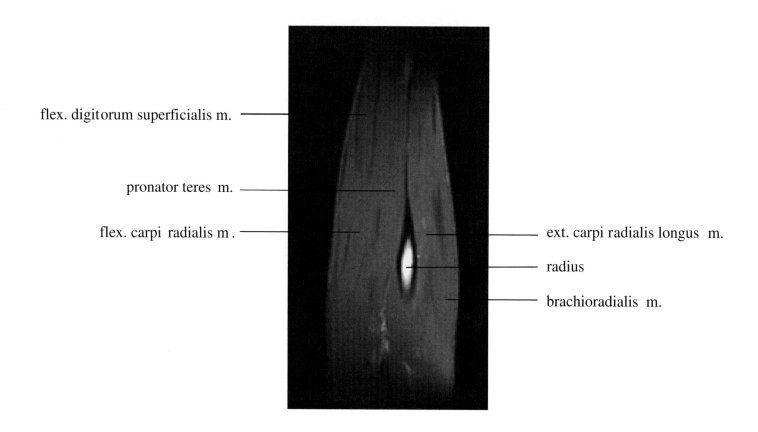

flex. digitorum superficialis m. ————

pronator teres m. ————

flex. carpi radialis m. ————

———— ext. carpi radialis longus m.

———— radius

———— brachioradialis m.

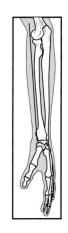

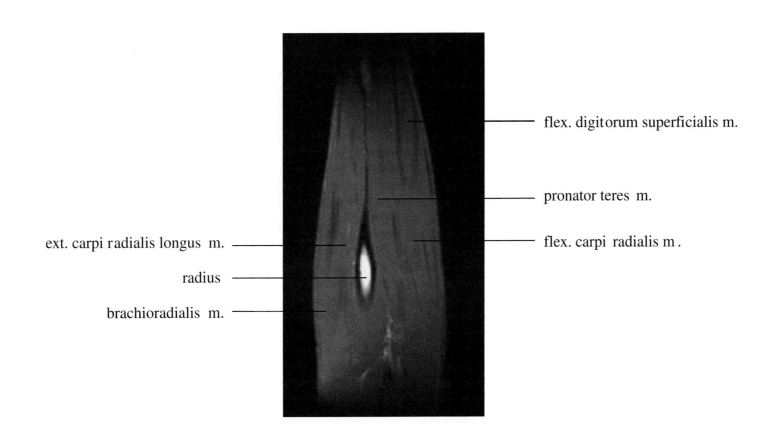

flex. digitorum superficialis m.

pronator teres m.

ext. carpi radialis longus m. ———————— flex. carpi radialis m.

radius

brachioradialis m.

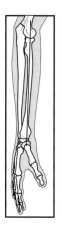

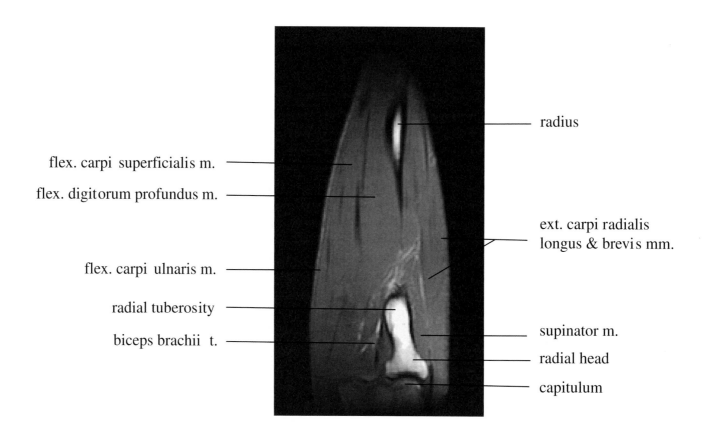

flex. carpi superficialis m. —————

flex. digitorum profundus m. —————

flex. carpi ulnaris m. —————

radial tuberosity —————

biceps brachii t. —————

————— radius

ext. carpi radialis
longus & brevis mm.

supinator m.

radial head

capitulum

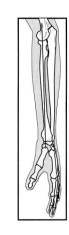

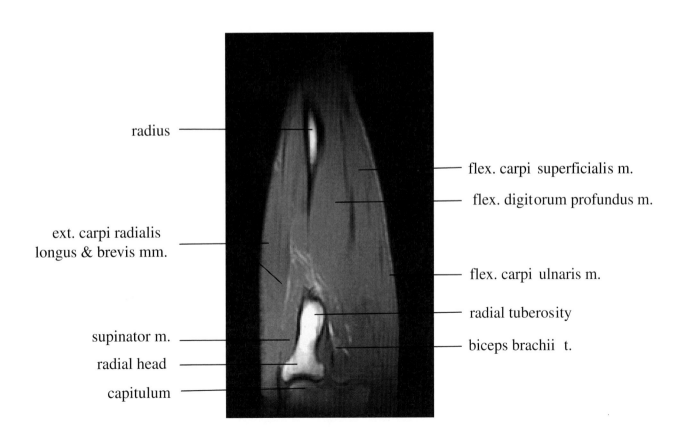

radius

flex. carpi superficialis m.

flex. digitorum profundus m.

ext. carpi radialis
longus & brevis mm.

flex. carpi ulnaris m.

radial tuberosity

supinator m.

biceps brachii t.

radial head

capitulum

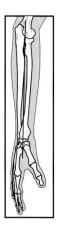

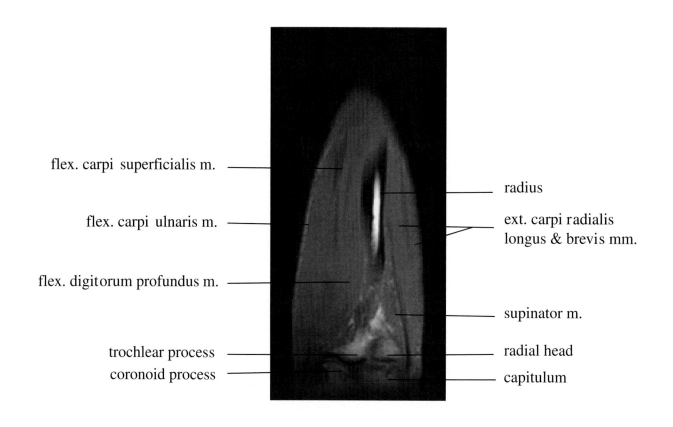

flex. carpi superficialis m. —

flex. carpi ulnaris m. —

flex. digitorum profundus m. —

trochlear process —

coronoid process —

— radius

— ext. carpi radialis
longus & brevis mm.

— supinator m.

— radial head

— capitulum

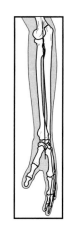

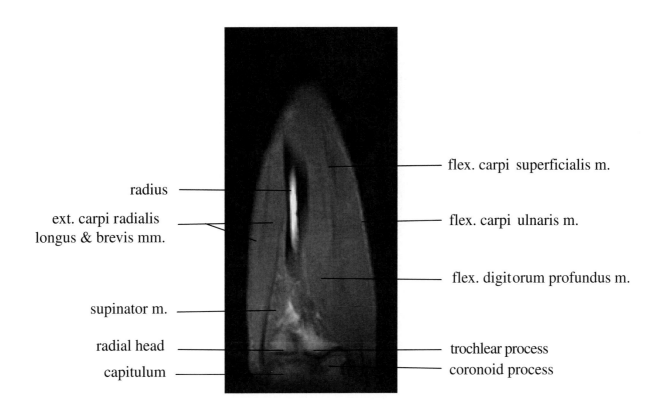

radius

ext. carpi radialis
longus & brevis mm.

supinator m.

radial head

capitulum

flex. carpi superficialis m.

flex. carpi ulnaris m.

flex. digitorum profundus m.

trochlear process

coronoid process

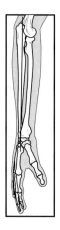

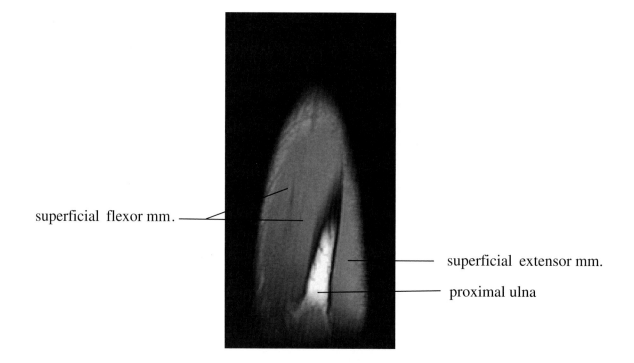

superficial flexor mm.

superficial extensor mm.

proximal ulna

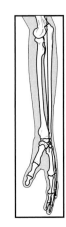

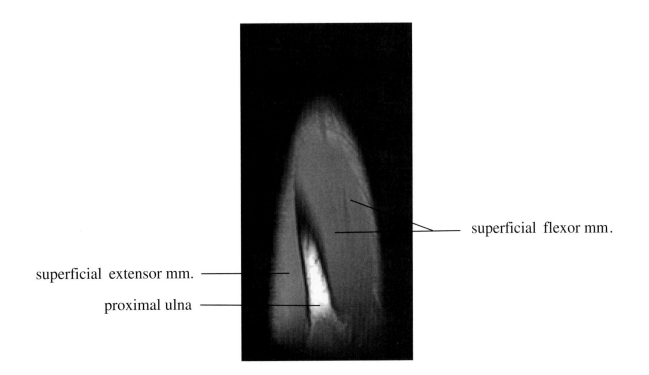

superficial flexor mm.

superficial extensor mm. ⎯⎯⎯⎯⎯⎯

proximal ulna ⎯⎯⎯⎯⎯

4

THE WRIST AND HAND

The wrist and the hand are "small parts" of the body. MR imaging has not been used as often in these areas because of the technical challenges they present. However, newer developments in surface coils and gradient hardware have allowed more accurate imaging of the wrist, hand, ankle, and foot because of faster data acquisition, smaller fields of view, and thinner slices. The major indications for wrist examination are suspected abnormalities of tendons and ligaments (especially the lunatotriquetral and scapholunate), presumed compressive neuropathies (especially of the median nerve), suspected avascular necrosis (particularly of the lunate, as in Kienböck's syndrome), and soft-tissue masses (especially ganglia) and soft-tissue or bony tumors. Rarely, MR imaging may be necessary to delineate the extent of infection in this region.

PRACTICAL PROTOCOL CONSIDERATIONS

The wrist and hand may be imaged by using the "head" or "knee" coils, but MR imaging with a dedicated circumferential quadrature or phased array coil is best. Use of the dedicated coils optimizes signal-to-noise ratio and allows the imager to produce high-resolution images with very small fields of view. The other advantage of the dedicated coils is that the patient may lie in the supine position with the arm at rest along the side. The hand and wrist should be placed in the neutral position without radial or ulnar deviation to maintain the alignment of the carpus and in pronation with the fingers held in extension. Although this is the ideal positioning, this technique may be modified according to the clinical indications for the study and the needs of the individual patient.

In general, it is best to use the smallest field of view that can be acquired (usually 6–8 cm) given the other parameters of the scan. Spin-echo images usually require a 256×256 matrix, and gradient-echo images may require alteration of the flip angle to optimize the T2-like contrast. Fat saturation may be used to increase the detection of fluid or edema. Some researchers have used the intravenous administration of gadolinium to study inflammatory arthritides or the intraarticular administration of MR contrast agents to study ligamentous disruptions. However, this is not standard technique at most institutions. In addition, kinematic studies of the wrist and hand are performed mainly for research purposes at this time.

Menu of Protocols: Wrist and Hand

Plane	Pulse Sequence	FA (degrees)	TR (msec)	TE (msec)	TI (msec)	FOV (cm)	Matrix (256×-)	ST/G (mm)	NEX	Comments
Localizer (coronal, transaxial, sagittal)	SE		600	20		8	128	3/1	2	Either is acceptable
Transaxial	SE, double echo		2250	20/80		8	128	3/1	2	Either is acceptable
Transaxial	FSE		2500	10		8–10	256	3/1	2	
Transaxial	FSE, FS		4000	108		8–10	192	3/1.5	2	
Transaxial	3D, GRE	30	45	10		6–8	192	1/0	1	
Sagittal	SE		450	20		8	128	3/1	2	Either is acceptable
Sagittal	SE, double echo		2500	30/90		8–10	128	3/1	2	
Sagittal	FSE, double echo		3000	20/100		8–10	192	3/1	1	
Sagittal	FSE, FS		4000	18		8–10	192	3/1.5	2	
Coronal	SE, double echo		2000	20/80		8	8128	3/1	2	Either is acceptable
Coronal	3D, GRE	30	45	9		8	192	VAR/0	2	
Coronal	3D, GRE	20	30	12		8–12	128	1.2/0	2	
Coronal	GRE	25	600	20		8–10	192	3/1.5	2	
Coronal	FMPIR		3000	51	150	12	128	4/1	1	
Pre-GAD (axial, coronal, sagittal)	SE (±FS)		600	20		8–10	192	3/1 3/1	2	Depends on site of abnormalities
Post-GAD (axial, coronal, sagittal)	SE (±FS)		600	20		8–10	192		2	Intraarticular GAD for ligaments, intravenous GAD for tumors, cysts, infection

MAJOR OSTEOCHONDRAL STRUCTURES/LANDMARKS

Wrist

- Distal radius
  - Articular cartilage
  - Styloid process
  - Ulnar (sigmoid) notch
  - Dorsal tubercle

- Distal ulna
  - Articular cartilage
  - Styloid process
  - Ulnar head
- Carpus
  - Scaphoid
  - Lunate
  - Triquetrum (and its tubercle)
  - Pisiform (sesamoid of flexor carpi ulnaris tendon)
  - Hamate (and its hamulus)
  - Capitate
  - Trapezoid (lesser multangular)
  - Trapezium (greater multangular)
  - Triangular fibrocartilage complex (TFCC)

Hand

- Metacarpals (I–V)
  - Metacarpal base
  - Metacarpal shaft
  - Metacarpal head
- Proximal phalanges
  - Base
  - Shaft
  - Head
- Distal phalanges
  - Base
  - Tuberosity (tuft)
- Sesamoids (variable)

MAJOR LIGAMENTS/TENDONS/BURSAE

Ligaments of the Wrist

The ligaments of the wrist provide for carpal and distal radioulnar stability. These ligaments are generally divided into two groups: extrinsic and intrinsic. The extrinsic ligaments extend from the radius, ulna, and metacarpals and bind the radius to the carpal bones. The intrinsic ligaments originate and insert within the carpus and bind the carpal bones together.

Radiocarpal Extrinsic Ligaments

- Volar (palmar) ligaments
  - Radioscaphocapitate
  - Long radiolunate (radiolunotriquetral)
  - Short radiolunate
  - Radioscapholunate
    - Radiolunate (ligament of Testut)
    - Radioscaphoid (ligament of Kuenz)
- Radial collateral ligament (from radial styloid tip to scaphoid waist on radial side)

Dorsal Extrinsic Ligaments

- Dorsal radioscapholunotriquetral
- Scaphotriquetral

Ulnocarpal Extrinsic Ligaments (Triangular Fibrocartilage (TFCC) Ligaments)

- Volar radioulnar
- Dorsal radioulnar
- Ulnotriquetral
- Ulnolunate
- Ulnar collateral
- Meniscal homologue

Intrinsic (Intercarpal) Ligaments

- Dorsal intercarpal
- Volar intercarpal
- Interosseous
  - Scapholunate
  - Lunatotriquetral
  - Deltoid (arcuate)—(stabilizes distal carpal row on proximal row)
  - Trapezoid—capitate
  - Trapezium—trapezoid
  - Capitate—hamate

Tendons of the Wrist

Palmar Group

- Carpal tunnel (volar boundary: the "flexor retinaculum," which extends from the scaphoid tuberosity and inserts on the trapezium, the hook of the hamate, and the pisiform; dorsal boundary: the lunate and capitate bones)
  - Flexor pollicis longus
  - Flexor digitorum superficialis (four tendons)
  - Flexor digitorum profundus (four tendons)
- Other flexor tendons
  - Palmaris longus
  - Flexor carpi radialis
  - Flexor carpi ulnaris

Dorsal Group

- Extensors
  - Extensor carpi ulnaris
    - Extensor digiti minimi
    - Extensor digitorum
    - Extensor indicis
    - Extensor pollicis longus
    - Extensor carpi radialis brevis

  - Extensor carpi radialis longus
  - Extensor pollicis brevis
- Abductor
  – Abductor pollicis longus

Bursae of the Wrist

- Ulnar bursa (covers digital flexor tendons-variable)

Components of Guyon's Canal (Ulnopalmar aspect of wrist superficial to flexor retinaculum)

- Ulnar nerve
- Ulnar artery
- Anomalous muscles

Ligaments of the Hand

- Palmar metacarpal
- Palmar carpometacarpal
- Deep transverse metacarpal
- Palmar (palmar plates)
- Collateral

Tendons of the Hand

- Long extensor tendon
- Flexor digitorum profundus
- Flexor digitorum superficialis

MAJOR MUSCLES

Wrist

(See forearm)

Hand

(See forearm)

• Lumbricals (associated with flexor digitorum profundus tendons)

ORIGIN/INSERTION/INNERVATION OF MAJOR MUSCLES

Wrist

(See forearm)

Hand

(See forearm)

Lumbricals

Muscle	Origin	Insertion	Innervation
–Two lateral	Distal to flexor retinaculum from radial/palmar surfaces of flexor digitorum profundus muscle	Radial border of expansion of extensor digitorum muscle at level of proximal phalanx	Median N.
–Two medial	Contiguous sides of tendons for digits III/IV and IV/V	Radial border of expansion of extensor digitorum muscle at level of proximal phalanx	Deep branch of ulnar N.

WRIST AND HAND: AXIAL ANATOMY

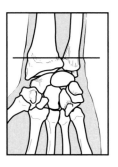

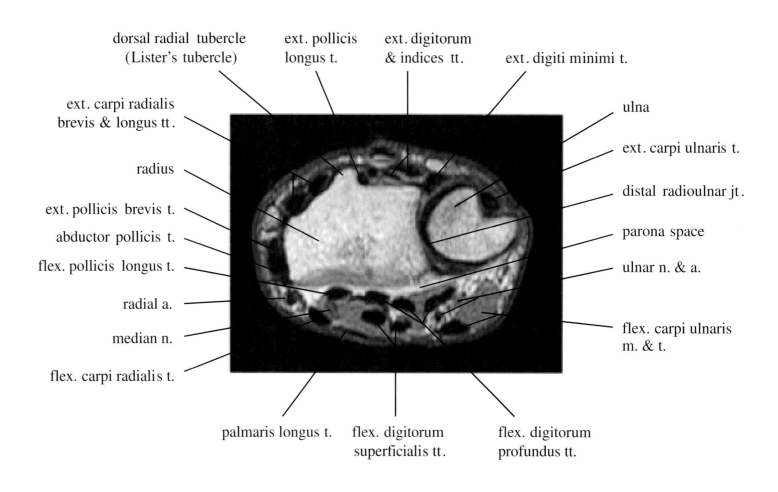

dorsal radial tubercle
(Lister's tubercle)

ext. pollicis
longus t.

ext. digitorum
& indices tt.

ext. digiti minimi t.

ext. carpi radialis
brevis & longus tt.

radius

ext. pollicis brevis t.

abductor pollicis t.

flex. pollicis longus t.

radial a.

median n.

flex. carpi radialis t.

ulna

ext. carpi ulnaris t.

distal radioulnar jt.

parona space

ulnar n. & a.

flex. carpi ulnaris
m. & t.

palmaris longus t.

flex. digitorum
superficialis tt.

flex. digitorum
profundus tt.

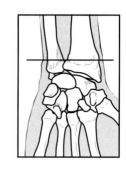

ext. digiti minimi t.

ext. digitorum
& indices tt.

ext. pollicis
longus t.

dorsal radial tubercle
(Lister's tubercle)

ulna

ext. carpi ulnaris t.

distal radioulnar jt.

parona space

ulnar n. & a.

flex. carpi ulnaris
m. & t.

ext. carpi radialis
brevis & longus tt.

radius

ext. pollicis brevis t.

abductor pollicis t.

flex. pollicis longus t.

radial a.

median n.

flex. carpi radialis t.

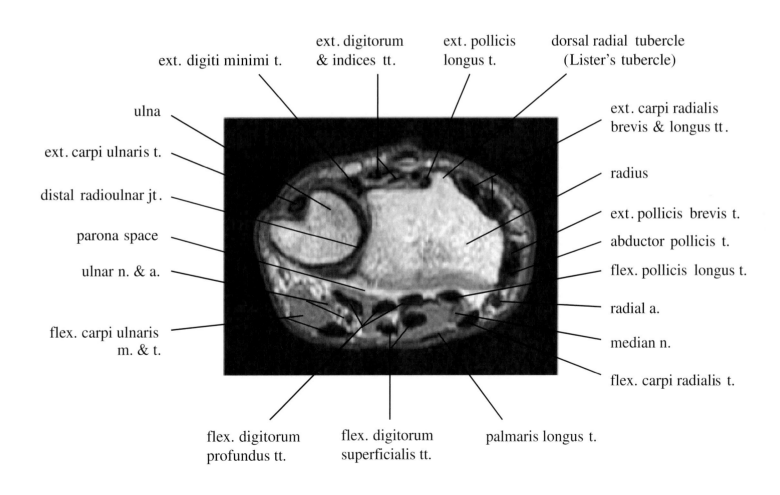

flex. digitorum
profundus tt.

flex. digitorum
superficialis tt.

palmaris longus t.

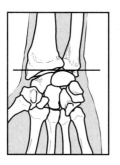

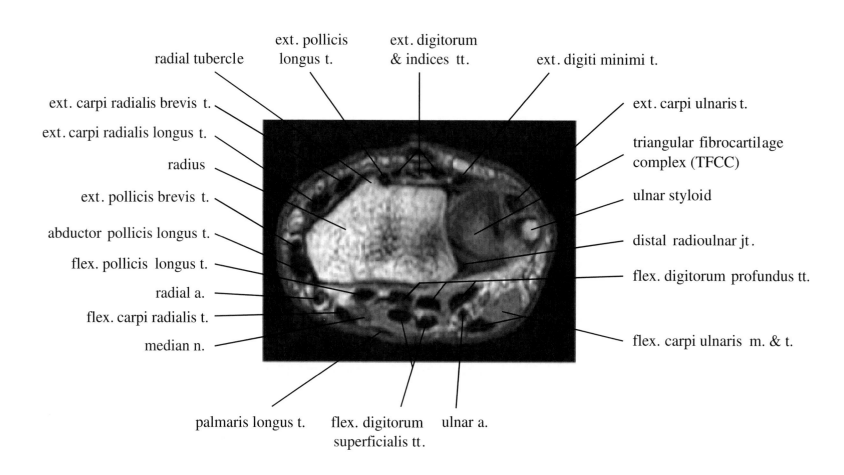

radial tubercle

ext. pollicis
longus t.

ext. digitorum
& indices tt.

ext. digiti minimi t.

ext. carpi radialis brevis t.

ext. carpi radialis longus t.

radius

ext. pollicis brevis t.

abductor pollicis longus t.

flex. pollicis longus t.

radial a.

flex. carpi radialis t.

median n.

ext. carpi ulnaris t.

triangular fibrocartilage
complex (TFCC)

ulnar styloid

distal radioulnar jt.

flex. digitorum profundus tt.

flex. carpi ulnaris m. & t.

palmaris longus t.

flex. digitorum
superficialis tt.

ulnar a.

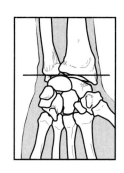

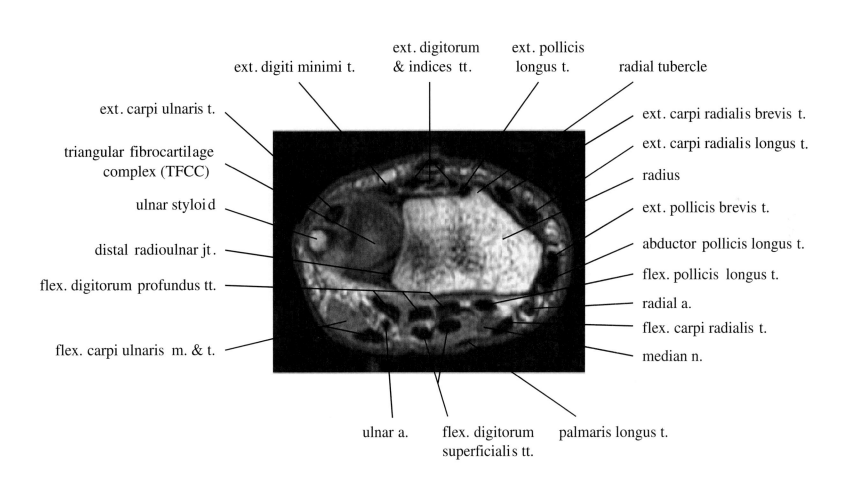

ext. digiti minimi t.

ext. digitorum
& indices tt.

ext. pollicis
longus t.

radial tubercle

ext. carpi ulnaris t.

triangular fibrocartilage
complex (TFCC)

ulnar styloid

distal radioulnar jt.

flex. digitorum profundus tt.

flex. carpi ulnaris m. & t.

ext. carpi radialis brevis t.

ext. carpi radialis longus t.

radius

ext. pollicis brevis t.

abductor pollicis longus t.

flex. pollicis longus t.

radial a.

flex. carpi radialis t.

median n.

ulnar a.

flex. digitorum
superficialis tt.

palmaris longus t.

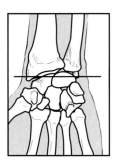

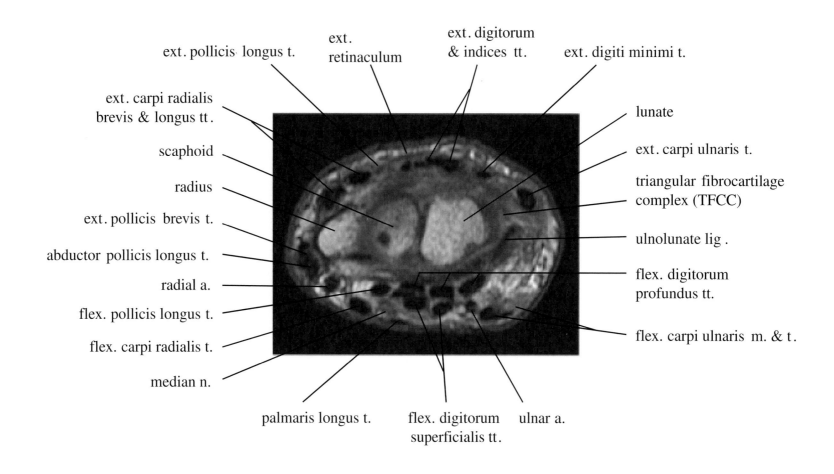

ext. pollicis longus t.

ext. retinaculum

ext. digitorum & indices tt.

ext. digiti minimi t.

ext. carpi radialis brevis & longus tt.

scaphoid

radius

ext. pollicis brevis t.

abductor pollicis longus t.

radial a.

flex. pollicis longus t.

flex. carpi radialis t.

median n.

lunate

ext. carpi ulnaris t.

triangular fibrocartilage complex (TFCC)

ulnolunate lig.

flex. digitorum profundus tt.

flex. carpi ulnaris m. & t.

palmaris longus t.

flex. digitorum superficialis tt.

ulnar a.

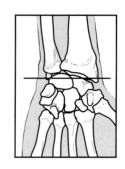

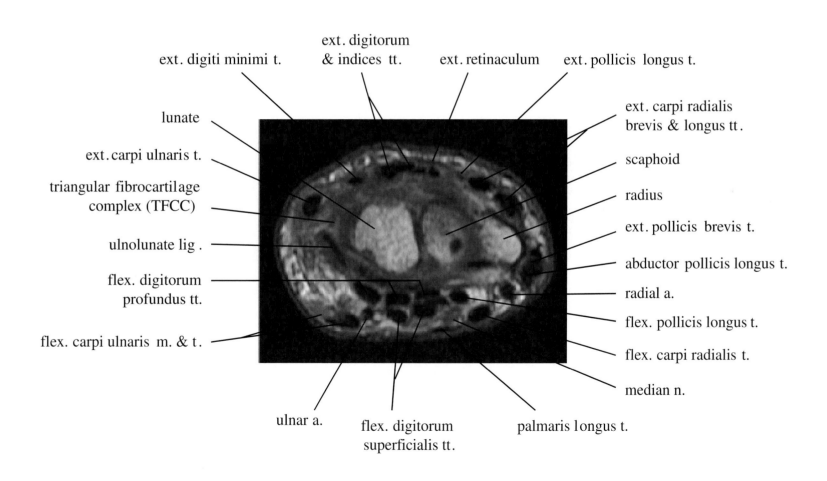

ext. digiti minimi t.

ext. digitorum
& indices tt.

ext. retinaculum

ext. pollicis longus t.

lunate

ext. carpi ulnaris t.

triangular fibrocartilage
complex (TFCC)

ulnolunate lig.

flex. digitorum
profundus tt.

flex. carpi ulnaris m. & t.

ext. carpi radialis
brevis & longus tt.

scaphoid

radius

ext. pollicis brevis t.

abductor pollicis longus t.

radial a.

flex. pollicis longus t.

flex. carpi radialis t.

median n.

ulnar a.

flex. digitorum
superficialis tt.

palmaris longus t.

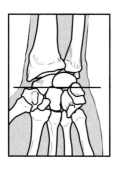

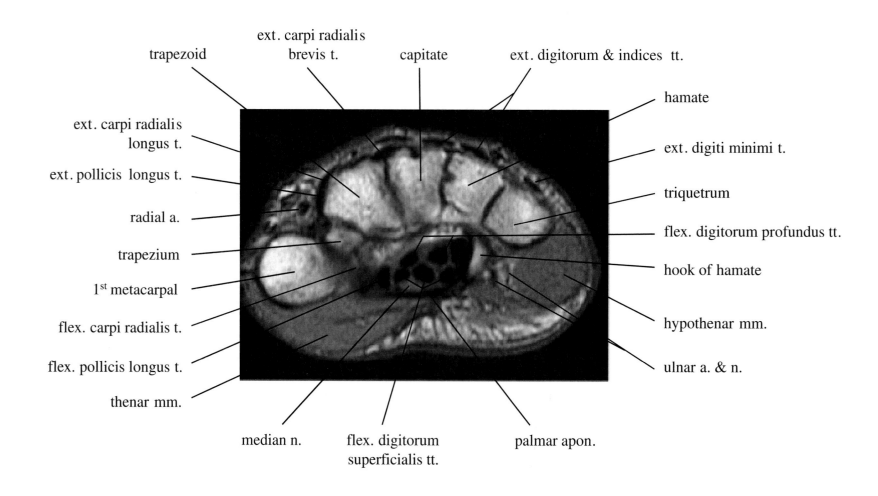

trapezoid

ext. carpi radialis
brevis t.

capitate

ext. digitorum & indices tt.

ext. carpi radialis
longus t.

ext. pollicis longus t.

radial a.

trapezium

1ˢᵗ metacarpal

flex. carpi radialis t.

flex. pollicis longus t.

thenar mm.

hamate

ext. digiti minimi t.

triquetrum

flex. digitorum profundus tt.

hook of hamate

hypothenar mm.

ulnar a. & n.

median n.

flex. digitorum
superficialis tt.

palmar apon.

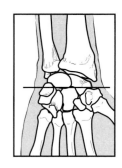

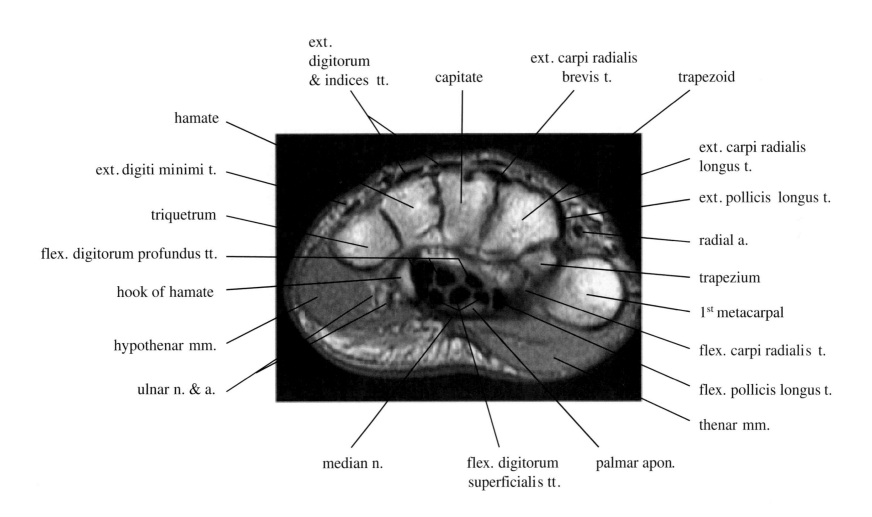

ext. digitorum & indices tt.

capitate

ext. carpi radialis brevis t.

trapezoid

hamate

ext. digiti minimi t.

triquetrum

flex. digitorum profundus tt.

hook of hamate

hypothenar mm.

ulnar n. & a.

ext. carpi radialis longus t.

ext. pollicis longus t.

radial a.

trapezium

1st metacarpal

flex. carpi radialis t.

flex. pollicis longus t.

thenar mm.

median n.

flex. digitorum superficialis tt.

palmar apon.

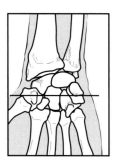

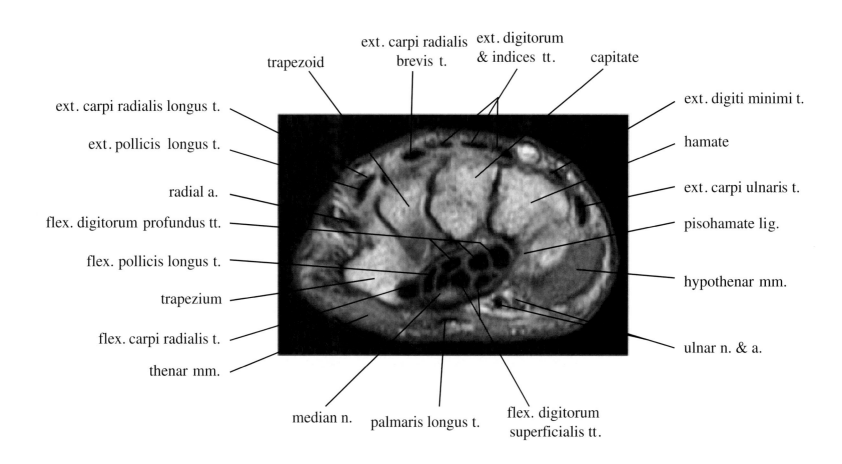

trapezoid

ext. carpi radialis
brevis t.

ext. digitorum
& indices tt.

capitate

ext. carpi radialis longus t.

ext. pollicis longus t.

radial a.

flex. digitorum profundus tt.

flex. pollicis longus t.

trapezium

flex. carpi radialis t.

thenar mm.

ext. digiti minimi t.

hamate

ext. carpi ulnaris t.

pisohamate lig.

hypothenar mm.

ulnar n. & a.

median n.

palmaris longus t.

flex. digitorum
superficialis tt.

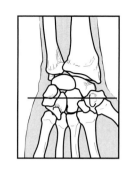

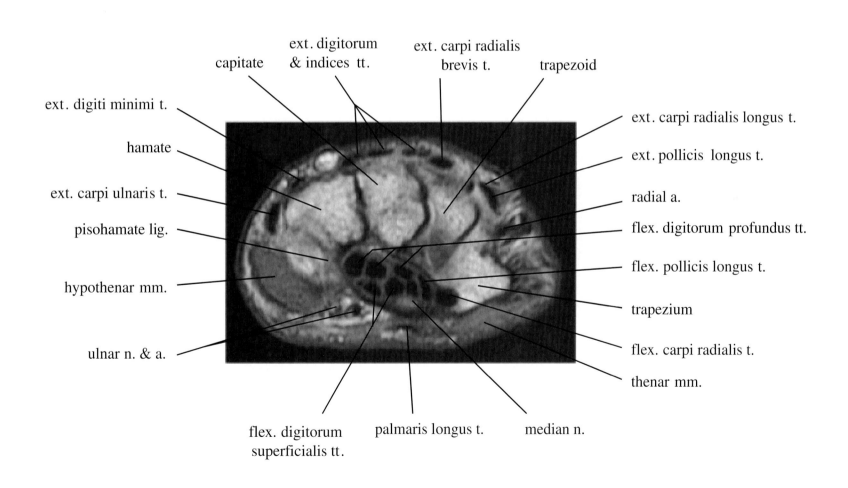

capitate

ext. digitorum
& indices tt.

ext. carpi radialis
brevis t.

trapezoid

ext. digiti minimi t.

ext. carpi radialis longus t.

hamate

ext. pollicis longus t.

ext. carpi ulnaris t.

radial a.

pisohamate lig.

flex. digitorum profundus tt.

flex. pollicis longus t.

hypothenar mm.

trapezium

ulnar n. & a.

flex. carpi radialis t.

thenar mm.

flex. digitorum
superficialis tt.

palmaris longus t.

median n.

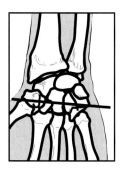

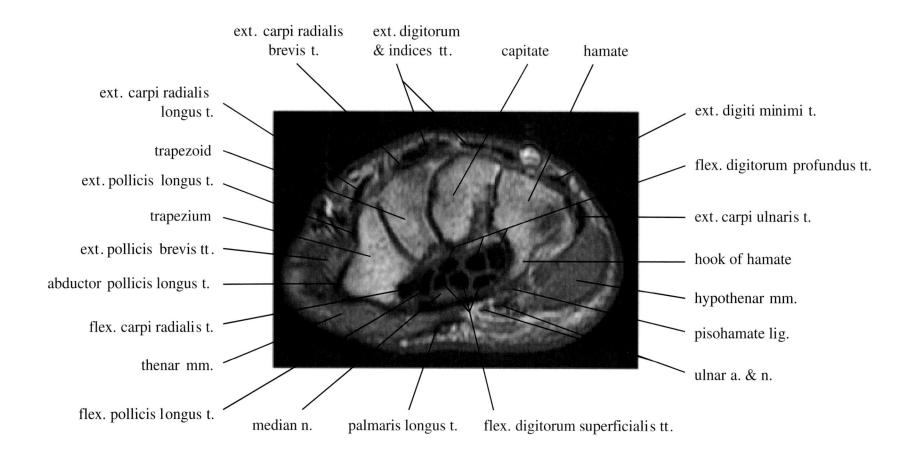

ext. carpi radialis
brevis t.

ext. digitorum
& indices tt.

capitate   hamate

ext. carpi radialis
longus t.

ext. digiti minimi t.

trapezoid

flex. digitorum profundus tt.

ext. pollicis longus t.

trapezium

ext. carpi ulnaris t.

ext. pollicis brevis tt.

hook of hamate

abductor pollicis longus t.

hypothenar mm.

flex. carpi radialis t.

pisohamate lig.

thenar mm.

ulnar a. & n.

flex. pollicis longus t.

median n.   palmaris longus t.   flex. digitorum superficialis tt.

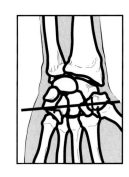

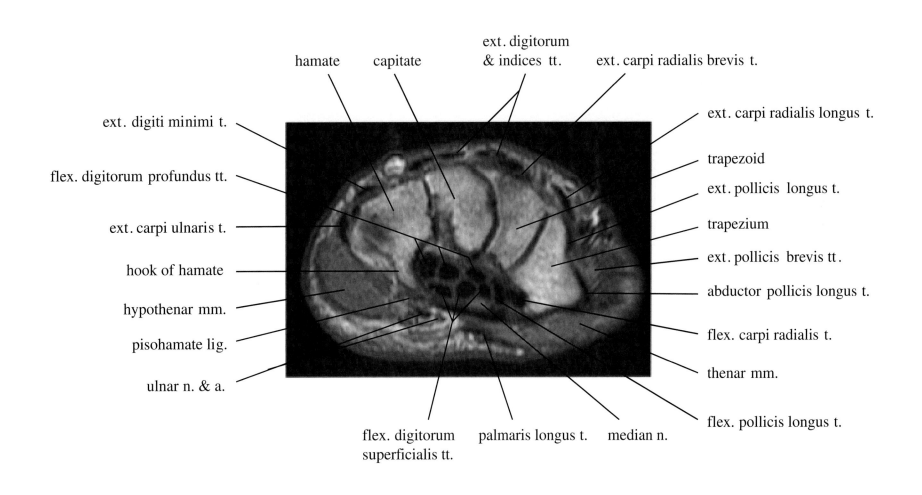

hamate

capitate

ext. digitorum
& indices tt.

ext. carpi radialis brevis t.

ext. carpi radialis longus t.

ext. digiti minimi t.

flex. digitorum profundus tt.

ext. carpi ulnaris t.

hook of hamate

hypothenar mm.

pisohamate lig.

ulnar n. & a.

trapezoid

ext. pollicis longus t.

trapezium

ext. pollicis brevis tt.

abductor pollicis longus t.

flex. carpi radialis t.

thenar mm.

flex. pollicis longus t.

flex. digitorum
superficialis tt.

palmaris longus t.

median n.

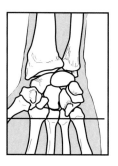

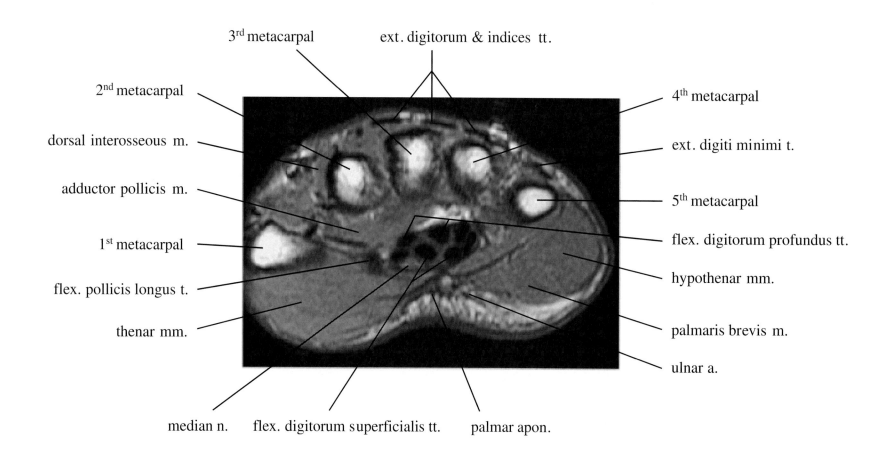

3rd metacarpal

ext. digitorum & indices tt.

2nd metacarpal

dorsal interosseous m.

adductor pollicis m.

1st metacarpal

flex. pollicis longus t.

thenar mm.

4th metacarpal

ext. digiti minimi t.

5th metacarpal

flex. digitorum profundus tt.

hypothenar mm.

palmaris brevis m.

ulnar a.

median n.   flex. digitorum superficialis tt.   palmar apon.

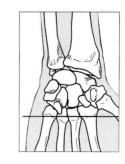

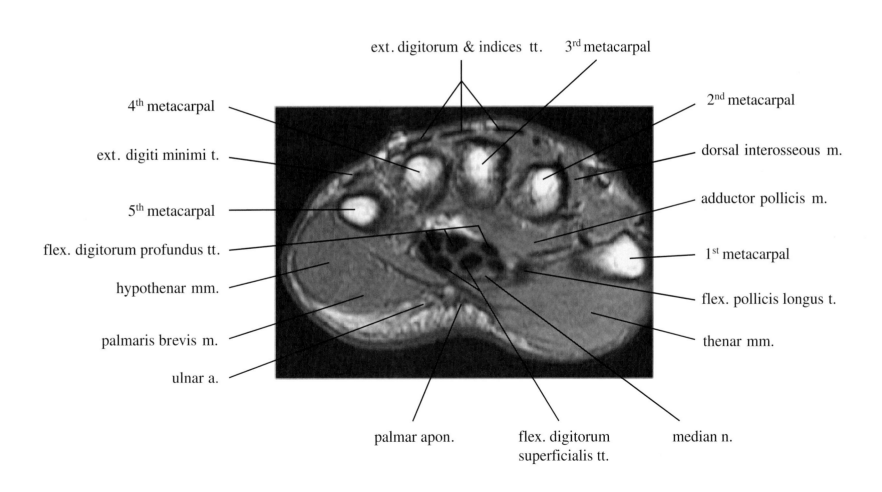

ext. digitorum & indices tt.   3rd metacarpal

4th metacarpal

2nd metacarpal

ext. digiti minimi t.

dorsal interosseous m.

5th metacarpal

adductor pollicis m.

flex. digitorum profundus tt.

1st metacarpal

hypothenar mm.

flex. pollicis longus t.

palmaris brevis m.

thenar mm.

ulnar a.

palmar apon.   flex. digitorum
superficialis tt.   median n.

THE WRIST AND HAND: SAGITTAL ANATOMY

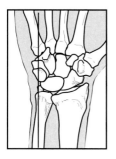

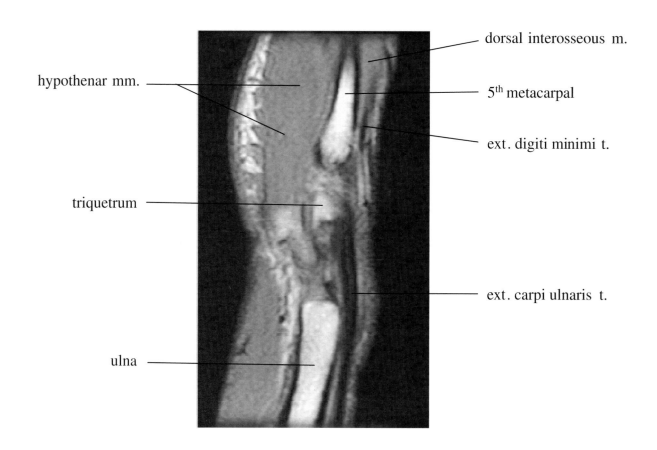

hypothenar mm.

triquetrum

ulna

dorsal interosseous m.

5th metacarpal

ext. digiti minimi t.

ext. carpi ulnaris t.

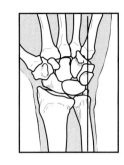

dorsal interosseous m.

5th metacarpal

ext. digiti minimi t.

ext. carpi ulnaris t.

hypothenar mm.

triquetrum

ulna

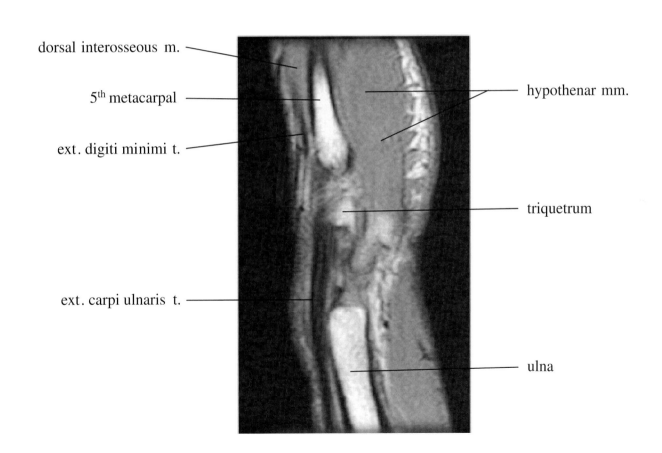

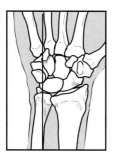

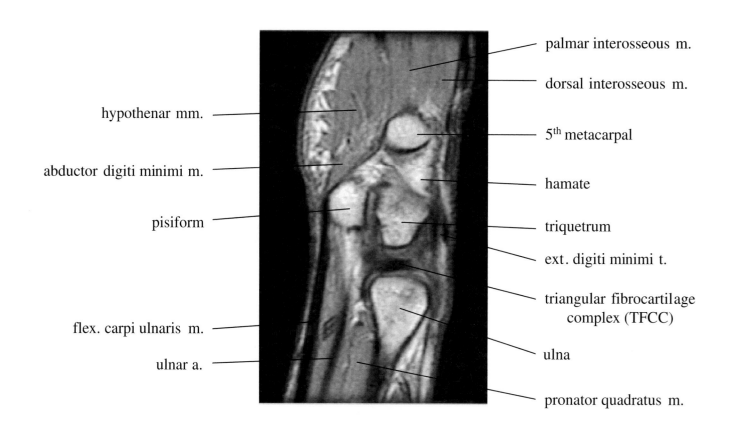

palmar interosseous m.

dorsal interosseous m.

hypothenar mm.

5th metacarpal

abductor digiti minimi m.

hamate

pisiform

triquetrum

ext. digiti minimi t.

triangular fibrocartilage complex (TFCC)

flex. carpi ulnaris m.

ulna

ulnar a.

pronator quadratus m.

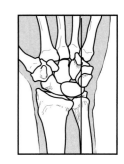

palmar interosseous m.

dorsal interosseous m.

5th metacarpal

hamate

triquetrum

ext. digiti minimi t.

triangular fibrocartilage
complex (TFCC)

ulna

pronator quadratus m.

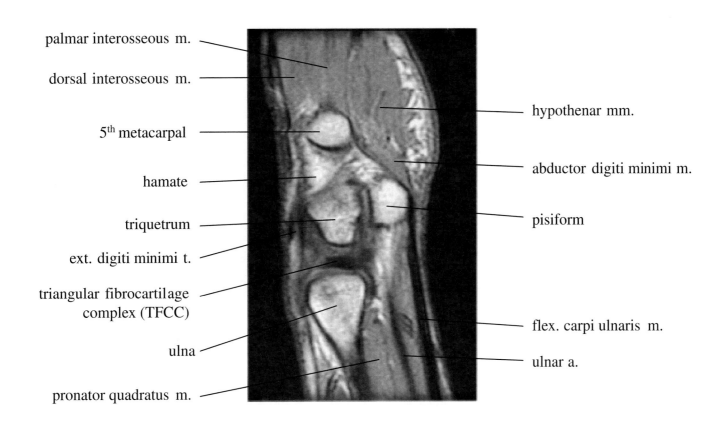

hypothenar mm.

abductor digiti minimi m.

pisiform

flex. carpi ulnaris m.

ulnar a.

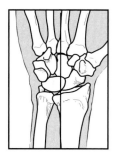

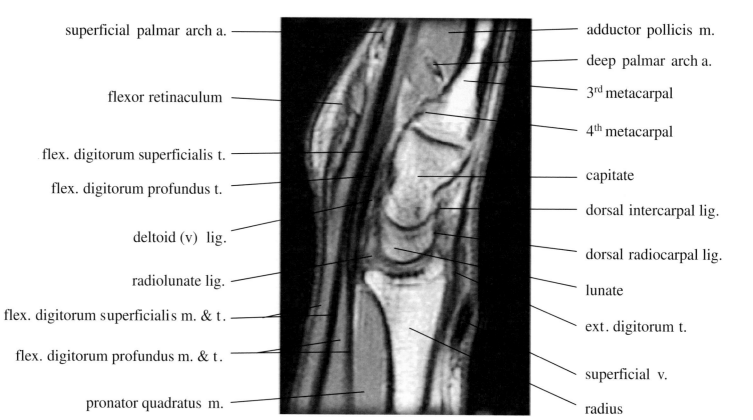

superficial palmar arch a.

flexor retinaculum

flex. digitorum superficialis t.

flex. digitorum profundus t.

deltoid (v) lig.

radiolunate lig.

flex. digitorum superficialis m. & t.

flex. digitorum profundus m. & t.

pronator quadratus m.

adductor pollicis m.

deep palmar arch a.

3rd metacarpal

4th metacarpal

capitate

dorsal intercarpal lig.

dorsal radiocarpal lig.

lunate

ext. digitorum t.

superficial v.

radius

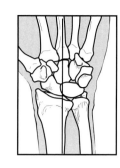

adductor pollicis m. —————

deep palmar arch a. —————

3rd metacarpal —————

4th metacarpal —————

capitate —————

dorsal intercarpal lig. —————

dorsal radiocarpal lig. —————

lunate —————

ext. digitorum t. —————

superficial v. —————

radius —————

————— superficial palmar arch a.

————— flexor retinaculum

————— flex. digitorum superficialis t.

————— flex. digitorum profundus t.

————— deltoid (v) lig.

————— radiolunate lig.

————— flex. digitorum superficialis m. & t.

————— flex. digitorum profundus m. & t.

————— pronator quadratus m.

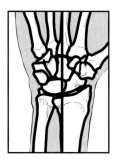

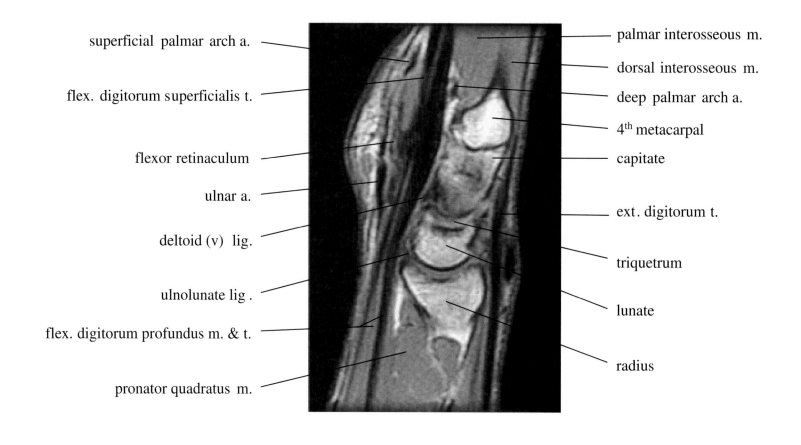

superficial palmar arch a.

palmar interosseous m.

dorsal interosseous m.

flex. digitorum superficialis t.

deep palmar arch a.

4th metacarpal

flexor retinaculum

capitate

ulnar a.

ext. digitorum t.

deltoid (v) lig.

triquetrum

ulnolunate lig .

lunate

flex. digitorum profundus m. & t.

radius

pronator quadratus m.

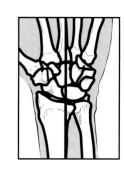

palmar interosseous m. —

dorsal interosseous m. —

deep palmar arch a. —

4th metacarpal —

capitate —

ext. digitorum t.—

triquetrum

lunate

radius

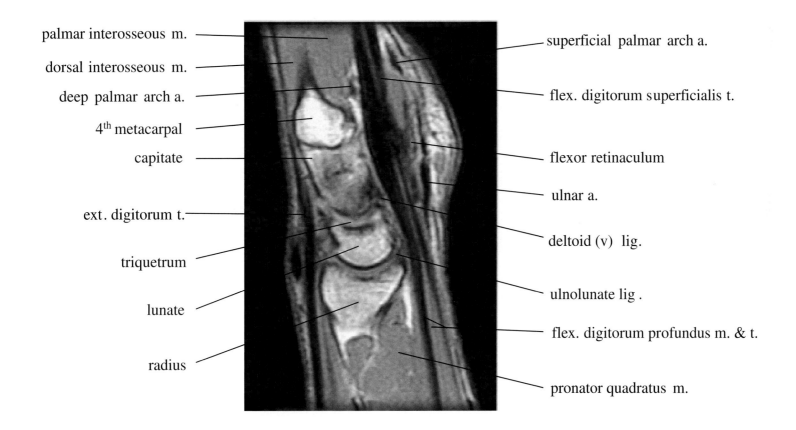

superficial palmar arch a.

flex. digitorum superficialis t.

flexor retinaculum

ulnar a.

deltoid (v) lig.

ulnolunate lig .

flex. digitorum profundus m. & t.

pronator quadratus m.

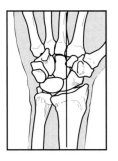

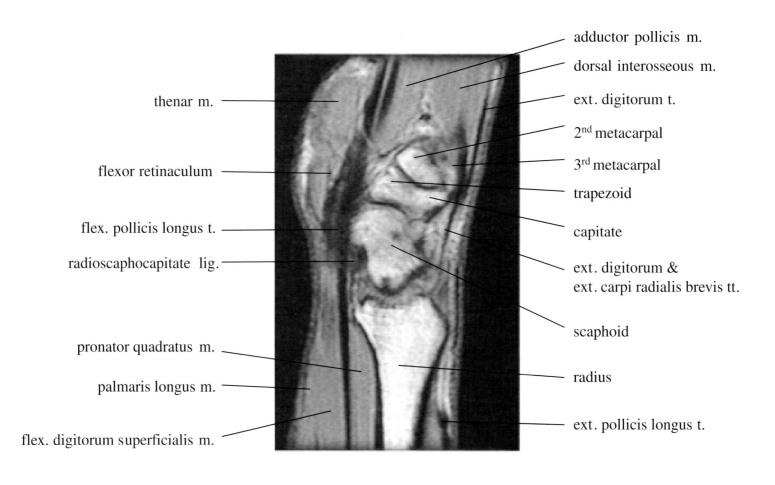

adductor pollicis m.

dorsal interosseous m.

ext. digitorum t.

thenar m.

2ⁿᵈ metacarpal

3ʳᵈ metacarpal

flexor retinaculum

trapezoid

flex. pollicis longus t.

capitate

radioscaphocapitate lig.

ext. digitorum &
ext. carpi radialis brevis tt.

scaphoid

pronator quadratus m.

radius

palmaris longus m.

flex. digitorum superficialis m.

ext. pollicis longus t.

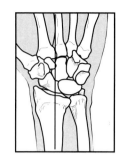

adductor pollicis m.

dorsal interosseous m.

ext. digitorum t.

2nd metacarpal

3rd metacarpal

trapezoid

capitate

ext. digitorum &
ext. carpi radialis brevis tt.

scaphoid

radius

ext. pollicis longus t.

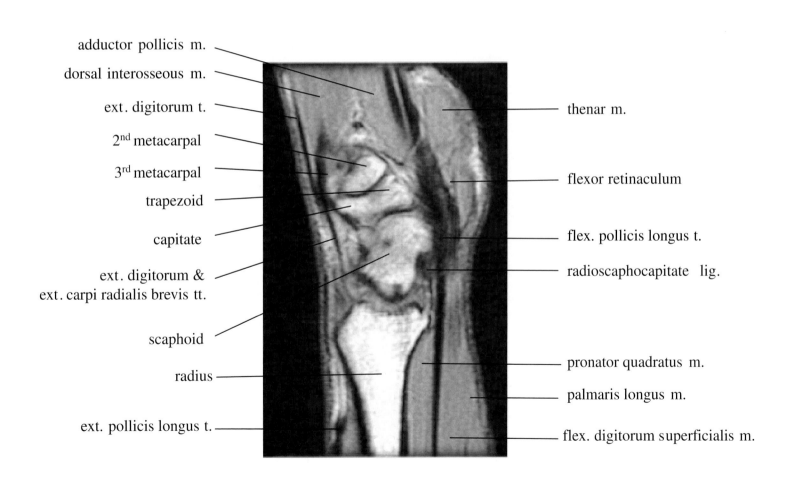

thenar m.

flexor retinaculum

flex. pollicis longus t.

radioscaphocapitate lig.

pronator quadratus m.

palmaris longus m.

flex. digitorum superficialis m.

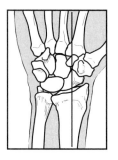

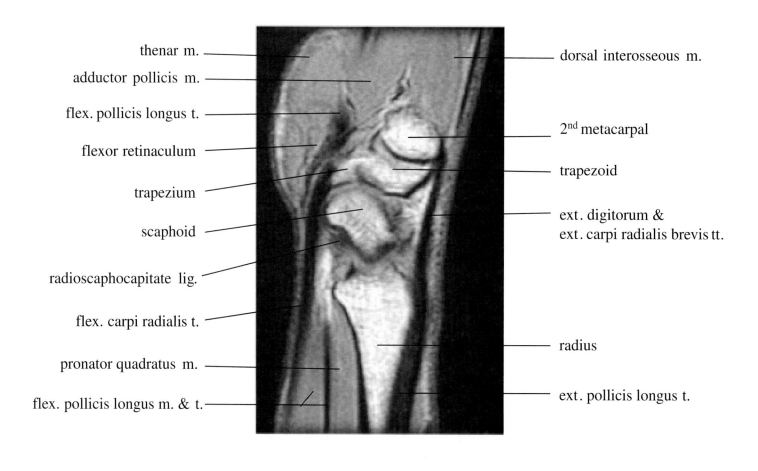

thenar m.

adductor pollicis m.

flex. pollicis longus t.

flexor retinaculum

trapezium

scaphoid

radioscaphocapitate lig.

flex. carpi radialis t.

pronator quadratus m.

flex. pollicis longus m. & t.

dorsal interosseous m.

2nd metacarpal

trapezoid

ext. digitorum &
ext. carpi radialis brevis tt.

radius

ext. pollicis longus t.

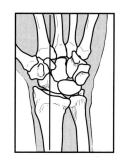

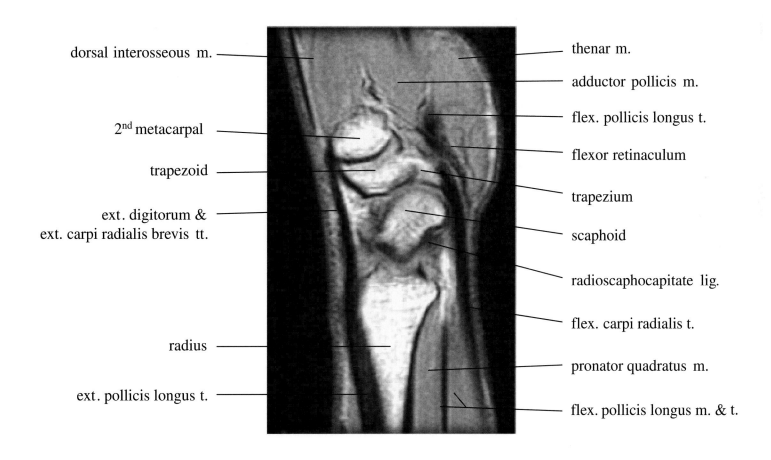

dorsal interosseous m. ——

2nd metacarpal ——

trapezoid ——

ext. digitorum &
ext. carpi radialis brevis tt. ——

radius ——

ext. pollicis longus t. ——

—— thenar m.

—— adductor pollicis m.

—— flex. pollicis longus t.

—— flexor retinaculum

—— trapezium

—— scaphoid

—— radioscaphocapitate lig.

—— flex. carpi radialis t.

—— pronator quadratus m.

—— flex. pollicis longus m. & t.

THE WRIST AND HAND: CORONAL ANATOMY

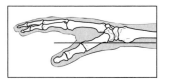

5th metacarpal ——————

hypothenar mm. ——————

pisiform ——————

flexor digitorum
profundus tt. ——————

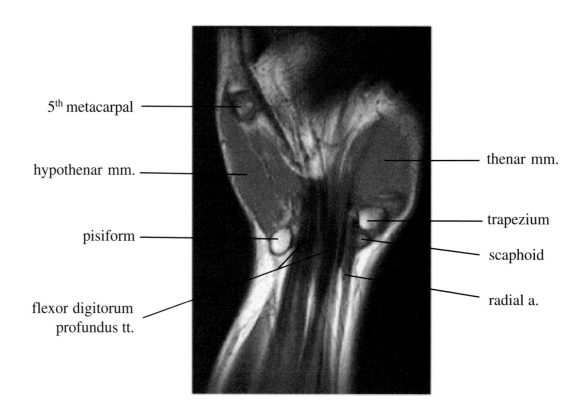

————— thenar mm.

————— trapezium

————— scaphoid

————— radial a.

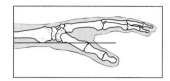

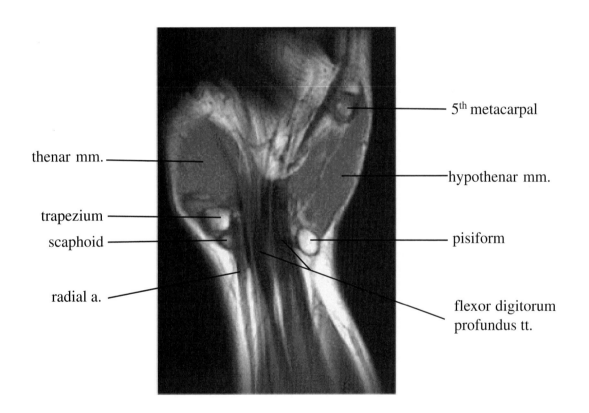

thenar mm.

5th metacarpal

trapezium

hypothenar mm.

scaphoid

pisiform

radial a.

flexor digitorum profundus tt.

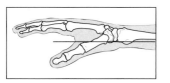

5th metacarpal

interosseous mm.

hypothenar mm.

hook of
hamate

pisohamate lig.

pisiform

lunate

ulna

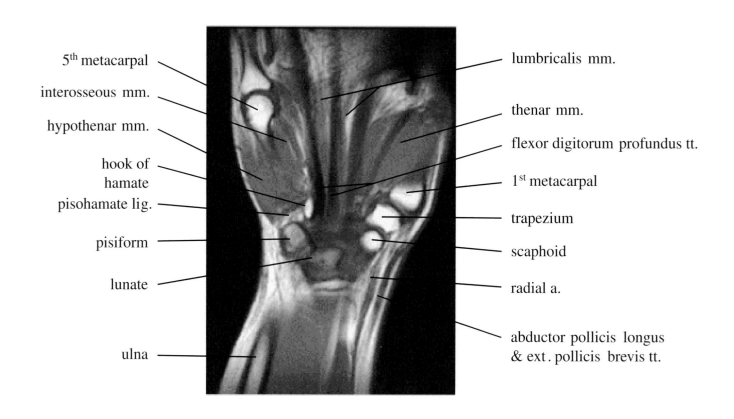

lumbricalis mm.

thenar mm.

flexor digitorum profundus tt.

1st metacarpal

trapezium

scaphoid

radial a.

abductor pollicis longus
& ext. pollicis brevis tt.

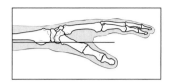

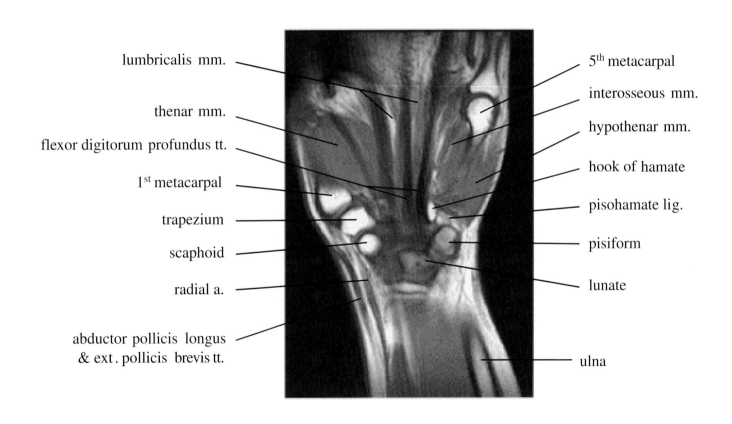

lumbricalis mm.

thenar mm.

flexor digitorum profundus tt.

1st metacarpal

trapezium

scaphoid

radial a.

abductor pollicis longus
& ext. pollicis brevis tt.

5th metacarpal

interosseous mm.

hypothenar mm.

hook of hamate

pisohamate lig.

pisiform

lunate

ulna

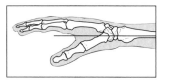

3rd metacarpal

interosseous mm.

4th metacarpal

hamate

ext. carpi ulnaris t.

triquetrum

lunotriquetral lig.

triangular fibrocartilage
complex (TFCC)

lunate

ulna

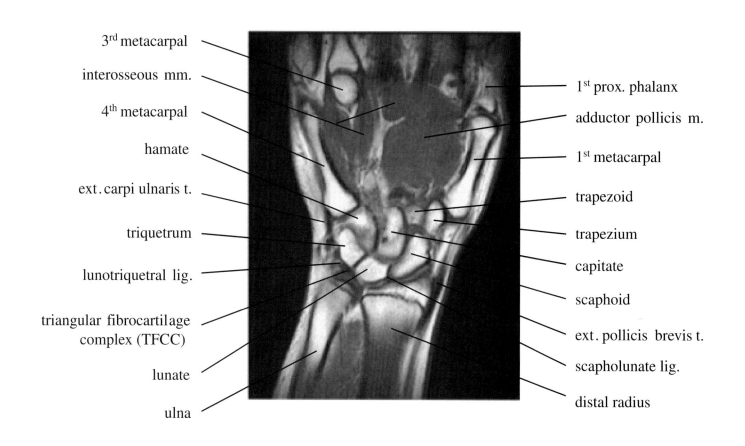

1st prox. phalanx

adductor pollicis m.

1st metacarpal

trapezoid

trapezium

capitate

scaphoid

ext. pollicis brevis t.

scapholunate lig.

distal radius

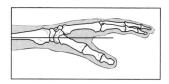

1st prox. phalanx —————

adductor pollicis m. —————

1st metacarpal —————

trapezoid —————

trapezium —————

capitate —————

scaphoid —————

ext. pollicis brevis t. —————

scapholunate lig. —————

distal radius —————

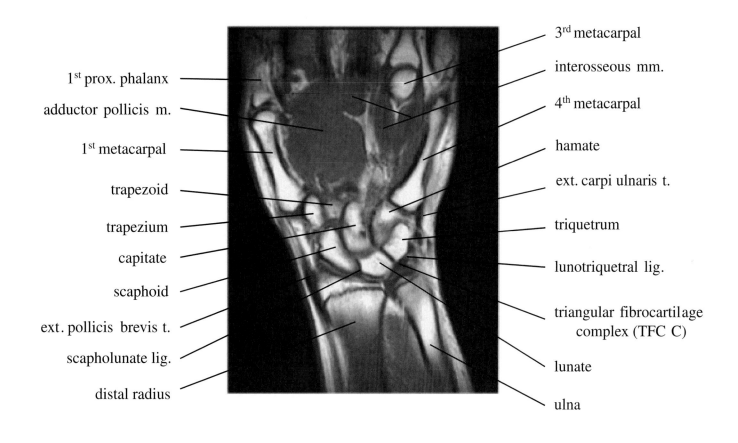

————— 3rd metacarpal

————— interosseous mm.

————— 4th metacarpal

————— hamate

————— ext. carpi ulnaris t.

————— triquetrum

————— lunotriquetral lig.

————— triangular fibrocartilage complex (TFC C)

————— lunate

————— ulna

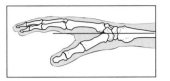

3rd metacarpal

4th metacarpal

hamate

triquetrum

lunotriquetral lig.

triangular fibrocartilage
complex (TFCC)

ext. carpi ulnaris t.

lunate

ulna

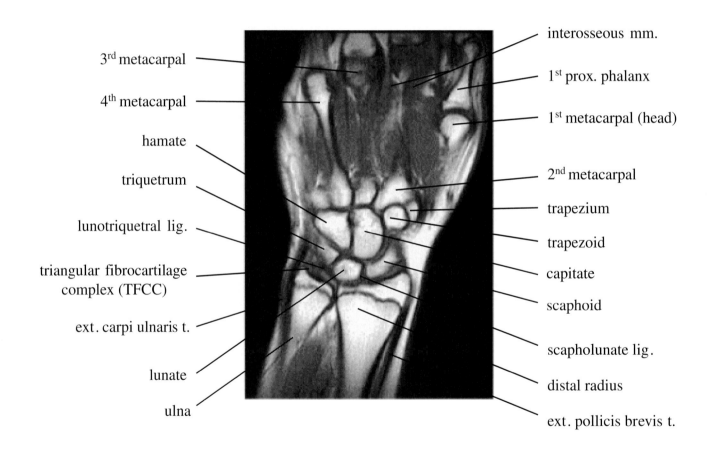

interosseous mm.

1st prox. phalanx

1st metacarpal (head)

2nd metacarpal

trapezium

trapezoid

capitate

scaphoid

scapholunate lig.

distal radius

ext. pollicis brevis t.

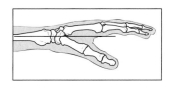

interosseous mm.

1ˢᵗ prox. phalanx

1ˢᵗ metacarpal (head)

2ⁿᵈ metacarpal

trapezium

trapezoid

capitate

scaphoid

scapholunate lig.

distal radius

ext. pollicis brevis t.

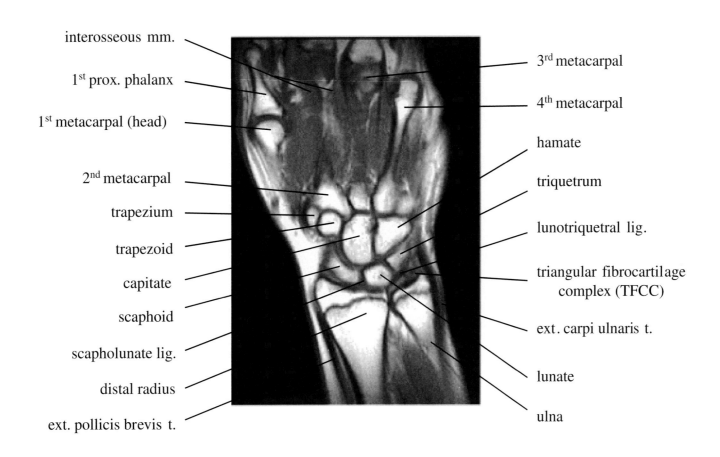

3ʳᵈ metacarpal

4ᵗʰ metacarpal

hamate

triquetrum

lunotriquetral lig.

triangular fibrocartilage
complex (TFCC)

ext. carpi ulnaris t.

lunate

ulna

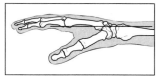

Wrist and Hand:
Oblique Coronal

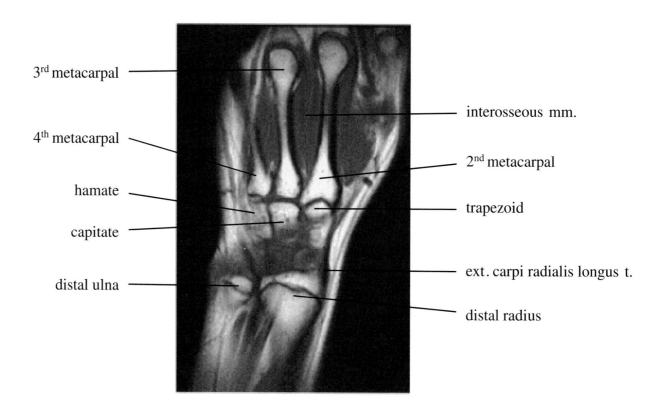

3rd metacarpal

4th metacarpal

hamate

capitate

distal ulna

interosseous mm.

2nd metacarpal

trapezoid

ext. carpi radialis longus t.

distal radius

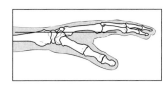

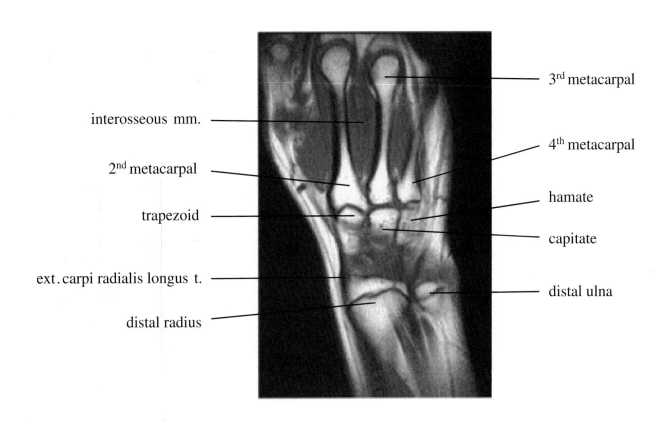

3rd metacarpal

interosseous mm.

4th metacarpal

2nd metacarpal

hamate

trapezoid

capitate

ext. carpi radialis longus t.

distal ulna

distal radius

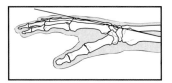

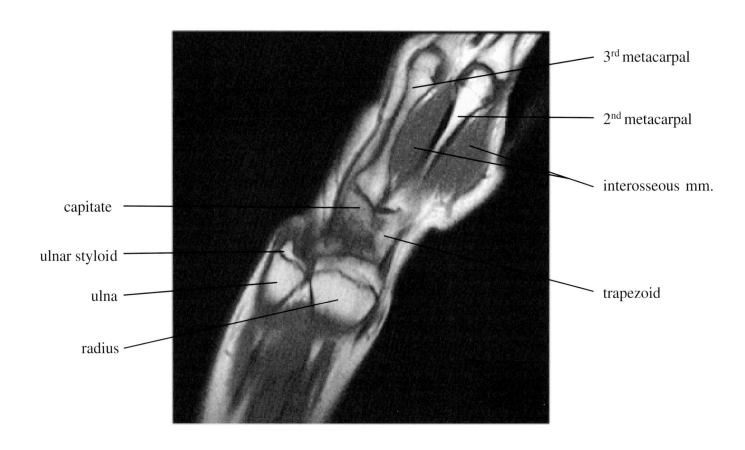

3rd metacarpal

2nd metacarpal

interosseous mm.

capitate

ulnar styloid

ulna

radius

trapezoid

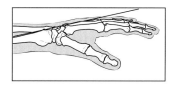

3rd metacarpal

2nd metacarpal

interosseous mm.

trapezoid

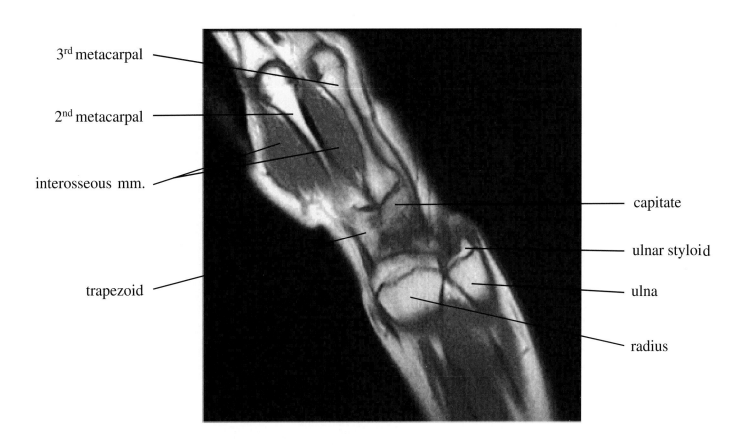

capitate

ulnar styloid

ulna

radius

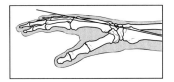

4th metacarpal

3rd metacarpal

capitate

2nd prox. phalanx

hamate

interosseous m.

triquetrum

2nd metacarpal

lunate

trapezoid

triangular fibrocartilage
complex (TFCC)

scaphoid

distal ulna

scapholunate lig.

distal radius

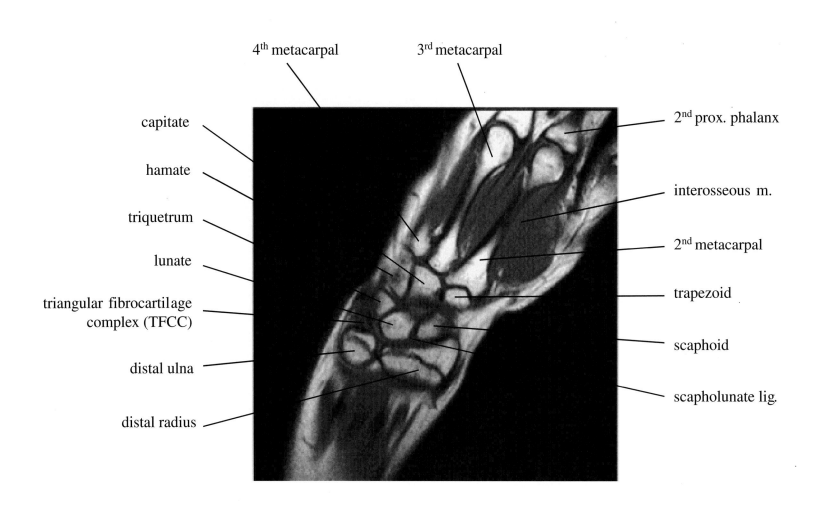

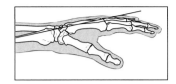

3rd metacarpal

4th metacarpal

2nd prox. phalanx

capitate

interosseous m.

hamate

2nd metacarpal

triquetrum

trapezoid

lunate

scaphoid

triangular fibrocartilage complex (TFCC)

scapholunate lig.

distal ulna

distal radius

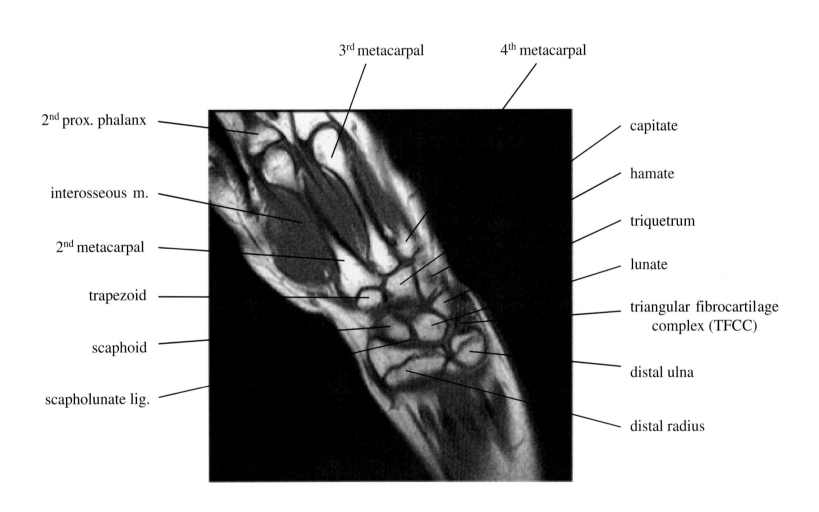

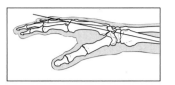

4th metacarpal

3rd metacarpal

prox. phalanges

capitate

interosseous mm.

1st prox. phalanx

hamate

1st metacarpal (head)

ext. carpi ulnaris t.

2nd metacarpal

triquetrum

trapezoid

triangular
fibrocartilage
complex (TFCC)

trapezium

lunotriquetral lig.

scaphoid

lunate

ext. pollicis brevis t.

distal radius

scapholunate lig.

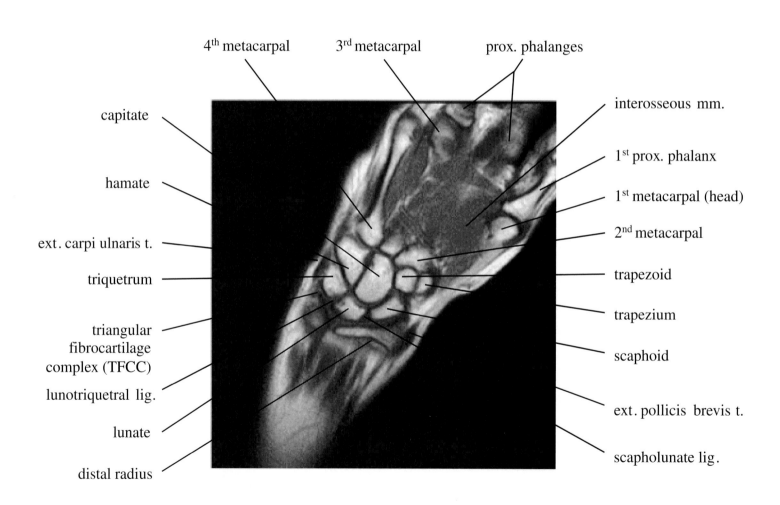

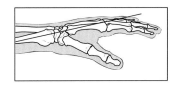

prox. phalanges   3rd metacarpal   4th metacarpal

interosseous mm.

capitate

1st prox. phalanx

1st metacarpal (head)

hamate

2nd metacarpal

ext. carpi ulnaris t.

trapezoid

triquetrum

trapezium

scaphoid

triangular fibrocartilage complex (TFCC)

lunotriquetral lig.

ext. pollicis brevis t.

lunate

scapholunate lig .

distal radius

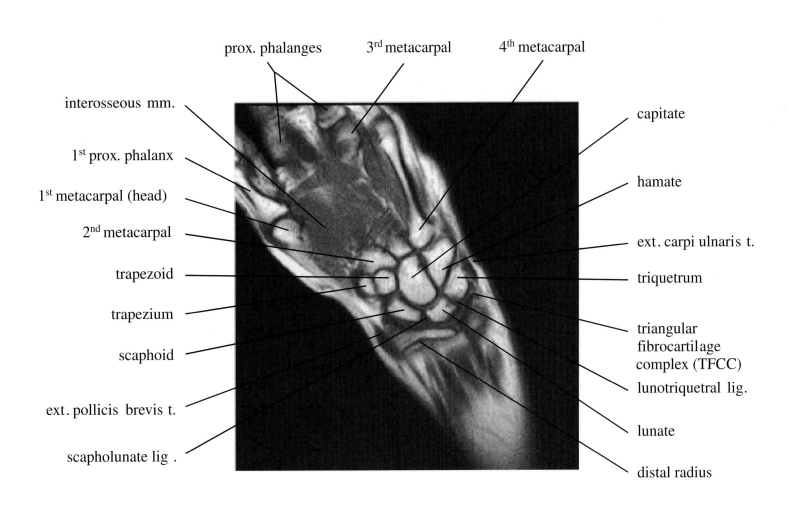

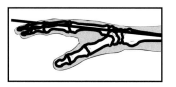

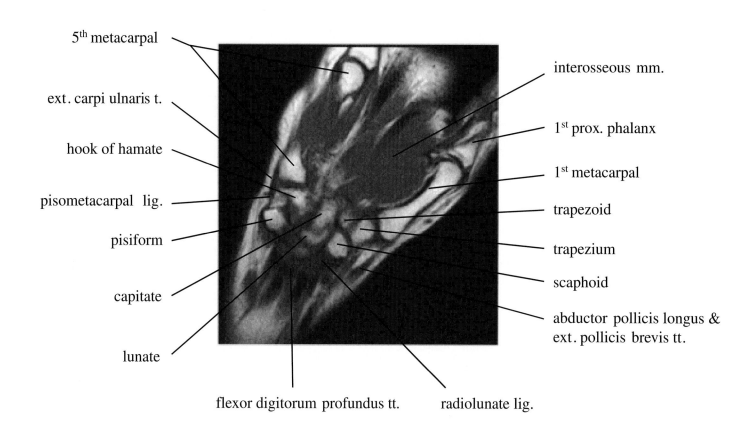

5th metacarpal

ext. carpi ulnaris t.

hook of hamate

pisometacarpal lig.

pisiform

capitate

lunate

interosseous mm.

1st prox. phalanx

1st metacarpal

trapezoid

trapezium

scaphoid

abductor pollicis longus &
ext. pollicis brevis tt.

flexor digitorum profundus tt.   radiolunate lig.

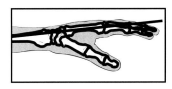

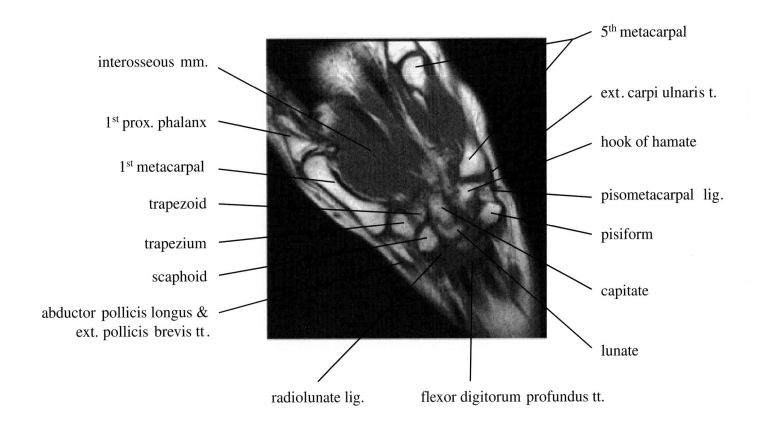

interosseous mm.

1st prox. phalanx

1st metacarpal

trapezoid

trapezium

scaphoid

abductor pollicis longus &
ext. pollicis brevis tt.

5th metacarpal

ext. carpi ulnaris t.

hook of hamate

pisometacarpal lig.

pisiform

capitate

lunate

radiolunate lig.

flexor digitorum profundus tt.

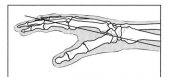

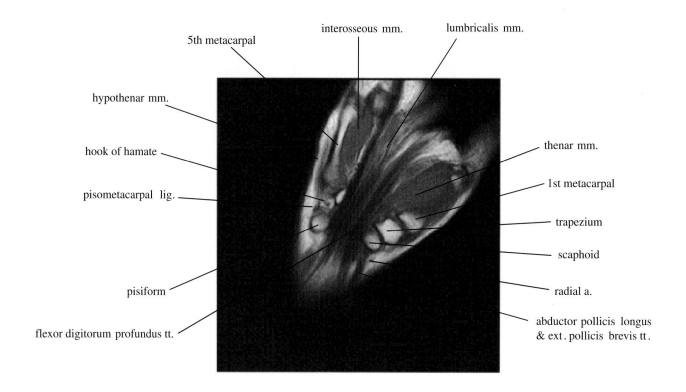

interosseous mm.

lumbricalis mm.

5th metacarpal

hypothenar mm.

thenar mm.

hook of hamate

1st metacarpal

pisometacarpal lig.

trapezium

scaphoid

radial a.

pisiform

abductor pollicis longus
& ext. pollicis brevis tt.

flexor digitorum profundus tt.

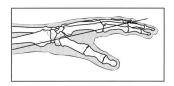

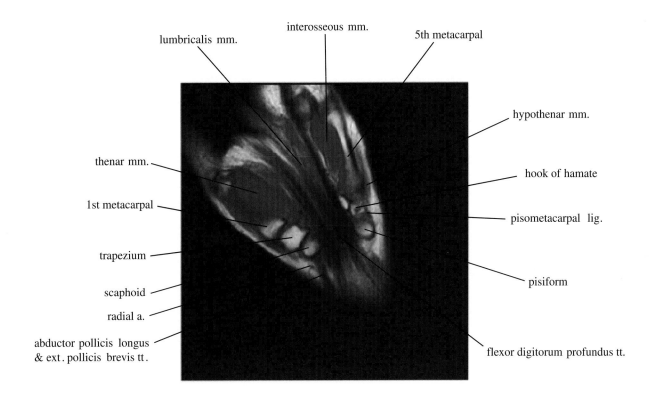

lumbricalis mm.

interosseous mm.

5th metacarpal

hypothenar mm.

thenar mm.

hook of hamate

1st metacarpal

pisometacarpal lig.

trapezium

pisiform

scaphoid

radial a.

abductor pollicis longus
& ext. pollicis brevis tt.

flexor digitorum profundus tt.

5

THE HIPS AND THIGH

The major indications for MR imaging of the hip and thigh include suspected infection, avascular necrosis, metastatic disease, transient osteoporosis (bone marrow edema) of the hip, and insufficiency fractures which may not be apparent on plain film examination. Bone and soft-tissue tumors or posttraumatic conditions (e.g., acute hemorrhage) are major indications for MR imaging of the thigh. Generally, MR studies of the hip may be performed with a standard protocol, and the studies do not usually require monitoring. Suspected soft-tissue or osseous tumors should be monitored while the patient is in the scanner, and the images should be approved before the patient leaves the MR suite, if possible.

PRACTICAL PROTOCOL CONSIDERATIONS

For MR examination of the hip and thigh, the patient is placed in the supine position with the legs resting comfortably. If a palpable abnormality, surgical scar, or other suspicious area is present at physical examination, a bath oil bead or vitamin E tablet should be placed at the proximal and distal or medial and lateral ends, or both, of the suspected abnormal site. Both hips are done routinely, but if there is a soft-tissue or osseous mass on one side, only the affected side is imaged.

In general, the body coil is used unless the surface coil is required for closer evaluation of a soft-tissue or intraosseous lesion. If there is a suspicion of a femoral neck fracture and the plain films are normal, a limited protocol consisting of a coronal T1-weighted sequence and/ or a coronal inversion recovery sequence can be performed. Since this examination is "limited," the charge should be reduced if possible. Both hips can be imaged together for symmetry, and then dedicated images can be acquired. The atlas demonstrates both imaging methods.

Menu of Protocols

Hips

Plane	Pulse Sequence	FA (degrees)	TR (msec)	TE (msec)	TI (msec)	FOV (cm)	Matrix (256X-)	ST/G (mm)	NEX	Comments
Localizer (transaxial)	SPGR	30	8	2.2		VAR	128	10/0	1	Either is acceptable
Localizer (coronal)	FMPIR		3000	25	150	VAR	128	4/1	2	
Localizer (coronal)	SE		450	min		VAR	128	5/1	1	
Coronal	FSE		3000	102		VAR	192	4/1	2	Either is acceptable
Coronal	FMPIR		3000	51	150	VAR	128	4/1	2	
Coronal	FSE, double echo		4000	20/100		VAR	256	5/1	1	
Oblique coronal										Same choices as coronal
										Plane parallel to long axis of femoral neck
Transaxial	FSE, double echo, ±FS		4000	20/100		VAR	256	5/1	1	Either is acceptable
Transaxial	SE		300	min		VAR	192	4/1	2	
Sagittal	SE		850	20		VAR	192	3/1	1	Either is acceptable
Sagittal	FSE, double echo, ± FS		4000	20/100		VAR	192	5/1	2	
Sagittal	SPGR, FS	30	45	15		VAR	192	2/0	1	

Thigh

Plane	Pulse Sequence	FA (degrees)	TR (msec)	TE (msec)	TI (msec)	FOV (cm)	Matrix (256X-)	ST/G (mm)	NEX	Comments
Localizer (transaxial)	SE		500	min		VAR	192	5/1.5	1	
Coronal, sagittal	SE		500	min		VAR	192	5/1.5	1	
Coronal	SE		1000	min		VAR	192	5/1.5	2	
Coronal	FMPIR		2500	30	150	VAR	128	5/1.5	2	
Sagittal	SE		1000	min		VAR	192	5/1.5	2	
Sagittal	FMPIR		2500	30	150	VAR	128	5/1.5	2	
Axial	SE		600	20		VAR	192	4/1	2	
Axial, pre-GAD	SE		600	20		VAR	192	4/1	2	
Axial, pre-GAD	SE, FS		600	20		VAR	192	4/1	2	

MAJOR OSTEOCHONDRAL STRUCTURES/LANDMARKS

- Ilium/Acetabulum
  - Iliac crest
  - Anterior superior iliac spine
  - Anterior inferior iliac spine
  - Iliopectineal line
  - Hip joint
  - Triradiate cartilage
  - Anterior column
  - Posterior column
  - Acetabular labrum
- Ischium
  - Ischial ramus
  - Ischial tuberosity
- Pubis
  - Superior pubic ramus
  - Obturator crest
- Femur
  - Femoral articular cartilage
  - Femoral head
  - Fovea capitis of femoral head
  - Femoral neck
  - Greater trochanter
  - Lesser trochanter
  - Anterior intertrochanteric line
  - Posterior intertrochanteric line
  - Trochanteric fossa
  - Pectineal line
  - Linea aspera

MAJOR LIGAMENTS/TENDONS/BURSAE

Ligaments

(Hip ligaments are capsular thickenings)

- Iliofemoral ("Y" ligament of Bigelow)—strongest
- Ischiofemoral
- Pubofemoral
- Capitis femoris (intracapsular)
- Ligamentum teres (acetabular fossa to fovea capitis)
- Transverse acetabular ligament

Tendons

- Iliopsoas
- Rectus femoris
- Gluteal (maximus, intermedius, minimus)

Bursae

- Iliopsoas
- Iliopectineal
- Trochanteric

MAJOR MUSCLES

Compartments

The muscles of the hip and thigh are divided into four groups.

- Anterior compartment
  - Sartorius
  - Quadriceps femoris
    - Rectus femoris
    - Vastus lateralis
    - Vastus intermedius
    - Vastus medialis
  - Articularis genus
- Medial compartment
  - Gracilis
  - Pectineus
  - Adductor longus
  - Adductor brevis
  - Adductor magnus
  - Obturator externus
- Posterior compartment (the "hamstrings")
  - Semitendinosus
  - Semimembranosus
  - Biceps femoris
- Lateral compartment
  - Gluteus maximus
  - Gluteus medius
  - Gluteus minimus
  - Tensor fasciae latae
  - Obturator internus
  - Superior gemellus
  - Inferior gemellus
  - Quadratus femoris
  - Piriformis

- Other hip/thigh muscles
  - Psoas major
  - Iliacus

ORIGIN/INSERTION/INNERVATION OF MAJOR MUSCLES

Muscle	Origin	Insertion	Innervation
– Sartorius	Anterior superior iliac spine (ASIS)	Tibial medial surface near tuberosity and neighboring fascia	Femoral N.
– Rectus femoris	Straight head—anterior inferior iliac spine Reflected head—groove above acetabulum	Across patellar ligament surface to tibial tuberosity	Femoral N.
– Articularis genus	Upper shaft of femur along margin of greater trochanter, above gluteal tuberosity, and upper portion of linea aspera	Proximal aspect of patella and anterior aspect of lateral condyle of tibia	Femoral N.

Medial Compartment

Muscle	Origin	Insertion	Innervation
– Gracilis	Pubic symphysis and inferior ramus of pubic bone	Upper shaft of tibial shaft between sartorius and semitendinosus tendons	Anterior division of obturator N.

(continued)

ORIGIN/INSERTION/INNERVATION OF MAJOR MUSCLES (*CONTINUED*)

Muscle	Origin	Insertion	Innervation
– Pectineus	Pectin of pubis, pectineal fascia, anterior margin of obturator sulcus, and pubofemoral ligament	Upper half of pectineal line of femur behind lesser trochanter	Femoral N. Rarely from accessory obturator or obturator N.
– Adductor longus	Medial portion of superior pubic ramus	Middle third of medial tip of linea aspera	Anterior division of obturator N. and occasionally branch from femoral N.
– Adductor brevis	Inferior pubic ramus between origin of gracilis and obturator externus	Distal two-thirds of pectineal line of femur and upper one-third of linea aspera	Anterior (or posterior) branch of obturator N.
– Adductor magnus	Lower part of inferior pubic ramus	Medial gluteal ridge and superior aspect of linea aspera by a tendon from distal three-fourths of linea aspera. Adductor tubercle at distal end of medial supracondylar ridge	Posterior branch of obturator N. and a branch from tibial division of sciatic N. (L4, S1)
– Obturator externus	External aspect of superior and inferior pubic ramus and ischial ramus	Trochanteric fossa of femur	Branch of obturator N. (L3, L4)

(*continued*)

ORIGIN/INSERTION/INNERVATION OF MAJOR MUSCLES (*CONTINUED*)

Muscle	Origin	Insertion	Innervation
Posterior Compartment (Hamstring Group)			
– Semi-tendinosus	Lower and medial aspect of ischial tuberosity in common with long head of biceps femoris muscle	Upper part of medial surface of tibia behind and distal to gracilis insertion	Two branches of tibial division of sciatic N. (L4, L5, S1, S2)
– Semi-membranosus	Upper and outer impression of ischial tuberosity	Horizontal groove on posteromedial aspect of medial tibial condyle—extension continues as oblique popliteal ligament of knee joint	Tibial division of sciatic N. (L4, L5, S1, S2)
– Biceps femoris, long head	Lower and medial impression of ischial tuberosity and sacrotuberous ligament	By a tendon that extends to lateral condyle of femur	Tibial division of sciatic N. (S1, S2, S2)
– Biceps femoris, short head	Lateral lip of linea aspera of femur, proximal two-thirds of supracondylar ridge, and lateral intermuscular septum	Lateral aspect of fibular head, lateral condyle of tibia, and into lateral fascia of leg	Branch of common peroneal division of sciatic N. (L5, S1, S2)

(continued)

ORIGIN/INSERTION/INNERVATION OF MAJOR MUSCLES (*CONTINUED*)

Muscle	*Origin*	*Insertion*	*Innervation*
Lateral Compartment			
– Gluteus maximus	Outer aspect of iliac crest, posterior gluteal line of ilium, thoracolumbar fascia between posteriosuperior ilium and side of sacrum, lateral parts of S4, S5, and coccygeal vertebrae, and posterior aspect of sacrotuberous ligament	Iliotibial tract, gluteal tuberosity of femur, adjacent part of tendinous origin of vastus lateralis	Inferior gluteal N. branches from sacral plexus (L5, S1, S2)
– Gluteus medius	External surface of ilium between anterior and posterior gluteal lines, and from gluteal aponeurosis	Posterosuperior angle of greater trochanter of femur	Superior gluteal N. (L4, L5, S1)
– Gluteus minimus	Ilium between anterior and inferior gluteal lines	Anterior border of greater trochanter of femur	Superior gluteal N. (L4, L5, S1)
– Tensor fasciae latae	Iliac crest and gluteus medius	Joins iliotibial tract about one-third of way down the thigh	Superior gluteal N. Lateral femoral circumflex (L4, L5, S1)
– Obturator internus	Pubic ramus near obturator foramen, ischium, obturator internus fascia	Medial side of greater trochanter of femur	Superior gluteal N. (L4, L5, S1)

(*continued*)

ORIGIN/INSERTION/INNERVATION OF MAJOR MUSCLES (*CONTINUED*)

Muscle	Origin	Insertion	Innervation
– Superior gamellus	Ischial spine and lesser sciatic notch	Unites with obturator internus tendon and inserts into medial side of greater trochanter	Superior gluteal N. (L4, L5, S1)
– Inferior gamellus	Ischial tuberosity	Greater trochanter of femur	Superior gluteal N. (L4, L5, S1)
– Quadratus femoris	Ischial tuberosity	Inferiorly and dorsally on greater trochanter	Medial femoral circumflex N.
– Piriformis	Front of sacrum between S1 and S4 foraminae, posterior border of greater sciatic notch, from sacrotuberous ligament near sacrum	Upper border of greater trochanter of femur	One or two branches of S1 or S2 N.

Outer Hip/Thigh Compartment

Muscle	Origin	Insertion	Innervation
– Psoas major	From T12 to L5 intervertebral disks and bodies, from L1 to L4 bodies and from ventral surfaces of lumbar transverse processes	Lesser trochanter of femur	Branches from L1, L2, L3, and L4 N.

(continued)

ORIGIN/INSERTION/INNERVATION OF MAJOR MUSCLES (*CONTINUED*)

Muscle	*Origin*	*Insertion*	*Innervation*
– Iliacus	Iliac crest, iliolumbar ligament, iliac fossa, anterior sacroiliac ligaments, sacral ala, and ventral border of ilium	Lateral aspect of the psoas tendon above inguinal ligament and onto femur distal to lesser trochanter; lateral portion is attached to tendon of rectus femoris and hip joint capsule	Femoral N. and L1 to L4 N.

THE HIPS: AXIAL ANATOMY

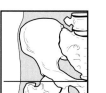

sartorius m.   femoral a. & v.   pectineus m.

rectus femoris m.

iliopsoas m.

tensor fasciae latae m.

vastus lateralis m.

iliotibial tract

femur

quadratus femoris m.

gluteus maximus m.

adductor longus m.

adductor brevis m.

obturator externus m.

obturator internus m.

ischium

biceps femoris & semitendinosus tt.

subcutaneous fat

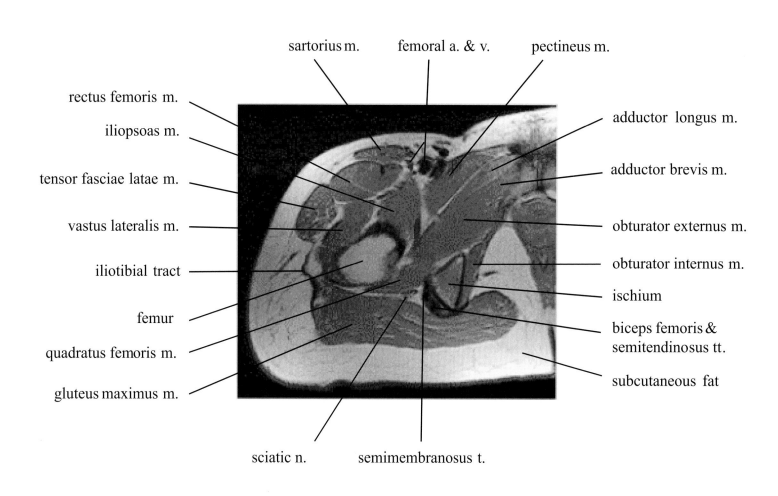

sciatic n.   semimembranosus t.

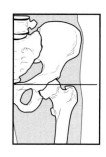

pectineus m.

femoral a. & v.

sartorius m.

adductor longus m.

adductor brevis m.

obturator externus m.

obturator internus m.

ischium

biceps femoris &
semitendinosus tt.

subcutaneous fat

rectus femoris m.

iliopsoas m.

tensor fasciae latae m.

vastus lateralis m.

iliotibial tract

femur

quadratus femoris m.

gluteus maximus m.

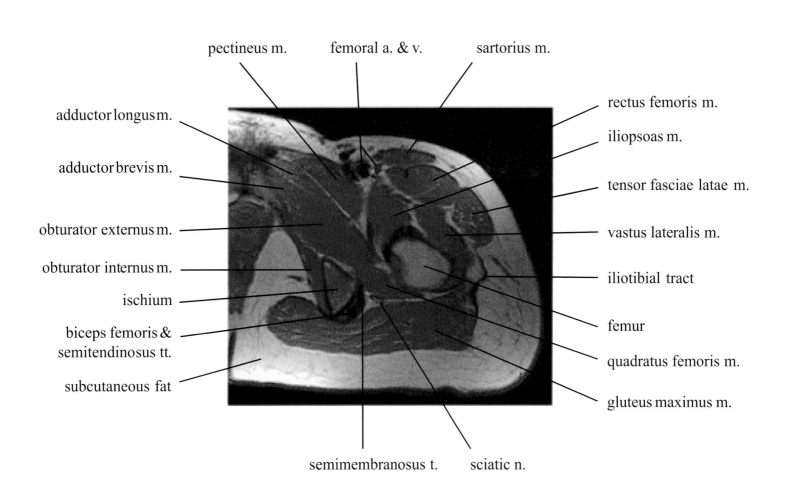

semimembranosus t.

sciatic n.

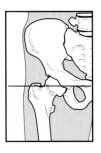

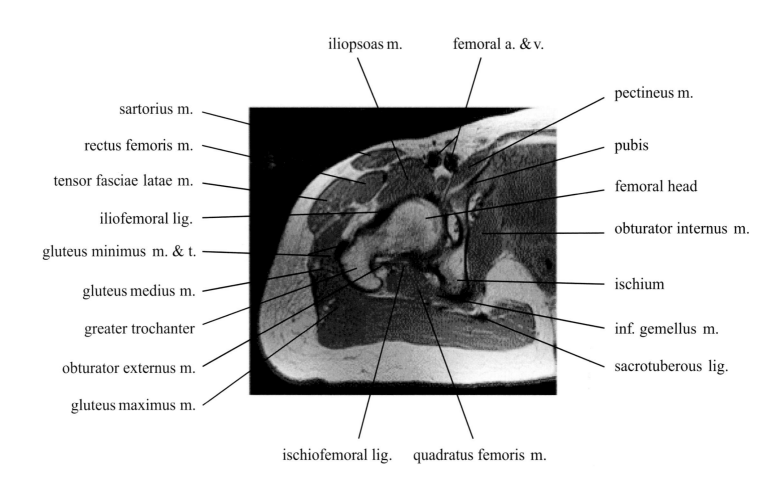

iliopsoas m.

femoral a. & v.

pectineus m.

sartorius m.

pubis

rectus femoris m.

femoral head

tensor fasciae latae m.

iliofemoral lig.

obturator internus m.

gluteus minimus m. & t.

gluteus medius m.

ischium

greater trochanter

inf. gemellus m.

obturator externus m.

sacrotuberous lig.

gluteus maximus m.

ischiofemoral lig.

quadratus femoris m.

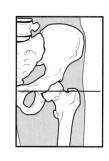

femoral a. & v.   iliopsoas m.

pectineus m.

pubis

femoral head

obturator internus m.

ischium

inf. gemellus m.

sacrotuberous lig.

sartorius m.

rectus femoris m.

tensor fasciae latae m.

iliofemoral lig.

gluteus minimus m. & t.

gluteus medius m.

greater trochanter

obturator externus m.

gluteus maximus m.

quadratus femoris m.   ischiofemoral lig.

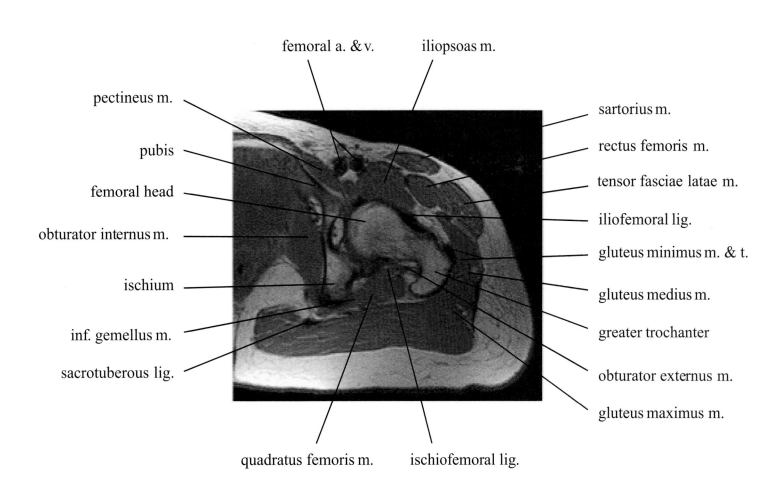

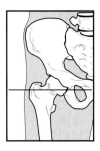

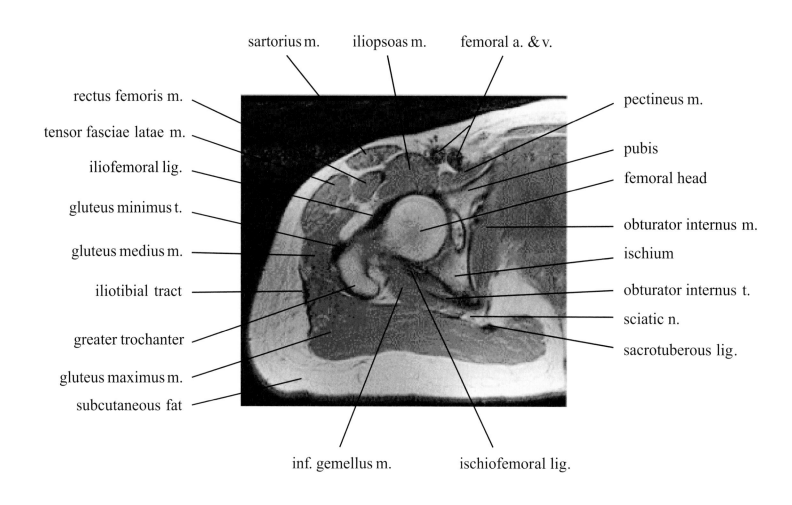

sartorius m.   iliopsoas m.   femoral a. & v.

rectus femoris m.

tensor fasciae latae m.

iliofemoral lig.

gluteus minimus t.

gluteus medius m.

iliotibial tract

greater trochanter

gluteus maximus m.

subcutaneous fat

pectineus m.

pubis

femoral head

obturator internus m.

ischium

obturator internus t.

sciatic n.

sacrotuberous lig.

inf. gemellus m.   ischiofemoral lig.

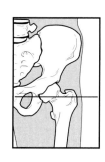

femoral a. & v.   iliopsoas m.   sartorius m.

pectineus m.

pubis

femoral head

obturator internus m.

ischium

obturator internus t.

sciatic n.

sacrotuberous lig.

rectus femoris m.

tensor fasciae latae m.

iliofemoral lig.

gluteus minimus t.

gluteus medius m.

iliotibial tract

greater trochanter

gluteus maximus m.

subcutaneous fat

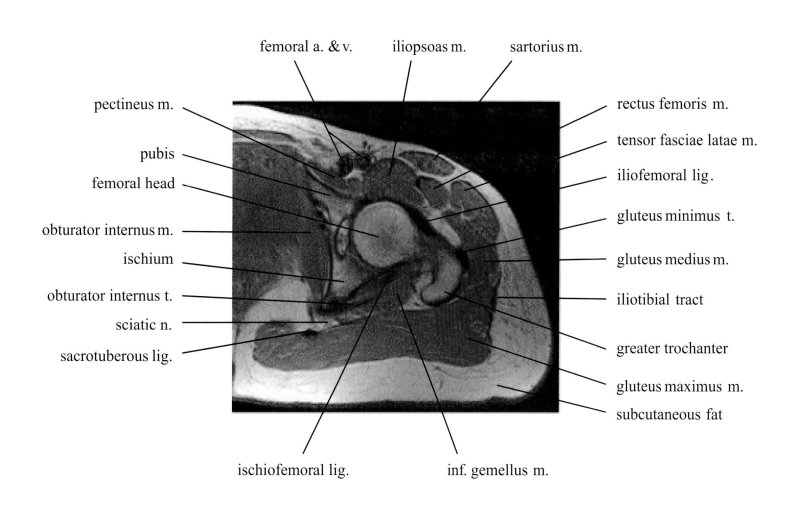

ischiofemoral lig.   inf. gemellus m.

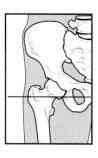

iliopsoas m.   ant. acetabular labrum   femoral a. & v.

sartorius m.

rectus femoris m.

iliofemoral lig.

tensor fasciae latae m.

gluteus minimus m.

gluteus medius m.

greater trochanter

gluteus maximus m.

pectineus m.

femoral head

ligamentum teres

obturator internus m.

ischial spine

inf. gluteal a.

sacrotuberous lig.

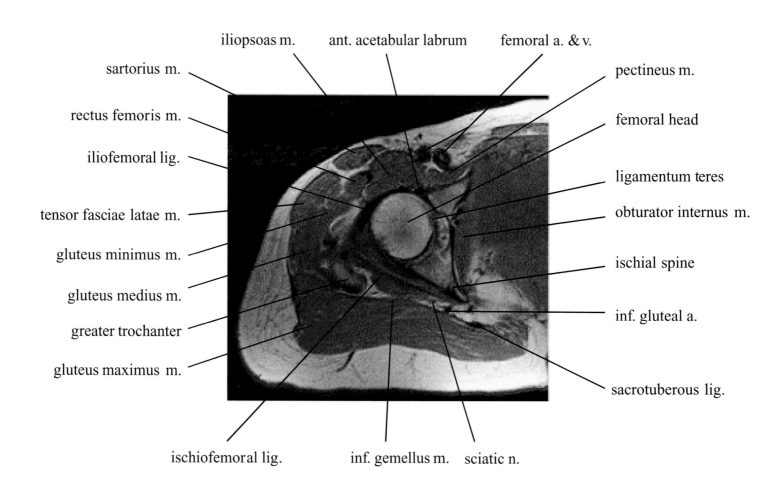

ischiofemoral lig.   inf. gemellus m.   sciatic n.

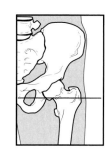

femoral a. & v.   iliopsoas m & t.

pectineus m.

ligamentum teres

femoral head

obturator internus m.

post. acetabular labrum

ischial spine

inf. gluteal a.

sciatic n.

sacrotuberous lig.

sartorius m.

rectus femoris m.

iliofemoral lig.

tensor fasciae latae m.

gluteus minimus m.

gluteus medius m. & t.

iliotibial tract

gluteus maximus m.

subcutaneous fat

piriformis m.   ischiofemoral lig.

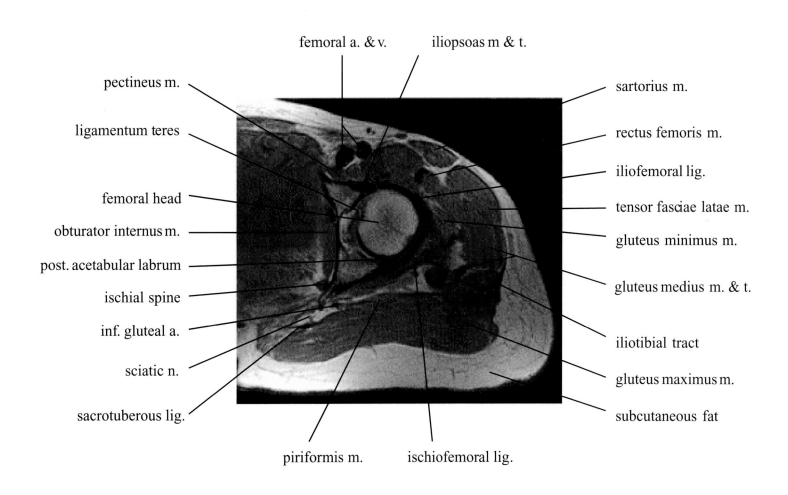

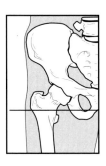

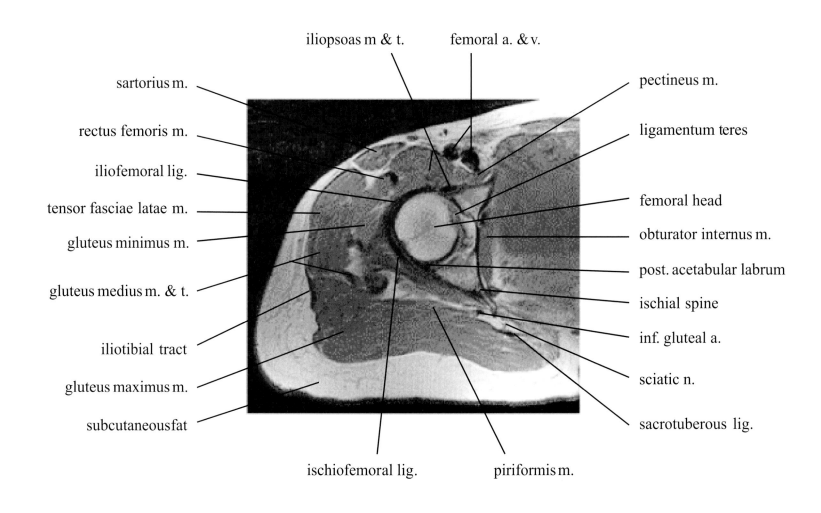

iliopsoas m & t.

femoral a. & v.

pectineus m.

sartorius m.

rectus femoris m.

ligamentum teres

iliofemoral lig.

femoral head

tensor fasciae latae m.

obturator internus m.

gluteus minimus m.

post. acetabular labrum

gluteus medius m. & t.

ischial spine

iliotibial tract

inf. gluteal a.

gluteus maximus m.

sciatic n.

subcutaneousfat

sacrotuberous lig.

ischiofemoral lig.

piriformis m.

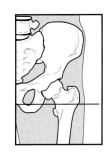

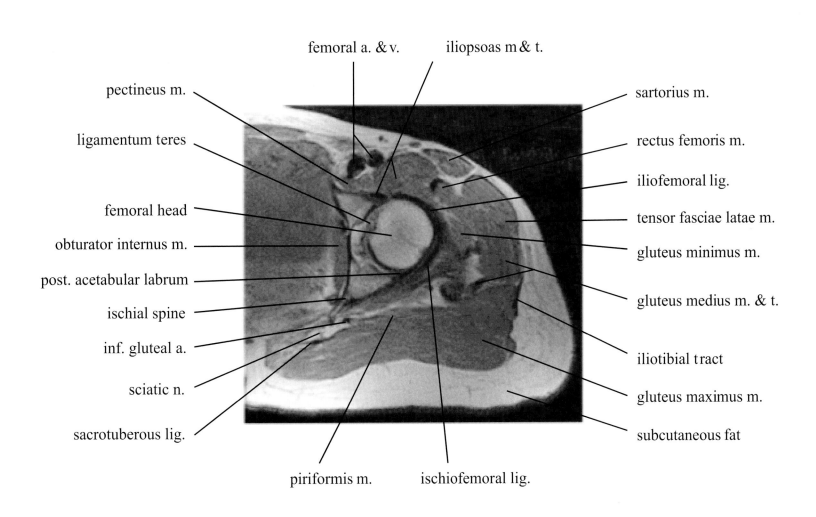

femoral a. & v.

iliopsoas m & t.

pectineus m.

sartorius m.

ligamentum teres

rectus femoris m.

iliofemoral lig.

femoral head

tensor fasciae latae m.

obturator internus m.

gluteus minimus m.

post. acetabular labrum

ischial spine

gluteus medius m. & t.

inf. gluteal a.

sciatic n.

iliotibial tract

gluteus maximus m.

sacrotuberous lig.

subcutaneous fat

piriformis m.

ischiofemoral lig.

THE HIPS: SAGITTAL ANATOMY

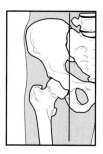

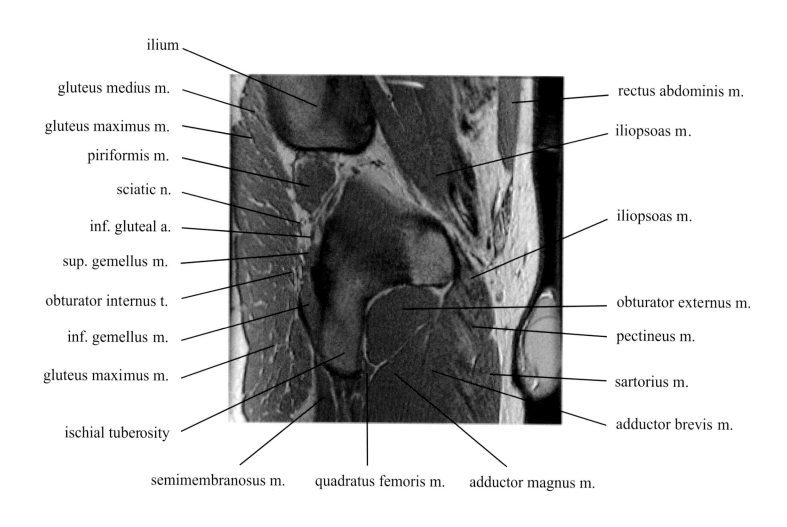

ilium

gluteus medius m.

gluteus maximus m.

piriformis m.

sciatic n.

inf. gluteal a.

sup. gemellus m.

obturator internus t.

inf. gemellus m.

gluteus maximus m.

ischial tuberosity

rectus abdominis m.

iliopsoas m.

iliopsoas m.

obturator externus m.

pectineus m.

sartorius m.

adductor brevis m.

semimembranosus m.   quadratus femoris m.   adductor magnus m.

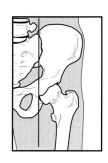

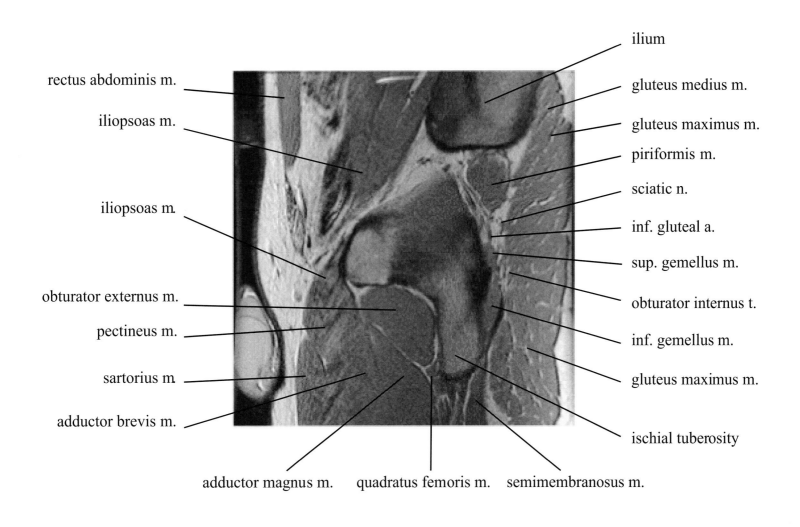

rectus abdominis m.

iliopsoas m.

iliopsoas m.

obturator externus m.

pectineus m.

sartorius m

adductor brevis m.

ilium

gluteus medius m.

gluteus maximus m.

piriformis m.

sciatic n.

inf. gluteal a.

sup. gemellus m.

obturator internus t.

inf. gemellus m.

gluteus maximus m.

ischial tuberosity

adductor magnus m.   quadratus femoris m.   semimembranosus m.

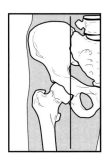

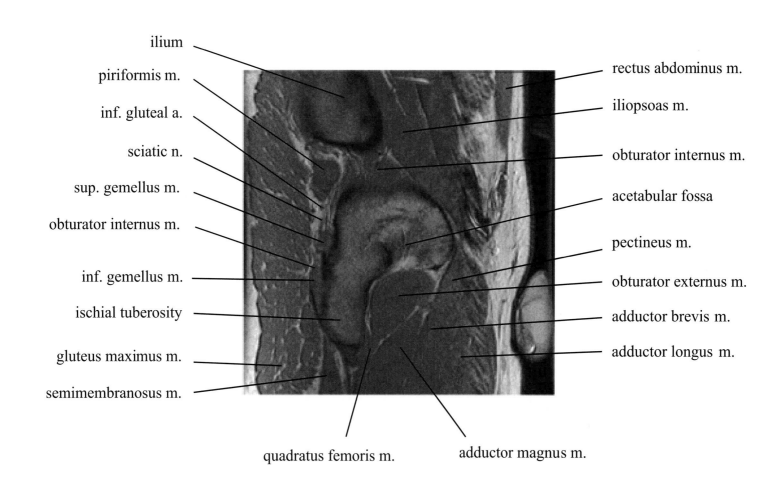

ilium

piriformis m.

inf. gluteal a.

sciatic n.

sup. gemellus m.

obturator internus m.

inf. gemellus m.

ischial tuberosity

gluteus maximus m.

semimembranosus m.

rectus abdominus m.

iliopsoas m.

obturator internus m.

acetabular fossa

pectineus m.

obturator externus m.

adductor brevis m.

adductor longus m.

quadratus femoris m.

adductor magnus m.

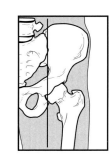

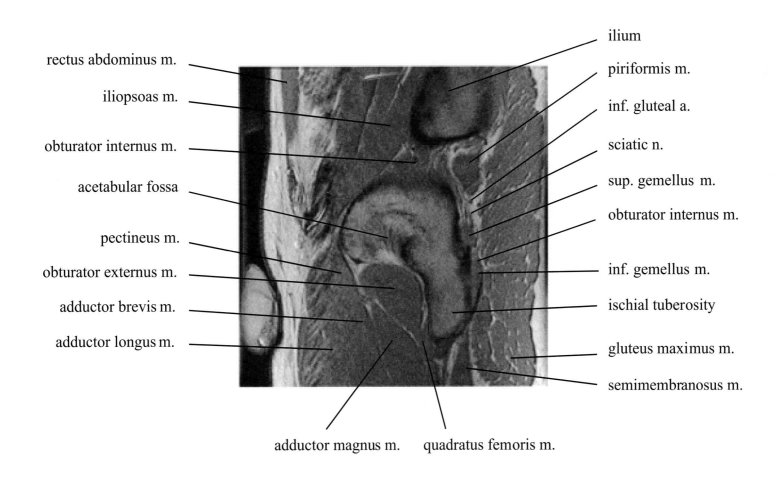

ilium

rectus abdominus m.

piriformis m.

iliopsoas m.

inf. gluteal a.

obturator internus m.

sciatic n.

acetabular fossa

sup. gemellus m.

obturator internus m.

pectineus m.

obturator externus m.

inf. gemellus m.

adductor brevis m.

ischial tuberosity

adductor longus m.

gluteus maximus m.

semimembranosus m.

adductor magnus m.   quadratus femoris m.

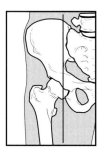

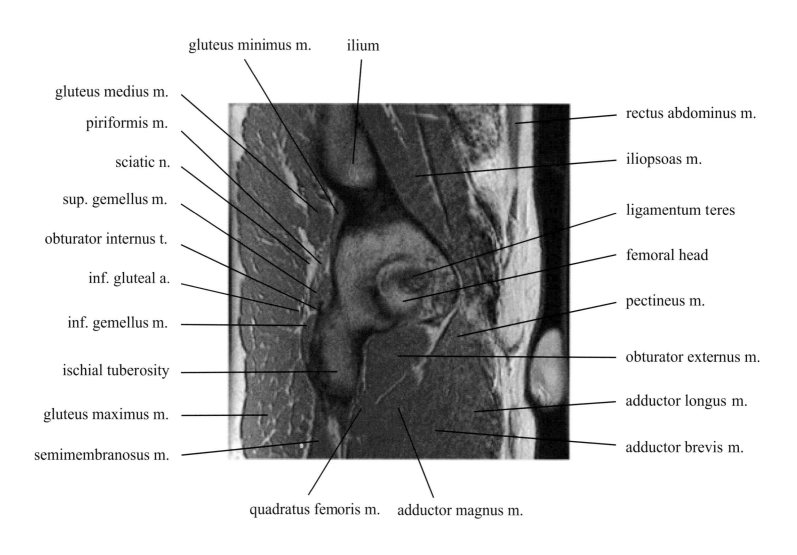

gluteus minimus m.

ilium

gluteus medius m.

piriformis m.

sciatic n.

sup. gemellus m.

obturator internus t.

inf. gluteal a.

inf. gemellus m.

ischial tuberosity

gluteus maximus m.

semimembranosus m.

rectus abdominus m.

iliopsoas m.

ligamentum teres

femoral head

pectineus m.

obturator externus m.

adductor longus m.

adductor brevis m.

quadratus femoris m.   adductor magnus m.

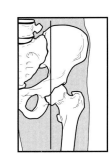

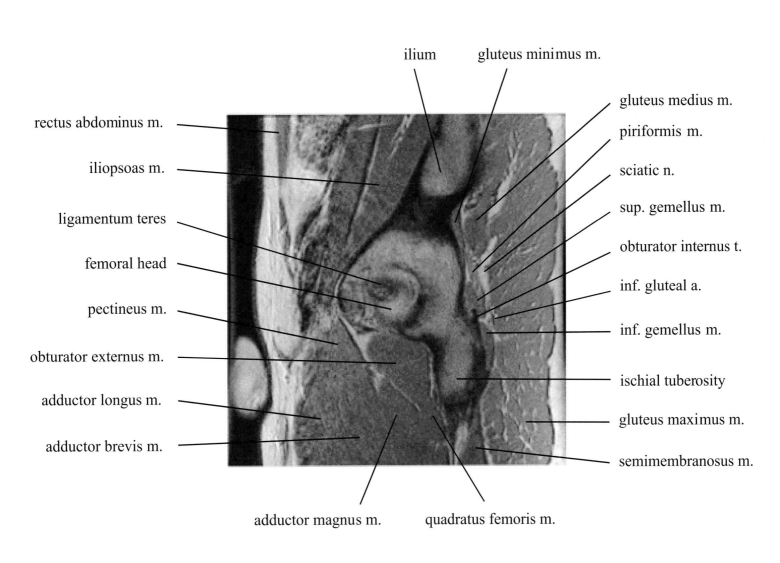

ilium

gluteus minimus m.

rectus abdominus m.

iliopsoas m.

ligamentum teres

femoral head

pectineus m.

obturator externus m.

adductor longus m.

adductor brevis m.

gluteus medius m.

piriformis m.

sciatic n.

sup. gemellus m.

obturator internus t.

inf. gluteal a.

inf. gemellus m.

ischial tuberosity

gluteus maximus m.

semimembranosus m.

adductor magnus m.

quadratus femoris m.

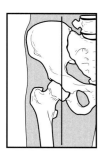

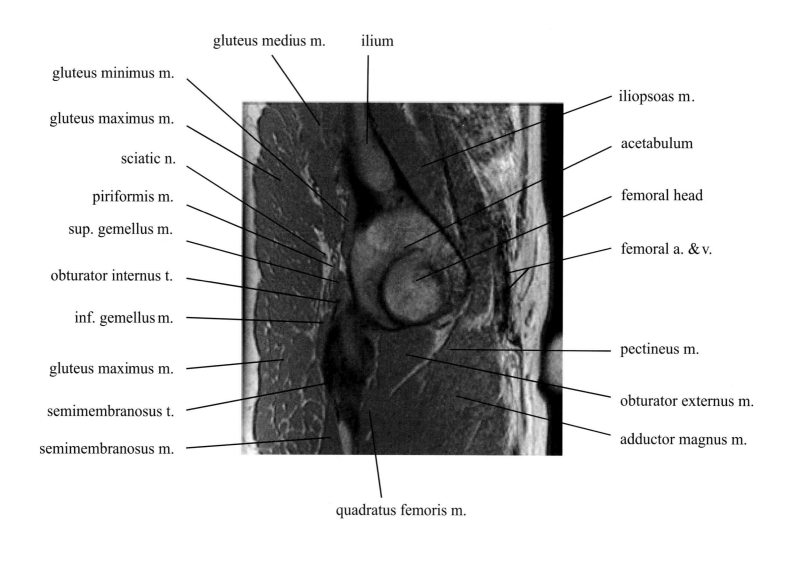

gluteus medius m.

ilium

gluteus minimus m.

gluteus maximus m.

sciatic n.

piriformis m.

sup. gemellus m.

obturator internus t.

inf. gemellus m.

gluteus maximus m.

semimembranosus t.

semimembranosus m.

iliopsoas m.

acetabulum

femoral head

femoral a. & v.

pectineus m.

obturator externus m.

adductor magnus m.

quadratus femoris m.

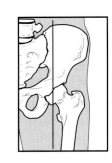

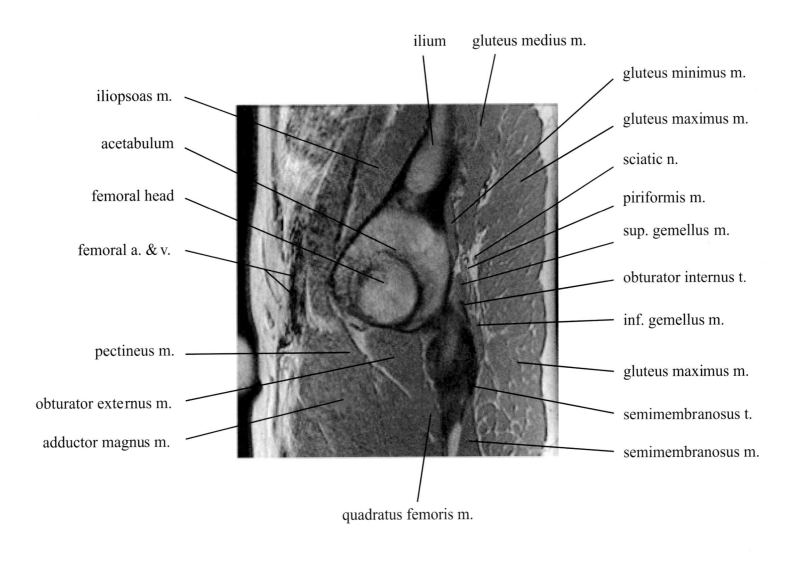

ilium   gluteus medius m.

iliopsoas m.

acetabulum

femoral head

femoral a. & v.

pectineus m.

obturator externus m.

adductor magnus m.

gluteus minimus m.

gluteus maximus m.

sciatic n.

piriformis m.

sup. gemellus m.

obturator internus t.

inf. gemellus m.

gluteus maximus m.

semimembranosus t.

semimembranosus m.

quadratus femoris m.

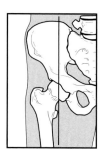

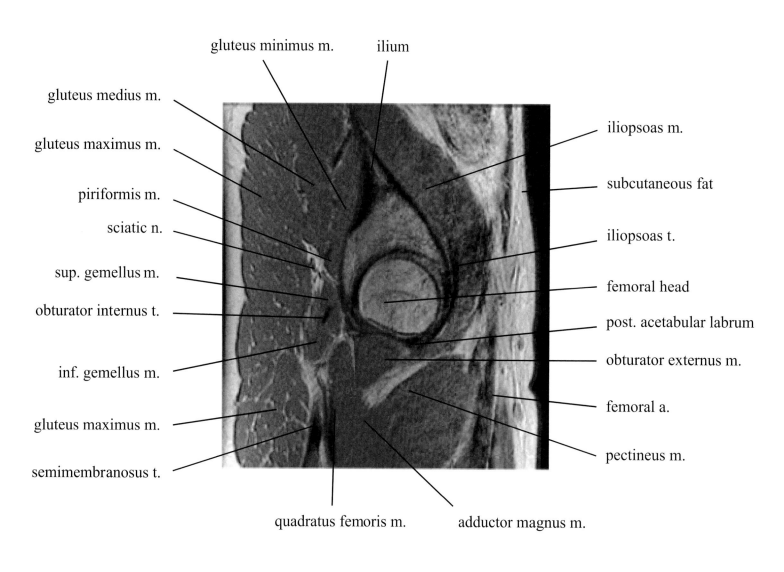

gluteus minimus m.   ilium

gluteus medius m.

gluteus maximus m.

piriformis m.

sciatic n.

sup. gemellus m.

obturator internus t.

inf. gemellus m.

gluteus maximus m.

semimembranosus t.

iliopsoas m.

subcutaneous fat

iliopsoas t.

femoral head

post. acetabular labrum

obturator externus m.

femoral a.

pectineus m.

quadratus femoris m.   adductor magnus m.

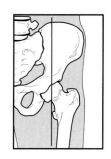

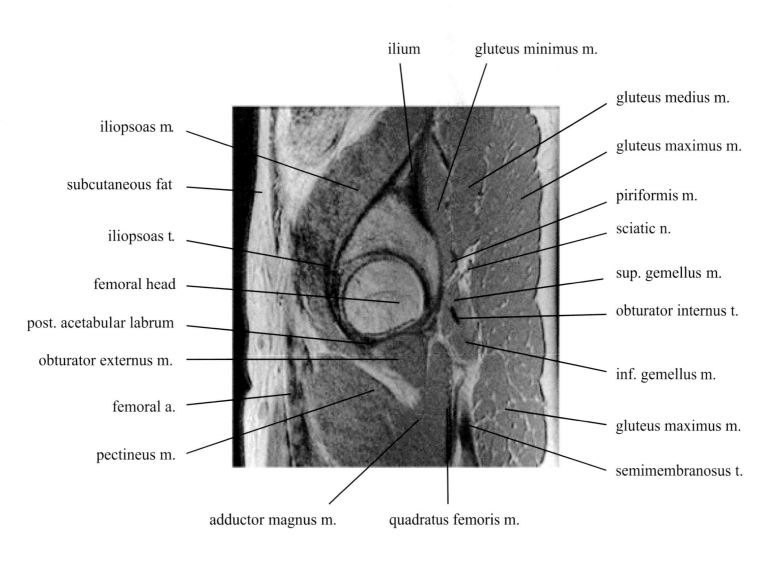

ilium

gluteus minimus m.

gluteus medius m.

iliopsoas m.

gluteus maximus m.

subcutaneous fat

piriformis m.

iliopsoas t.

sciatic n.

femoral head

sup. gemellus m.

post. acetabular labrum

obturator internus t.

obturator externus m.

femoral a.

inf. gemellus m.

pectineus m.

gluteus maximus m.

semimembranosus t.

adductor magnus m.

quadratus femoris m.

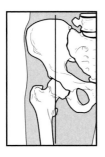

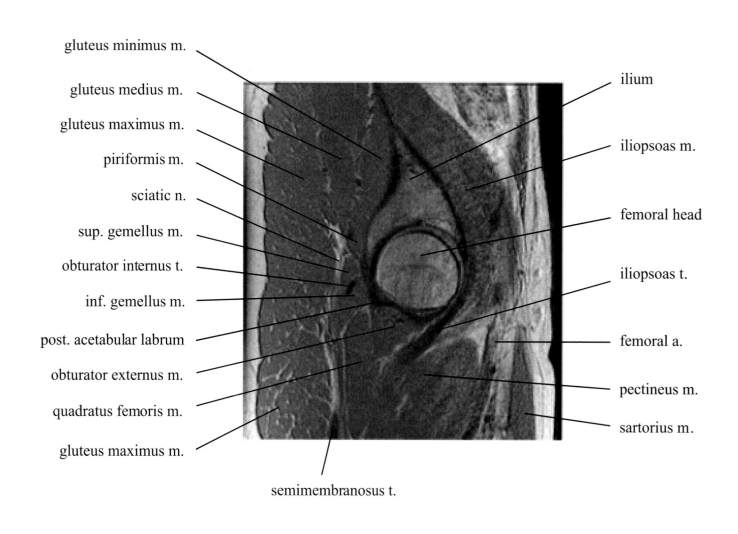

gluteus minimus m.

gluteus medius m.

gluteus maximus m.

piriformis m.

sciatic n.

sup. gemellus m.

obturator internus t.

inf. gemellus m.

post. acetabular labrum

obturator externus m.

quadratus femoris m.

gluteus maximus m.

semimembranosus t.

ilium

iliopsoas m.

femoral head

iliopsoas t.

femoral a.

pectineus m.

sartorius m.

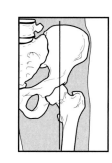

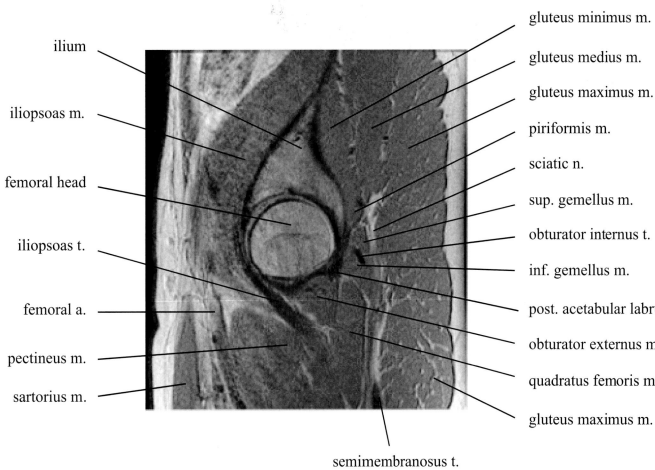

ilium

iliopsoas m.

femoral head

iliopsoas t.

femoral a.

pectineus m.

sartorius m.

gluteus minimus m.

gluteus medius m.

gluteus maximus m.

piriformis m.

sciatic n.

sup. gemellus m.

obturator internus t.

inf. gemellus m.

post. acetabular labrum

obturator externus m.

quadratus femoris m.

gluteus maximus m.

semimembranosus t.

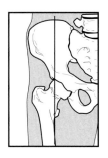

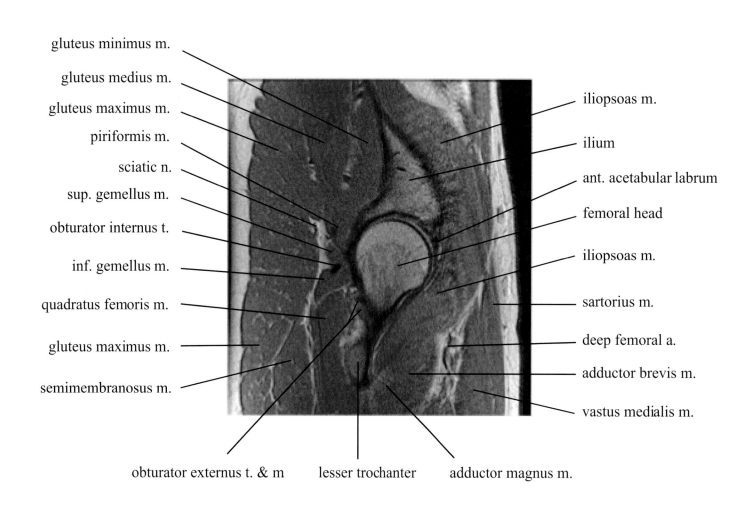

gluteus minimus m.

gluteus medius m.

gluteus maximus m.

piriformis m.

sciatic n.

sup. gemellus m.

obturator internus t.

inf. gemellus m.

quadratus femoris m.

gluteus maximus m.

semimembranosus m.

iliopsoas m.

ilium

ant. acetabular labrum

femoral head

iliopsoas m.

sartorius m.

deep femoral a.

adductor brevis m.

vastus medialis m.

obturator externus t. & m   lesser trochanter   adductor magnus m.

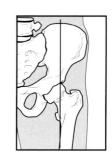

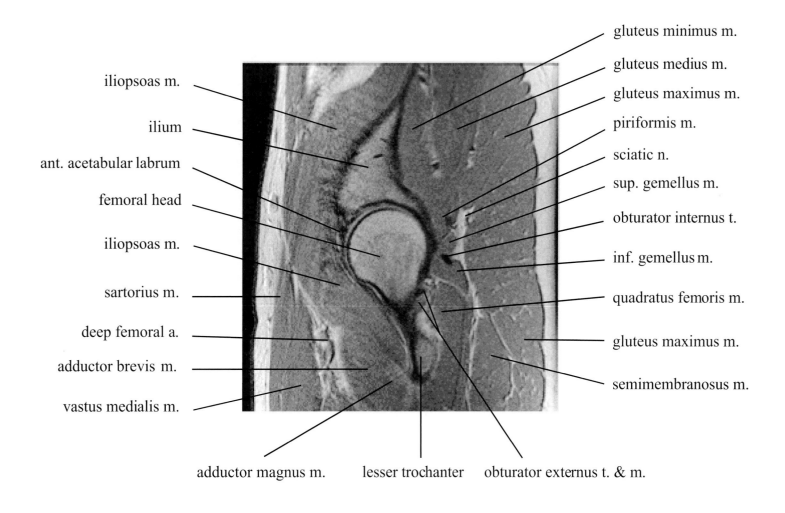

iliopsoas m.

ilium

ant. acetabular labrum

femoral head

iliopsoas m.

sartorius m.

deep femoral a.

adductor brevis m.

vastus medialis m.

gluteus minimus m.

gluteus medius m.

gluteus maximus m.

piriformis m.

sciatic n.

sup. gemellus m.

obturator internus t.

inf. gemellus m.

quadratus femoris m.

gluteus maximus m.

semimembranosus m.

adductor magnus m.   lesser trochanter   obturator externus t. & m.

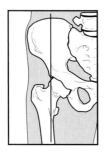

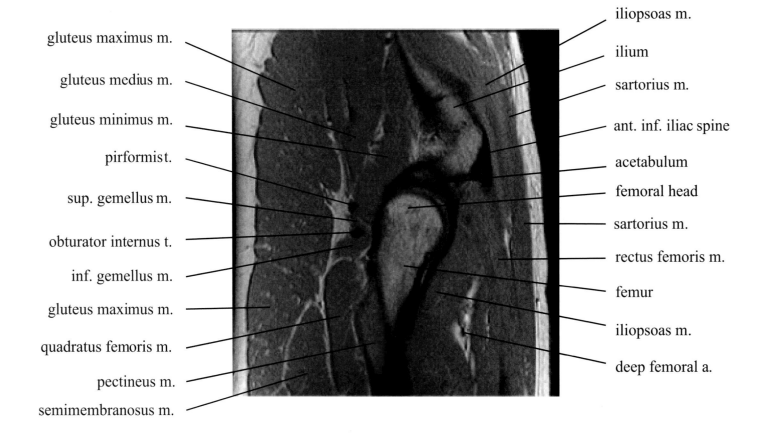

gluteus maximus m.

gluteus medius m.

gluteus minimus m.

pirformist.

sup. gemellus m.

obturator internus t.

inf. gemellus m.

gluteus maximus m.

quadratus femoris m.

pectineus m.

semimembranosus m.

iliopsoas m.

ilium

sartorius m.

ant. inf. iliac spine

acetabulum

femoral head

sartorius m.

rectus femoris m.

femur

iliopsoas m.

deep femoral a.

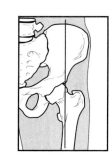

iliopsoas m.

ilium

sartorius m.

ant. inf. iliac spine

acetabulum

femoral head

sartorius m.

rectus femoris m.

femur

iliopsoas m.

deep femoral a.

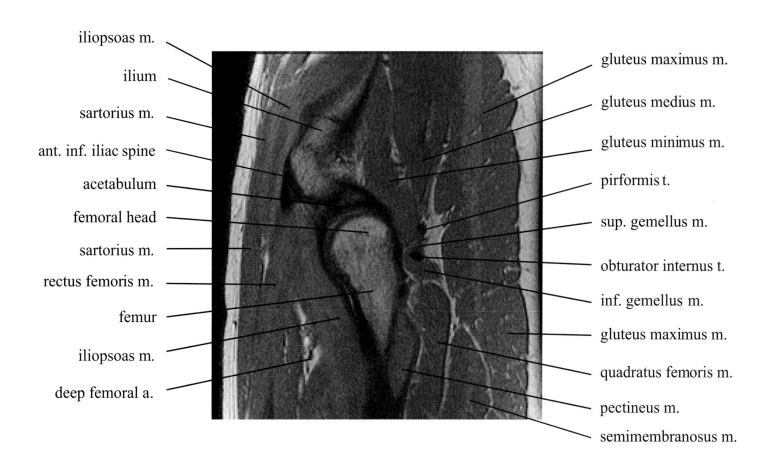

gluteus maximus m.

gluteus medius m.

gluteus minimus m.

pirformis t.

sup. gemellus m.

obturator internus t.

inf. gemellus m.

gluteus maximus m.

quadratus femoris m.

pectineus m.

semimembranosus m.

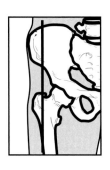

gluteus medius m.

gluteus medius t.

gluteus maximus m.

greater trochanter

obturator externus t.

quadratus femoris m.

gluteus maximus m.

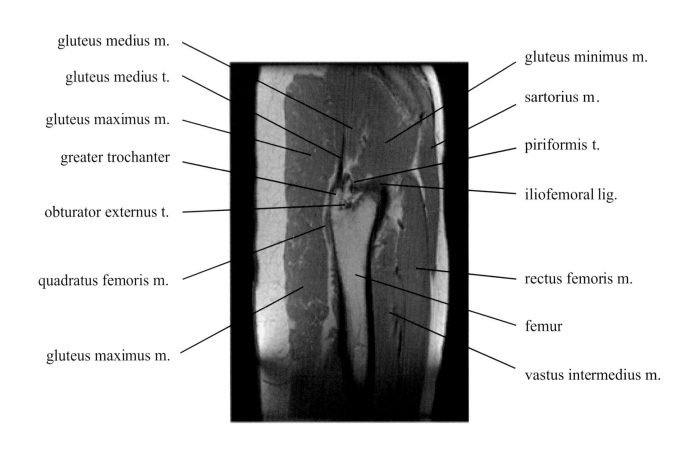

gluteus minimus m.

sartorius m.

piriformis t.

iliofemoral lig.

rectus femoris m.

femur

vastus intermedius m.

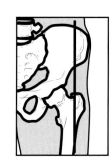

gluteus medius m.

gluteus medius t.

gluteus maximus m.

greater trochanter

obturator externus t.

quadratus femoris m.

gluteus maximus m.

gluteus minimus m.

sartorius m.

piriformis t.

iliofemoral lig.

rectus femoris m.

femur

vastus intermedius m.

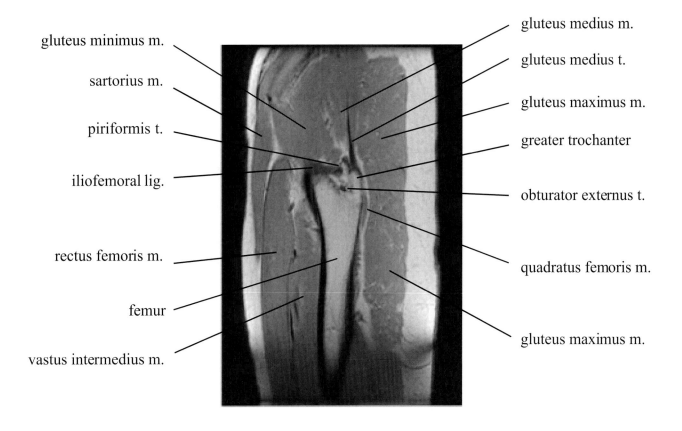

THE HIPS: CORONAL ANATOMY

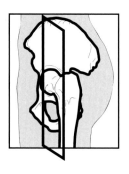

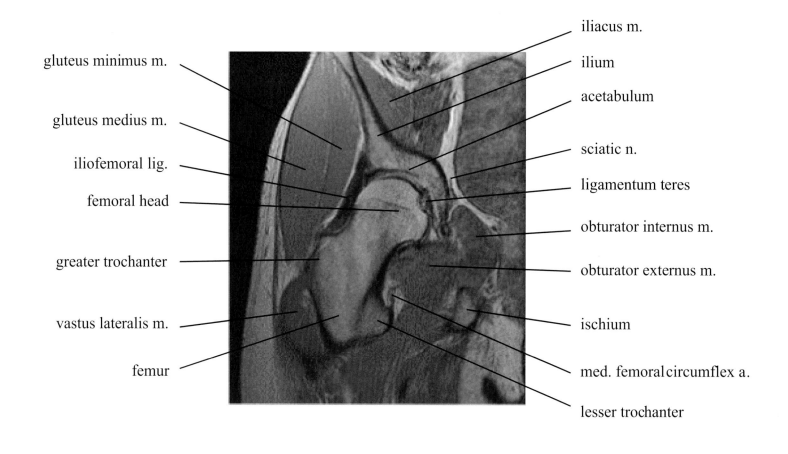

gluteus minimus m.

gluteus medius m.

iliofemoral lig.

femoral head

greater trochanter

vastus lateralis m.

femur

iliacus m.

ilium

acetabulum

sciatic n.

ligamentum teres

obturator internus m.

obturator externus m.

ischium

med. femoral circumflex a.

lesser trochanter

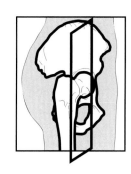

iliacus m.

ilium

acetabulum

sciatic n.

ligamentum teres

obturator internus m.

obturator externus m.

ischium

med. femoral circumflex a.

lesser trochanter

gluteus minimus m.

gluteus medius m.

iliofemoral lig.

femoral head

greater trochanter

vastus lateralis m.

femur

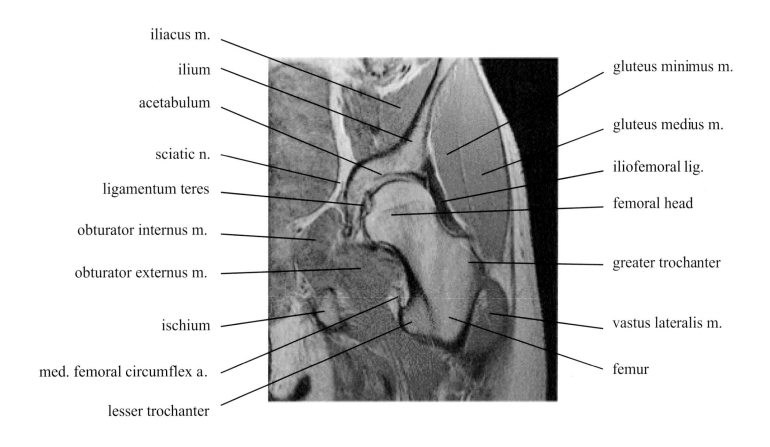

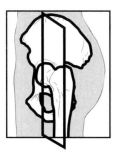

ilium

gluteus minimus m.

iliofemoral lig.

gluteus medius m.

gluteus minimus t.

greater trochanter

femur

vastus lateralis m.

lesser trochanter

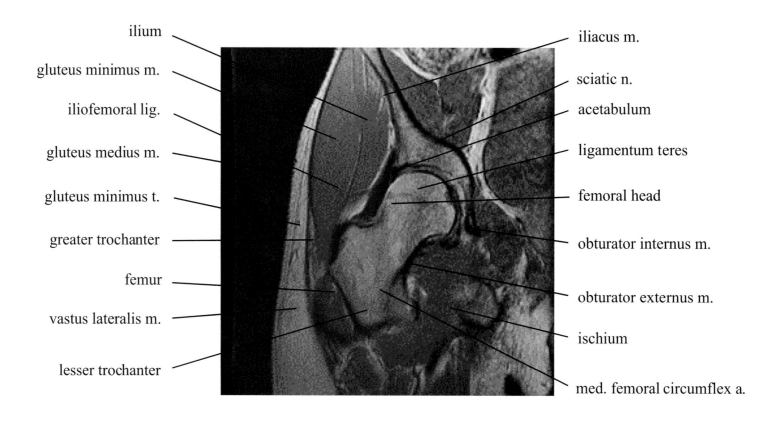

iliacus m.

sciatic n.

acetabulum

ligamentum teres

femoral head

obturator internus m.

obturator externus m.

ischium

med. femoral circumflex a.

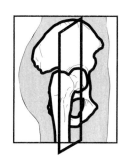

iliacus m.

sciatic n.

acetabulum

ligamentum teres

femoral head

obturator internus m.

obturator externus m.

ischium

med. femoral circumflex a.

ilium

gluteus minimus m.

iliofemoral lig.

gluteus medius m.

gluteus minimus t.

greater trochanter

femur

vastus lateralis m.

lesser trochanter

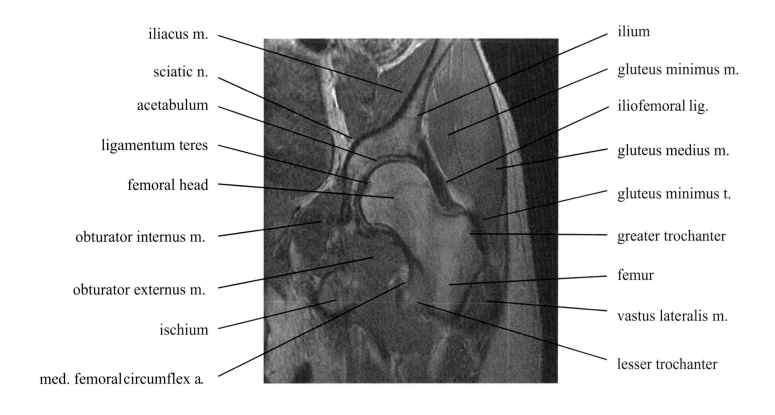

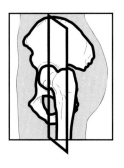

gluteus minimus m.

gluteus medius m.

sup. acetabular labrum

iliofemoral lig.

gluteus minimus t.

greater trochanter

femur

vastus lateralis m.

tensor fasciae latae m.

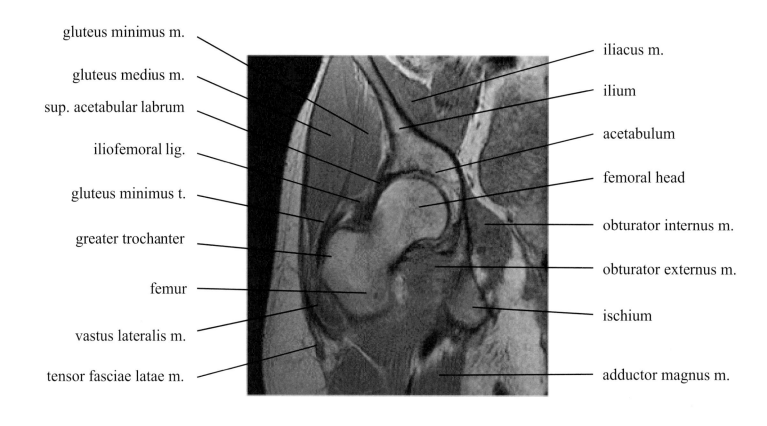

iliacus m.

ilium

acetabulum

femoral head

obturator internus m.

obturator externus m.

ischium

adductor magnus m.

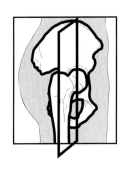

iliacus m.

ilium

acetabulum

femoral head

obturator internus m.

obturator externus m.

ischium

adductor magnus m.

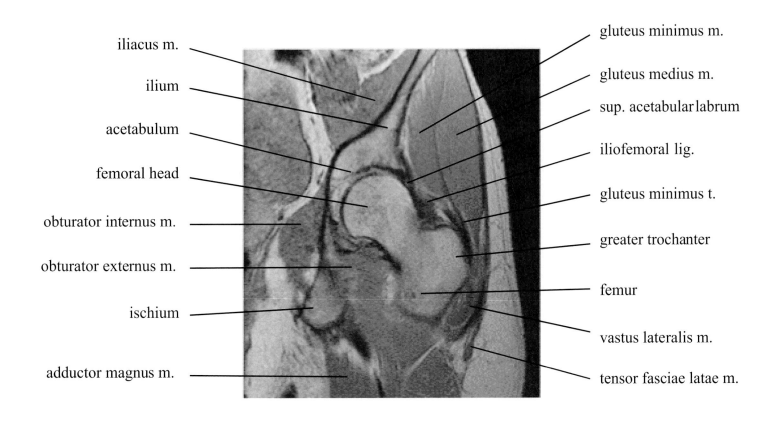

gluteus minimus m.

gluteus medius m.

sup. acetabular labrum

iliofemoral lig.

gluteus minimus t.

greater trochanter

femur

vastus lateralis m.

tensor fasciae latae m.

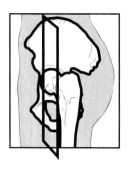

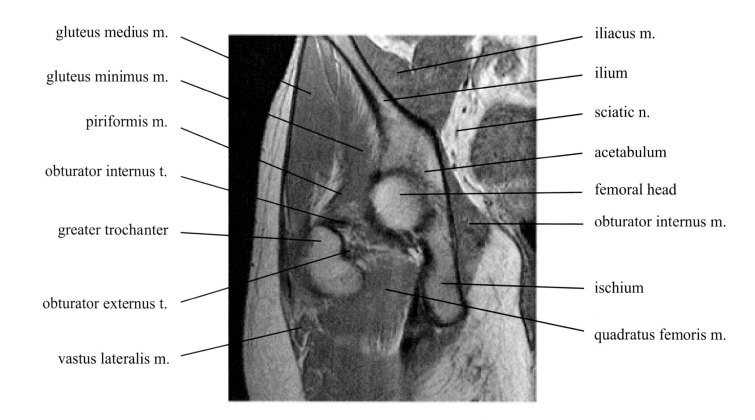

gluteus medius m.

gluteus minimus m.

piriformis m.

obturator internus t.

greater trochanter

obturator externus t.

vastus lateralis m.

iliacus m.

ilium

sciatic n.

acetabulum

femoral head

obturator internus m.

ischium

quadratus femoris m.

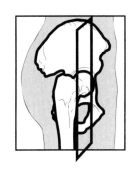

iliacus m.

ilium

sciatic n.

acetabulum

femoral head

obturator internus m.

ischium

quadratus femoris m.

gluteus medius m.

gluteus minimus m.

piriformis m.

obturator internus t.

greater trochanter

obturator externus t.

vastus lateralis m.

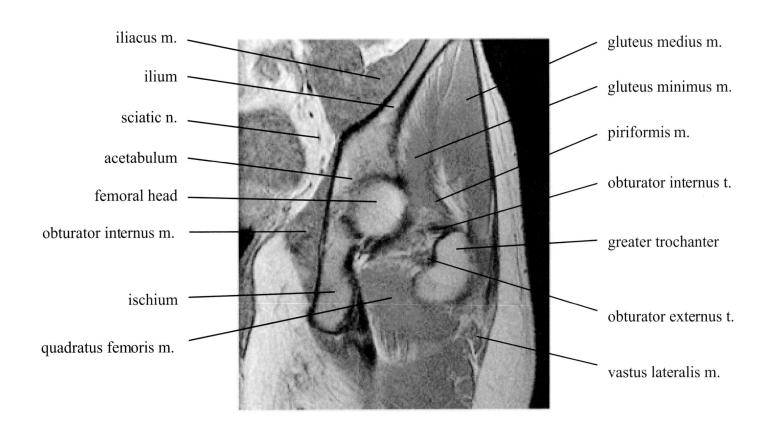

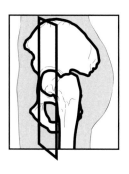

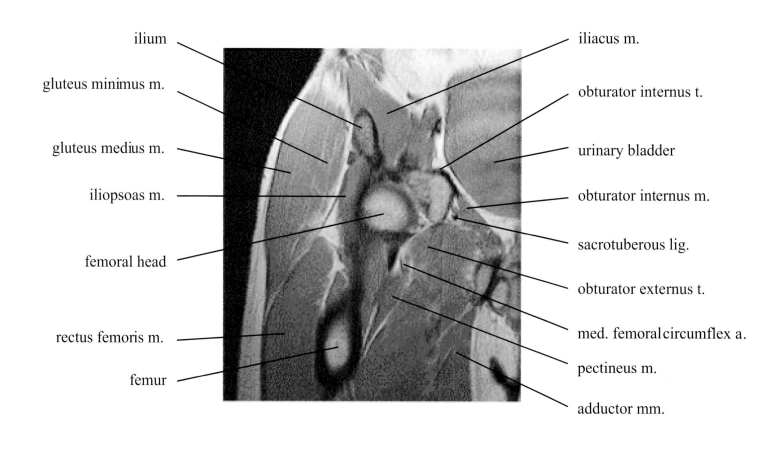

ilium

gluteus minimus m.

gluteus medius m.

iliopsoas m.

femoral head

rectus femoris m.

femur

iliacus m.

obturator internus t.

urinary bladder

obturator internus m.

sacrotuberous lig.

obturator externus t.

med. femoral circumflex a.

pectineus m.

adductor mm.

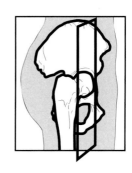

iliacus m.

obturator internus t.

urinary bladder

obturator internus m.

sacrotuberous lig.

obturator externus t.

med. femoral circumflex a.

pectineus m.

adductor mm.

ilium

gluteus minimus m.

gluteus medius m.

iliopsoas m.

femoral head

rectus femoris m.

femur

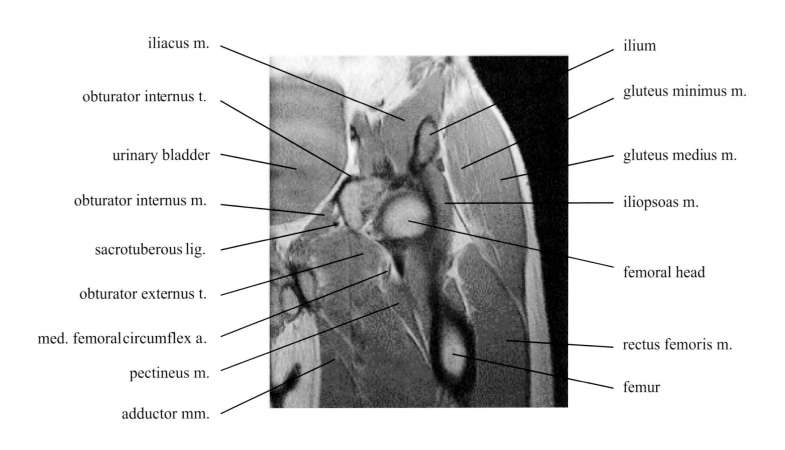

THE THIGH: AXIAL ANATOMY

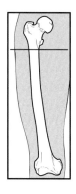

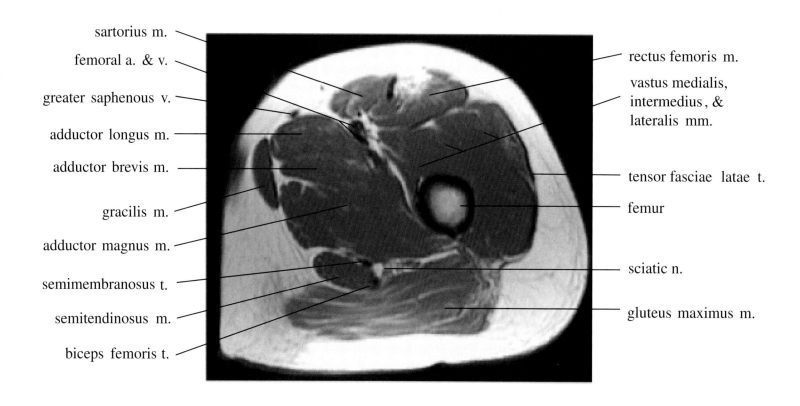

sartorius m.

femoral a. & v.

greater saphenous v.

adductor longus m.

adductor brevis m.

gracilis m.

adductor magnus m.

semimembranosus t.

semitendinosus m.

biceps femoris t.

rectus femoris m.

vastus medialis,
intermedius, &
lateralis mm.

tensor fasciae latae t.

femur

sciatic n.

gluteus maximus m.

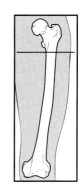

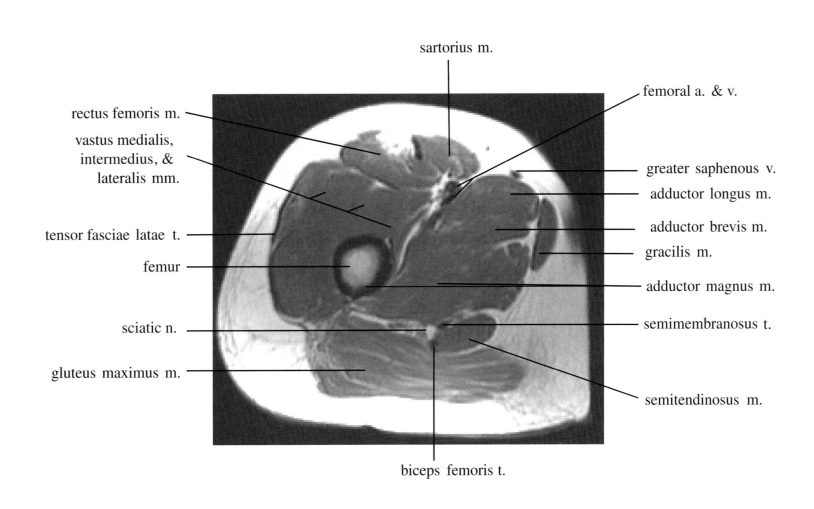

sartorius m.

femoral a. & v.

rectus femoris m.

vastus medialis,
intermedius, &
lateralis mm.

greater saphenous v.

adductor longus m.

tensor fasciae latae t.

adductor brevis m.

gracilis m.

femur

adductor magnus m.

sciatic n.

semimembranosus t.

gluteus maximus m.

semitendinosus m.

biceps femoris t.

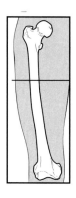

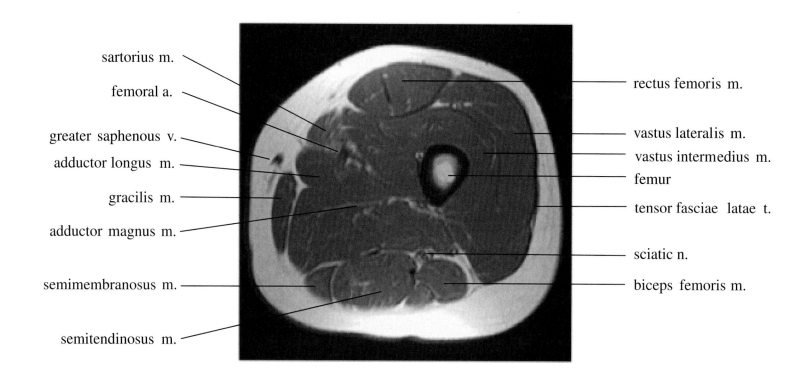

sartorius m.

femoral a.

greater saphenous v.

adductor longus m.

gracilis m.

adductor magnus m.

semimembranosus m.

semitendinosus m.

rectus femoris m.

vastus lateralis m.

vastus intermedius m.

femur

tensor fasciae latae t.

sciatic n.

biceps femoris m.

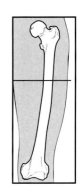

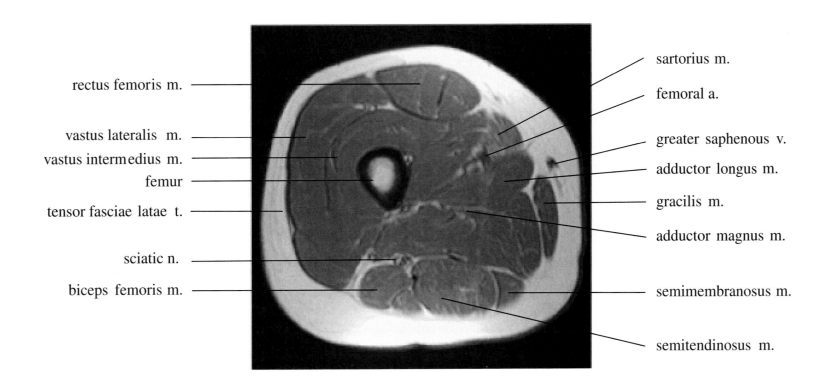

rectus femoris m.

vastus lateralis m.

vastus intermedius m.

femur

tensor fasciae latae t.

sciatic n.

biceps femoris m.

sartorius m.

femoral a.

greater saphenous v.

adductor longus m.

gracilis m.

adductor magnus m.

semimembranosus m.

semitendinosus m.

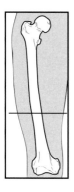

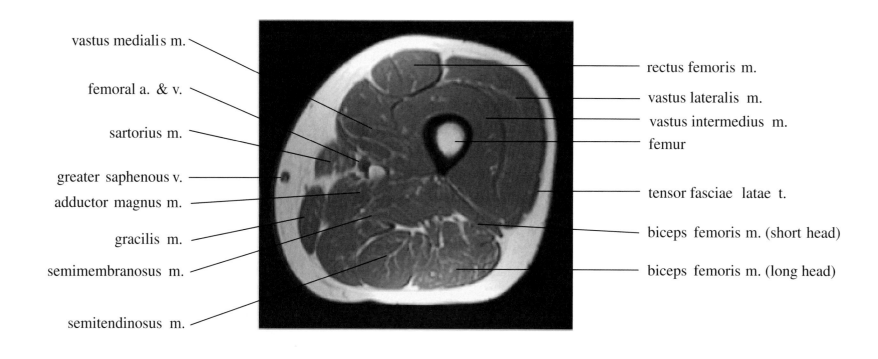

vastus medialis m.

femoral a. & v.

sartorius m.

greater saphenous v.

adductor magnus m.

gracilis m.

semimembranosus m.

semitendinosus m.

rectus femoris m.

vastus lateralis m.

vastus intermedius m.

femur

tensor fasciae latae t.

biceps femoris m. (short head)

biceps femoris m. (long head)

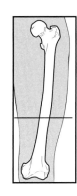

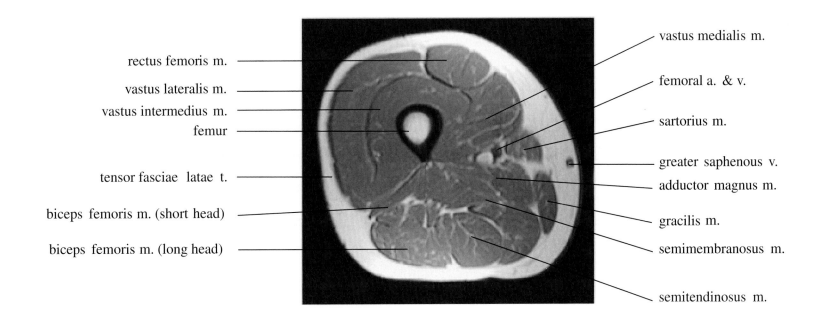

rectus femoris m.

vastus lateralis m.

vastus intermedius m.

femur

tensor fasciae latae t.

biceps femoris m. (short head)

biceps femoris m. (long head)

vastus medialis m.

femoral a. & v.

sartorius m.

greater saphenous v.

adductor magnus m.

gracilis m.

semimembranosus m.

semitendinosus m.

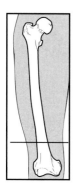

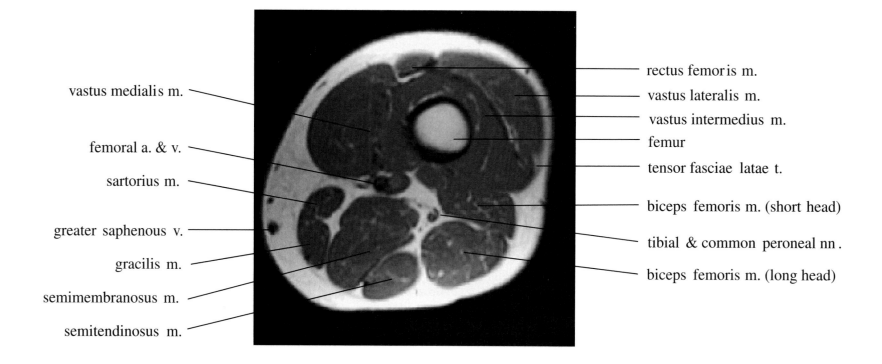

vastus medialis m.

femoral a. & v.

sartorius m.

greater saphenous v.

gracilis m.

semimembranosus m.

semitendinosus m.

rectus femoris m.

vastus lateralis m.

vastus intermedius m.

femur

tensor fasciae latae t.

biceps femoris m. (short head)

tibial & common peroneal nn.

biceps femoris m. (long head)

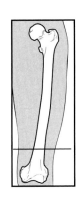

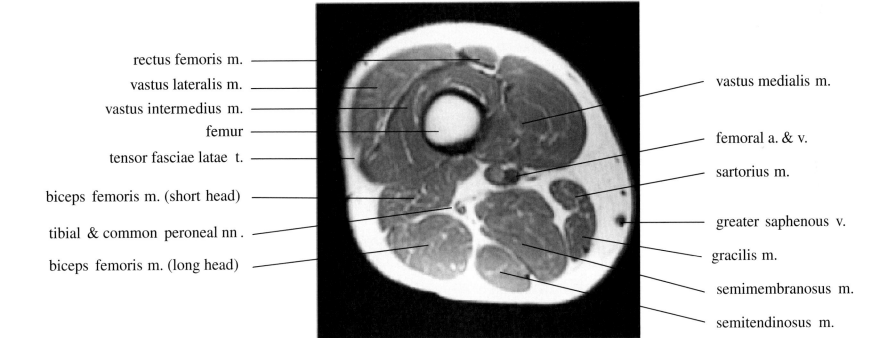

rectus femoris m.

vastus lateralis m.

vastus intermedius m.

femur

tensor fasciae latae t.

biceps femoris m. (short head)

tibial & common peroneal nn .

biceps femoris m. (long head)

vastus medialis m.

femoral a. & v.

sartorius m.

greater saphenous v.

gracilis m.

semimembranosus m.

semitendinosus m.

THE THIGH: SAGITTAL ANATOMY

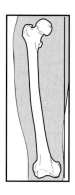

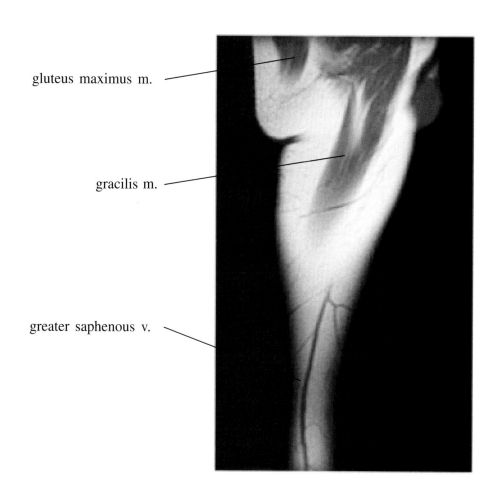

gluteus maximus m.

gracilis m.

greater saphenous v.

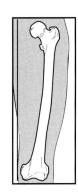

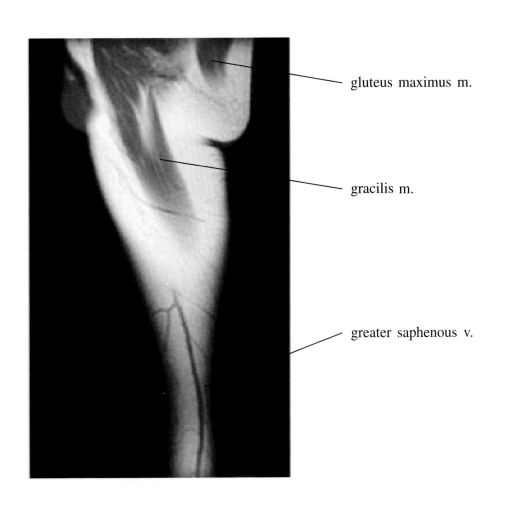

gluteus maximus m.

gracilis m.

greater saphenous v.

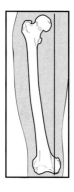

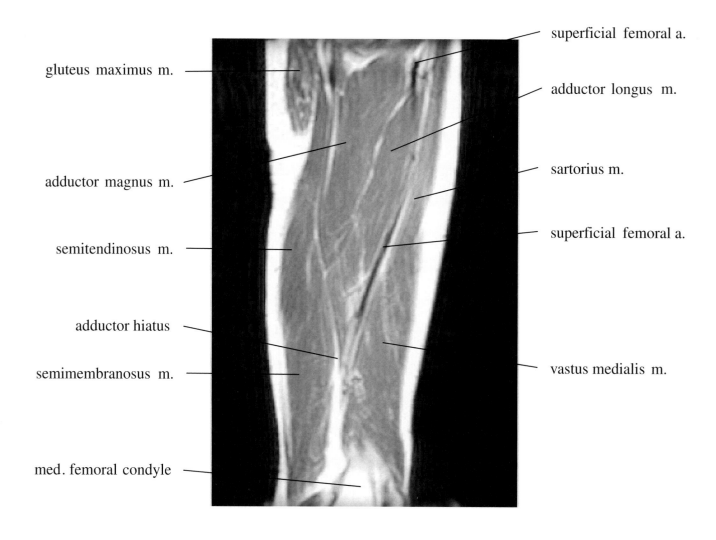

gluteus maximus m. —

adductor magnus m. —

semitendinosus m. —

adductor hiatus —

semimembranosus m. —

med. femoral condyle —

— superficial femoral a.

— adductor longus m.

— sartorius m.

— superficial femoral a.

— vastus medialis m.

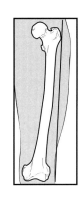

tensor fasciae latae m.——————————————— gluteus maximus m.

rectus femoris m.————————————

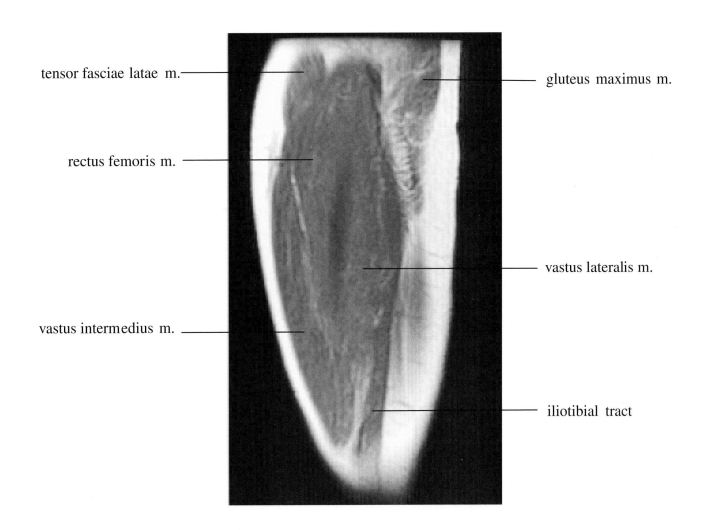

vastus lateralis m.

vastus intermedius m. ————————————

iliotibial tract

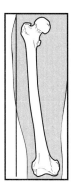

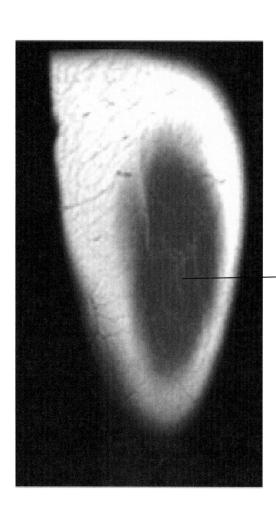

vastus lateralis m.

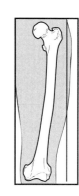

vastus lateralis m. —

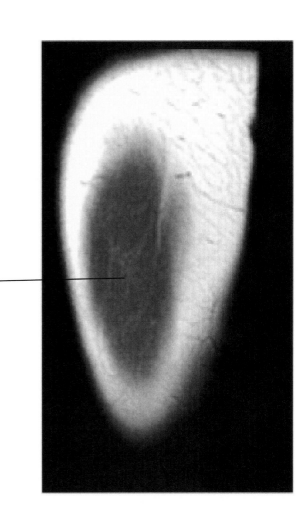

THE THIGH: CORONAL ANATOMY

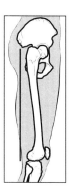

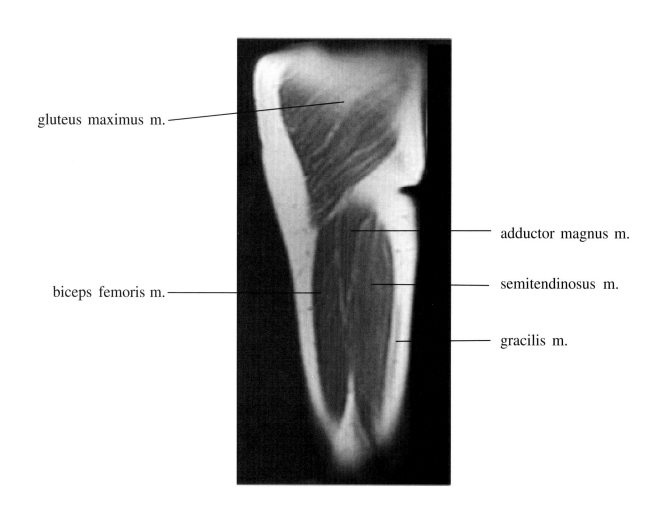

gluteus maximus m.

adductor magnus m.

semitendinosus m.

biceps femoris m.

gracilis m.

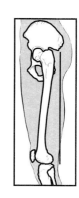

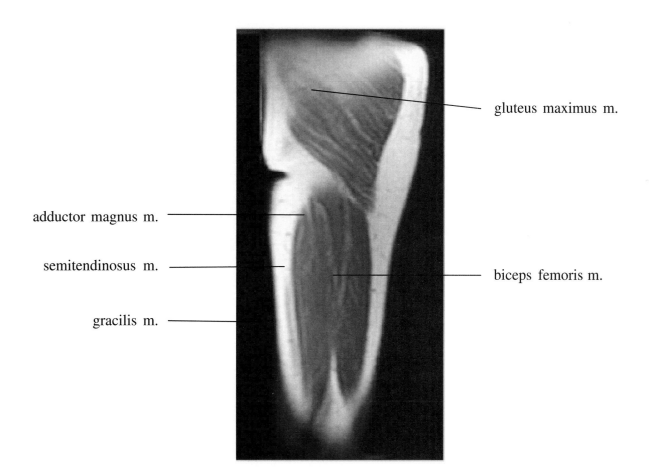

gluteus maximus m.

adductor magnus m.

semitendinosus m.

biceps femoris m.

gracilis m.

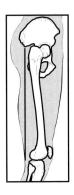

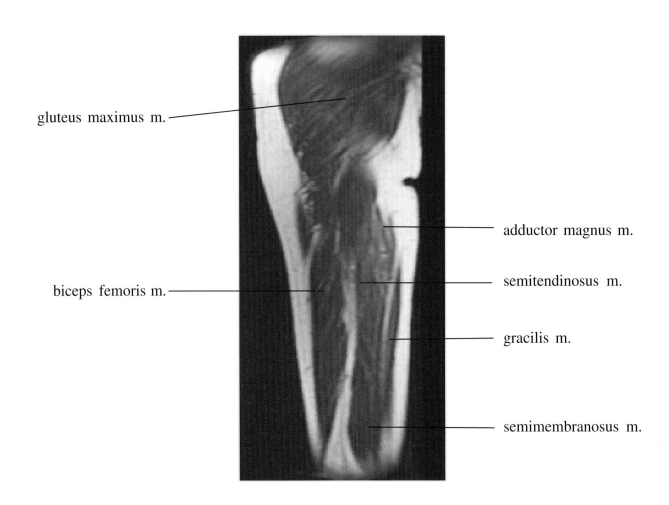

gluteus maximus m.

adductor magnus m.

semitendinosus m.

biceps femoris m.

gracilis m.

semimembranosus m.

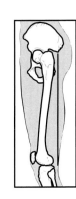

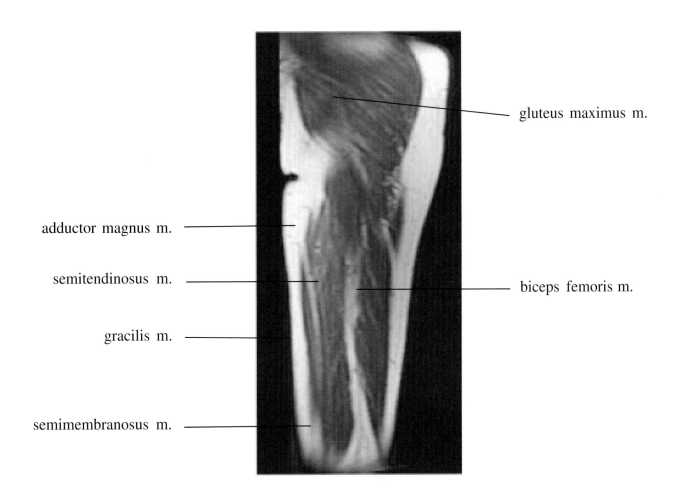

gluteus maximus m.

adductor magnus m.

semitendinosus m.

biceps femoris m.

gracilis m.

semimembranosus m.

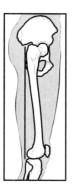

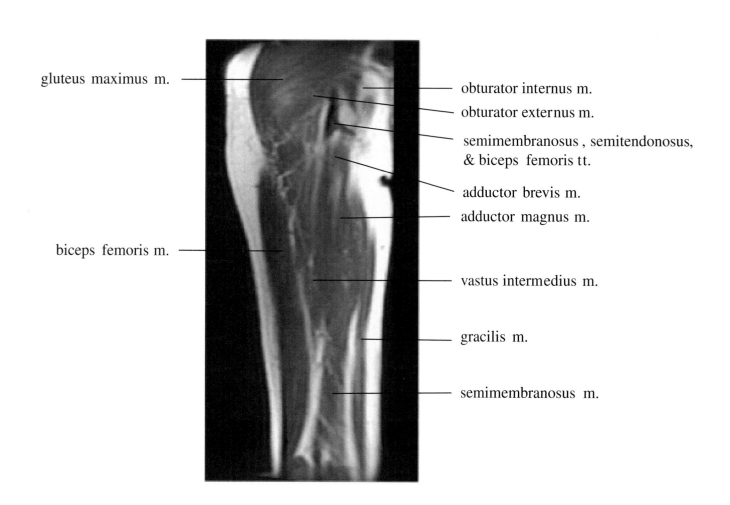

gluteus maximus m. —————

biceps femoris m. —————

————— obturator internus m.

————— obturator externus m.

————— semimembranosus , semitendonosus, & biceps femoris tt.

————— adductor brevis m.

————— adductor magnus m.

————— vastus intermedius m.

————— gracilis m.

————— semimembranosus m.

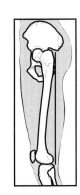

obturator internus m.

obturator externus m.

semimembranosus, semitendonosus,
& biceps femoris tt..

adductor brevis m.

adductor magnus m.

vastus intermedius m.

gracilis m.

semimembranosus m.

gluteus maximus m.

biceps femoris m.

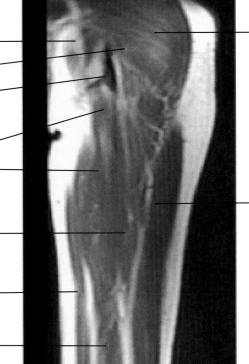

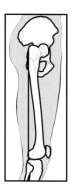

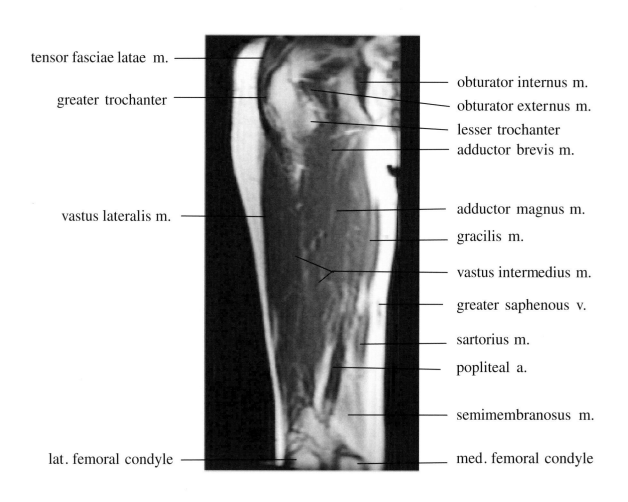

tensor fasciae latae m.

greater trochanter

vastus lateralis m.

lat. femoral condyle

obturator internus m.

obturator externus m.

lesser trochanter

adductor brevis m.

adductor magnus m.

gracilis m.

vastus intermedius m.

greater saphenous v.

sartorius m.

popliteal a.

semimembranosus m.

med. femoral condyle

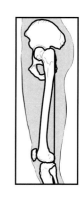

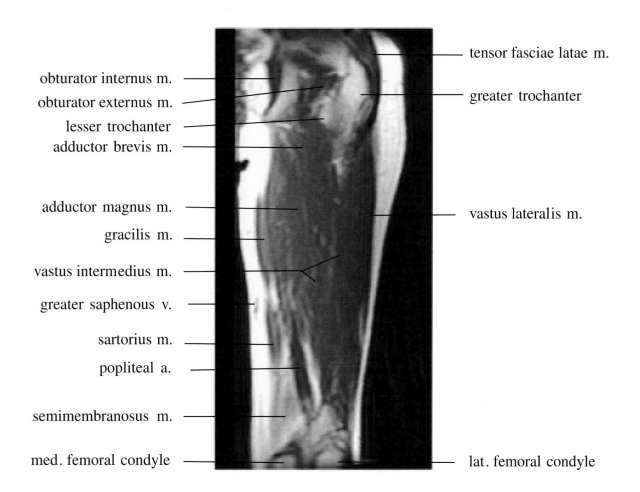

obturator internus m.

obturator externus m.

lesser trochanter

adductor brevis m.

adductor magnus m.

gracilis m.

vastus intermedius m.

greater saphenous v.

sartorius m.

popliteal a.

semimembranosus m.

med. femoral condyle

tensor fasciae latae m.

greater trochanter

vastus lateralis m.

lat. femoral condyle

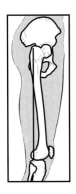

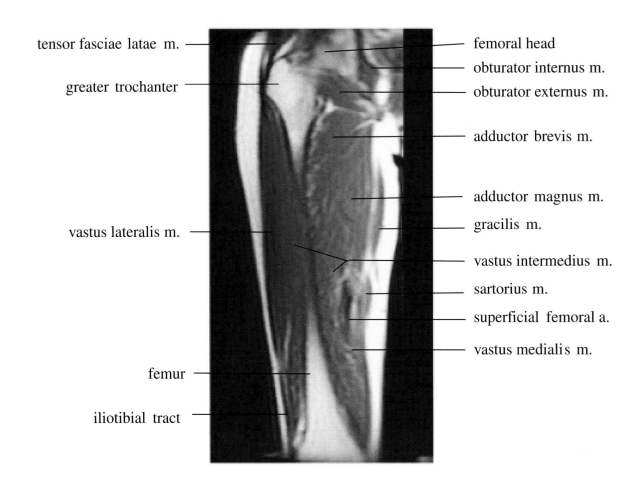

tensor fasciae latae m. ——

greater trochanter ——

vastus lateralis m. ——

femur ——

iliotibial tract ——

—— femoral head

—— obturator internus m.

—— obturator externus m.

—— adductor brevis m.

—— adductor magnus m.

—— gracilis m.

—— vastus intermedius m.

—— sartorius m.

—— superficial femoral a.

—— vastus medialis m.

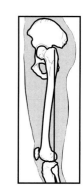

femoral head

obturator internus m.

obturator externus m.

adductor brevis m.

adductor magnus m.

gracilis m.

vastus intermedius m.

sartorius m.

superficial femoral a.

vastus medialis m.

tensor fasciae latae m.

greater trochanter

vastus lateralis m.

femur

iliotibial tract

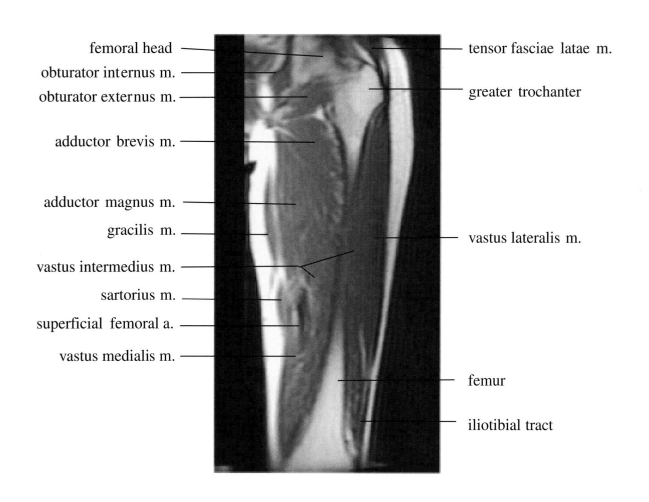

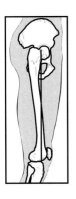

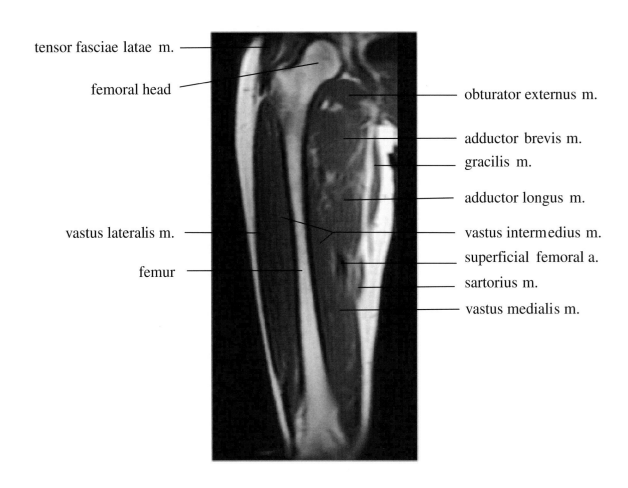

tensor fasciae latae m.

femoral head

obturator externus m.

adductor brevis m.

gracilis m.

adductor longus m.

vastus lateralis m.

vastus intermedius m.

superficial femoral a.

femur

sartorius m.

vastus medialis m.

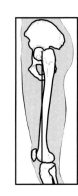

obturator externus m. —————

adductor brevis m. —————

gracilis m. —————

adductor longus m. —————

vastus intermedius m. —————

superficial femoral a. —————

sartorius m. —————

vastus medialis m. —————

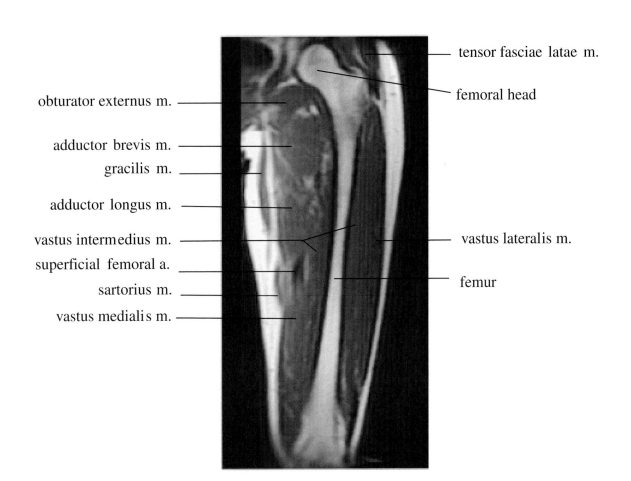

————— tensor fasciae latae m.

————— femoral head

————— vastus lateralis m.

————— femur

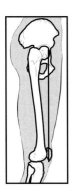

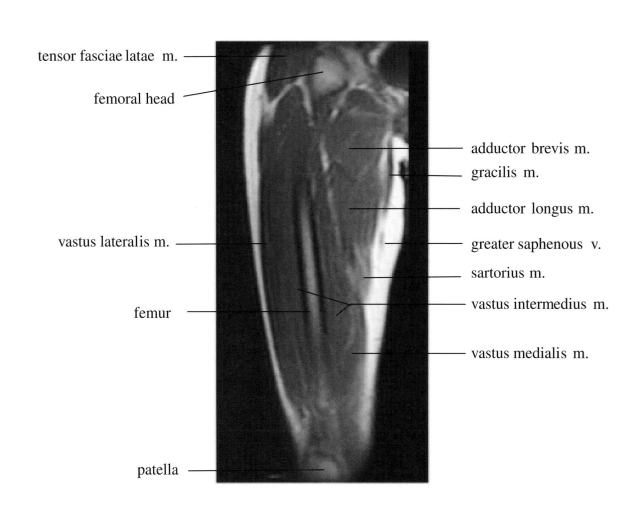

tensor fasciae latae m.

femoral head

adductor brevis m.

gracilis m.

adductor longus m.

vastus lateralis m.

greater saphenous v.

sartorius m.

vastus intermedius m.

femur

vastus medialis m.

patella

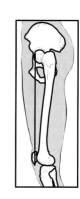

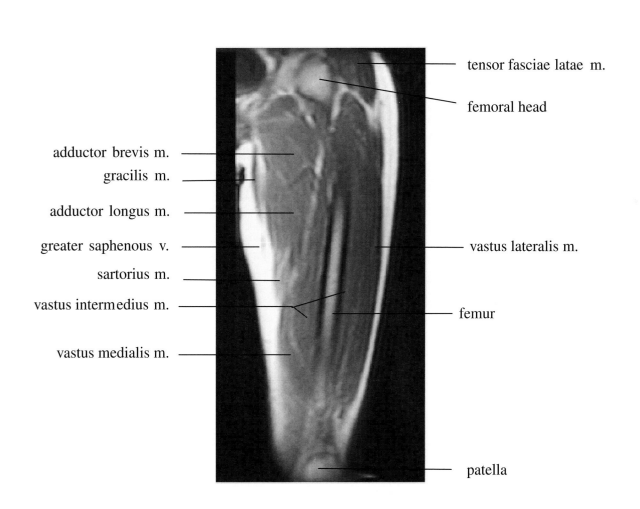

tensor fasciae latae m.

femoral head

adductor brevis m.

gracilis m.

adductor longus m.

greater saphenous v.

vastus lateralis m.

sartorius m.

vastus intermedius m.

femur

vastus medialis m.

patella

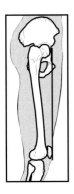

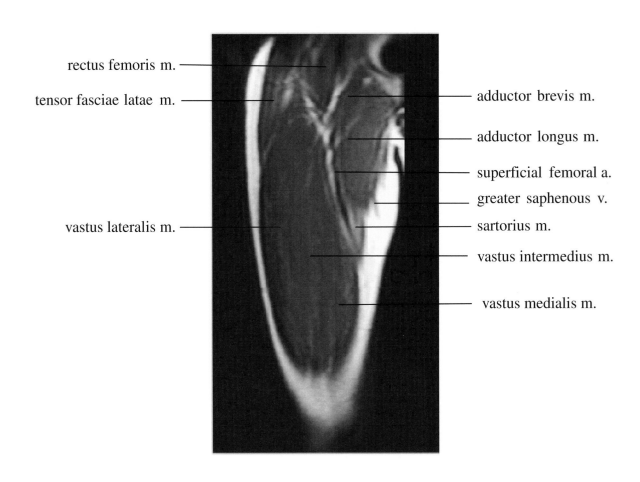

rectus femoris m. ——————

tensor fasciae latae m. ——————

—————— adductor brevis m.

—————— adductor longus m.

—————— superficial femoral a.

—————— greater saphenous v.

vastus lateralis m. ——————

—————— sartorius m.

—————— vastus intermedius m.

—————— vastus medialis m.

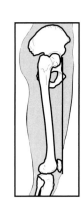

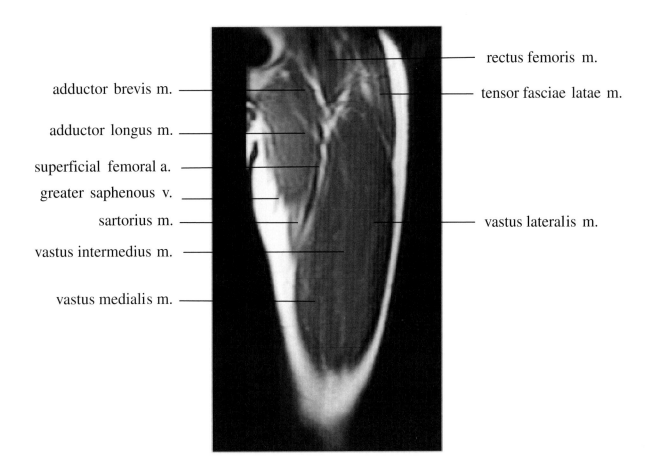

rectus femoris m.

adductor brevis m.

tensor fasciae latae m.

adductor longus m.

superficial femoral a.

greater saphenous v.

sartorius m.

vastus lateralis m.

vastus intermedius m.

vastus medialis m.

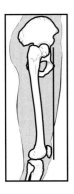

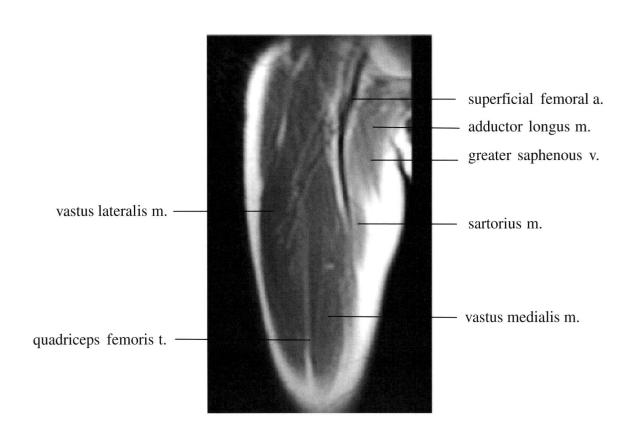

superficial femoral a.

adductor longus m.

greater saphenous v.

vastus lateralis m.

sartorius m.

vastus medialis m.

quadriceps femoris t.

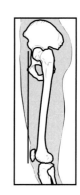

superficial femoral a. ——————

adductor longus m. ——————

greater saphenous v. ——————

sartorius m. ——————

vastus medialis m. ——————

vastus lateralis m. ——————

quadriceps femoris t. ——————

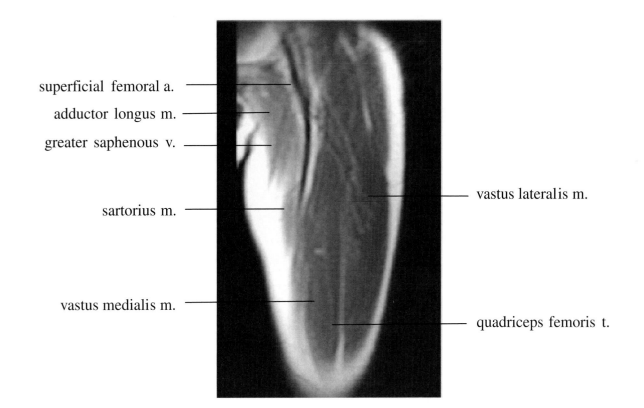

6

THE KNEE AND THE LOWER EXTREMITY

A. THE KNEE

The knee is the joint most commonly examined with MR imaging. The primary indications for the MR study are to delineate the sequelae of trauma or define chronic and unexplained knee pain. The major abnormalities encountered are meniscal tears, ligament or tendon injury or disruption, bone "bruises" (intramedullary contusions), and cartilage damage (either acute or remote).

PRACTICAL PROTOCOL CONSIDERATIONS

For MR imaging of the knee, the patient is placed in the supine position with the knee centered in the dedicated extremity (or preferably "knee") coil. The patient is asked to place the knee in a comfortable position, usually 15°–20° of external rotation with slight flexion (usually 5°–10°). This position is not only most comfortable for the patient but is convenient for visualization of the anterior cruciate ligament (ACL) on the sagittal images. The partial flexion also helps in the evaluation of the patellofemoral compartment and patellar alignment.

Below is a list of suggested protocol options accumulated from the literature. The choice of protocol may depend upon the type of equipment available and needs of the practice; therefore, this list is meant to be merely a practical outline. In many practices, standard spin-echo (SE) sequences, instead of fast spin-echo (FSE) sequences, are still used. This method is certainly acceptable, although slightly more time-consuming. Radial imaging and three-dimensional (3D) volumetric techniques are alternative protocols, but these are not routinely used today.

Menu of Protocols: Knee

Plane	Pulse Sequence	FA (degrees)	TR (msec)	TE (msec)	TI (msec)	FOV (cm)	Matrix (256X-)	ST/G (mm)	NEX	Comments
Localizer (sagittal)	FMPIR		2500	25	150	18	128	5/2.5	1	Sensitive to bone contusions
Localizer (transaxial)	2D SPGR	30	34	min		20	256	5/0	1	Either is acceptable
Localizer (transaxial)	SE		600	min		14	256	4/1	2	
Sagittal	SE, double echo		2000	20/80		14	192	4/1	1	Either is acceptable
Sagittal	FSE (±FS)		5500	85		16	192	4/0.5	1	
Sagittal	FSE, double echo		4000	20/100		12–14	256	3/1	1	
Coronal	FSE, FS		3000	20		14	192	4/0.5	2	Either is acceptable
Coronal	FSE, FS		5500	85		16	192	4/0.5	2	Sensitive to edema
Coronal	FSE (+1-FS)		4000	105		11	256	4/1	2	
Coronal	FMPIR		3000	51	150	16	128	4/1	2	Sensitive to edema
Transaxial	FSE, FS		3000	20		14	256	4/1	2	Excellent for patellar cartilage
Transaxial	3D GRE	20	40	13		16	128	1.2/0	2	
Transaxial	SPGR	30	34	3.3		20	128	5/2	1	

MAJOR OSTEOCARTILAGINOUS STRUCTURES/LANDMARKS

- Femur
  - Femoral condyles
  - Femoral condylar hyaline cartilage
  - Femoral trochlea
  - Femoral trochlear hyaline cartilage
- Lateral meniscus
- Medial meniscus
- Patella
- Patellar hyaline cartilage
- Tibia
  - Tibial plateaus (condyles)
  - Intercondylar eminence
  - Tibial condylar hyaline cartilage
  - Tibial condylar spines
  - Tibial tubercle (tuberosity)

MAJOR LIGAMENTS/TENDONS/BURSAE

Ligament	Origin	Insertion
• Anterior cruciate (ACL)	Inner aspect of lateral femoral condyle	Anterior tibia adjacent to anterior tibial spine
• Coronary (meniscofemoral and meniscotibial components)	Medial and lateral menisci	Femur/tibia
• Fibular collateral (FCL)	Lateral condyle of femur	Head of fibula
• Meniscofemoral (Humphrey's—crosses anterior to PCL) (Wrisberg—crosses posterior to PCL)	Posteromedial aspect of lateral meniscus	Inner aspect of medial femoral condyle
• Patellar	Inferior margin of patella	Anterior tibial spine
• Posterior cruciate (PCL)	Inner aspect of medial condyle	Posterior tibia femoral
• Tibial collateral (TCL)	Medial condyle of femur	Medial tibia (5–7 cm below joint line)
• Transverse meniscal	Anteromedial aspect of lateral meniscus	Anteromedial aspect of lateral meniscus

ORIGIN/INSERTION/INNERVATION OF MAJOR MUSCLES

Muscle	Origin	Insertion	Innervation
Extensor Group			
• Rectus femorus	Anterosuperior iliac spine	Patellar retinacula	Femoral N.
– Straight head			
– Reflected head	Upper margin of acetabulum and at joint capsule	Patellar retinaculum	Femoral N.
• Sartorius	Anterosuperior iliac spine	Medial tibia via pes anserinus	Femoral N.

(continued)

ORIGIN/INSERTION/INNERVATION OF MAJOR MUSCLES (*CONTINUED*)

Muscle	Origin	Insertion	Innervation
• Vastus medialis	Medial lip of linea aspera and terminal tendons of adductor longus/ magnus	Medial retinaculum	Femoral N.
• Vastus lateralis	Base of greater trochanter and lateral lip of the linea aspera aponeurosis	Patella retinaculum	Femoral N.
• Vastus intermedius	Anterolateral mid- to distal femur	Common terminal tendon	Femoral N.
Flexor Group			
• Biceps femoris			
– Long head	Posterior surface of ischial tuberosity	Head of fibula (portion to lateral condyle of tibia)	Tibialis component of sciatic N.
– Short head	Middle third of lateral lip of linea aspera		Peroneal division of sciatic N.
– Semi-membranosus	Ischial tuberosity of tibia	1. Medial condyle 2. Posterior wall of knee joint capsule 3. Fascia of popliteus tendon (via pes anserinus)	Tibialis component of sciatic N.
– Semi-tendinosus	Ischial tuberosity	Medial surface of proximal end of tibia and fascia of leg (via pes anserinus)	Tibialis component of sciatic N.

B. THE LOWER EXTREMITY

The major indications for MR imaging of the lower limb include suspected tumors, stress injuries, infection, or acute muscle and soft-tissue injuries such as acute hemorrhage and muscle tears. Before the patient arrives, study protocol should be determined according to the clinical indication, and, ideally, the examination should be monitored.

PRACTICAL PROTOCOL CONSIDERATIONS

For MR imaging of the lower limb, the patient is usually placed in the supine position with the extremity resting comfortably within the magnet. If the patient has a palpable abnormality or a surgical scar, a bath oil bead or vitamin E tablet should be placed at the upper and lower margins of the scar or the palpable mass. If the mass is large, these localizers should reflect the superior and inferior margins of the lesion.

The body coil can be used for the localizer, but torso or surface coils should be used if possible to provide better signal-to-noise ratio. Most of these examinations should be planned before the patient arrives, and the exact protocol will vary according to the indications for the study. The patient should be monitored during the examination to ensure that the areas of clinical concern are covered by the MR study. Spin echo, fast spin echo, and gradient echo techniques are used, and some of the more common ones will be outlined in the next section.

Menu of Protocols: Lower Extremity

Plane	Pulse Sequence	FA (degrees)	TR (msec)	TE (msec)	TI (msec)	FOV (cm)	Matrix (256X-)	ST/G (mm)	NEX	Comments
Localizer (transaxial)	SE		500	min		VAR	192	5/1.5	1	Mark area of concern
Coronal, sagittal	SE		500	min		VAR	192	5/1.5	1	
Coronal	SE		1000	min		VAR	192	5/1.5	2	Either is acceptable
Coronal	FMPIR		2500	30	150	VAR	128	5/1.5	1	
Sagittal	SE		1000	min		VAR	192	5/1.5	2	Either is acceptable
Sagittal	FMPIR		2500	30	150	VAR	128	5/1.5	2	
Transaxial	SE		600	20 VAR		VAR	192	4/1	2	
Transaxial, pre-GAD	SE		600	20		VAR	192	4/1	2	Repeat after GAD
Transaxial, pre-GAD	SE, FS		600	20		VAR	192	4/1	2	Repeat after GAD

MAJOR OSTEOCHONDRAL STRUCTURES/LANDMARKS

(See knee and ankle/foot)

MAJOR LIGAMENTS/TENDONS/BURSAE

(See knee and ankle/foot)

MAJOR MUSCLES

Compartments

The lower leg is divided into four main compartments by the interosseous membrane, the crural fascia, and the intermuscular septae.

- Anterior compartment muscles
  - Tibialis anterior
  - Extensor digitorum longus
  - Extensor hallucis longus
  - Peroneus tertius
- Lateral compartment muscles
  - Peroneus longus muscle
  - Peroneus brevis muscles
- Posterior compartment muscles
  - Superficial group
  - Plantaris
  - Soleus
  - Gastrocnemius
- Deep group
  - Popliteus
  - Flexor digitorum longus
  - Tibialis posterior
  - Flexor hallucis longus and popliteus

ORIGIN/INSERTION/INNERVATION OF MAJOR MUSCLES

Muscle	Origin	Insertion	Innervation
Anterior Compartment			
– Tibialis anterior	Lateral condyle of tibia, interosseous membrane, crural fascia and intramuscular septum	Medial surface of the medial cuneiform, base of first metatarsal	Branches from common peroneal N. and deep peroneal N.
– Extensor digitorum longus	Lateral condyle of tibia, anterior surface of fibula, intermuscular septum, and crural fascia near tibia	Tendon divides into two parts below superior ext. retinaculum. Four tendons then cross dorsal surface of each toe. Tendons divide into one central and two lateral slips; lateral slip inserts on base of distal phalanx, and central slip ends on dorsum of middle phalanx. Extensor expansions are formed over MTP joints, and lateral slips of tendon are jointed distally by interosseus tendons and lumbrical muscles.	Branches of deep peroneal N.

(continued)

ORIGIN/INSERTION/INNERVATION OF MAJOR MUSCLES (*CONTINUED*)

Muscle	Origin	Insertion	Innervation
– Extensor hallucis longus	Middle two-thirds of anterior surface of fibula and interosseous membrane	Base of distal phalanx of great toe	Deep peroneal N.
– Peroneus tertius (in essence, a lateral slip of extensor digitorum longus muscle and often merges with it except at its insertion)	Distal one-third of anterior surface of fibula, interosseous membrane, and anterior intermuscular septum	Dorsal shaft of fifth metatarsal	Distal nerve to extensor digitorum muscle (a branch of deep peroneal)

Lateral Compartment

– Peroneus longus	Fibula—head and upper two-thirds of lateral surface of body, anterior and posterior intermuscular septae, and crural fascia	Inferolateral lateral aspect of medial cuneiform, base and inferolateral surface of first metatarsal	Common peroneal N. primarily, partially by superficial peroneal

(continued)

ORIGIN/INSERTION/INNERVATION OF MAJOR MUSCLES (*CONTINUED*)

Muscle	*Origin*	*Insertion*	*Innervation*
– Peroneus brevis	Fibula—lower two-thirds of lateral surface, anterior and posterior intramuscular septae	Tuberosity of base of fifth metatarsal	Superficial peroneal N., less commonly off branch supplying peroneus longus

Superficial Posterior Compartment

Muscle	*Origin*	*Insertion*	*Innervation*
– Gastrocnemius			
• Medial head	Popliteal surface of femur just above medial femoral condyle	After aponeurotic fusion with tendon of soleus muscle it forms calcaneal tendon and inserts onto posterior and superior surface of calcaneus	Tibial portion of sciatic N.
• Lateral head	Upper and posterior portion of lateral surface of lateral femoral condyle at end of supracondylar line		
– Soleus	Posterior surfaces of fibular head, upper one-third of fibular shaft, intermuscular septum, medial border of middle third and soleus line of tibia	Fuses with tendon of gastrocnemius to form calcaneal tendon inserting onto posterior and superior surface of calcaneus	Tibial portion of sciatic N.

(*continued*)

ORIGIN/INSERTION/INNERVATION OF MAJOR MUSCLES (*CONTINUED*)

Muscle	Origin	Insertion	Innervation
– Plantaris	Lower lateral supracondylar femur just above lateral head of gastrocnemius muscle, oblique popliteal ligament	Via medial border of calcaneal tendon it inserts onto posterior and superior aspect of calcaneus	Tibial portion of sciatic N.

Deep Posterior Compartment

Muscle	Origin	Insertion	Innervation
– Popliteus	Anterior end of groove on lateral aspect of lateral femoral condyle	Shaft of tibia proximal to popliteal line of tibia	Tibial N. (separate branch or with nerve to posterior tibial muscle)
– Flexor hallucis longus	Lower two-thirds of posterior surface of fibular shaft and intramuscular septum	Bases of distal phalanx of second to fourth toes	Tibial N.
– Flexor digitorum longus	Medial side and posterior surface of midtibia and intermuscular septum	Bases of terminal phalanges of second to fourth toes	Tibial N.

(*continued*)

ORIGIN/INSERTION/INNERVATION OF MAJOR MUSCLES (*CONTINUED*)

Muscle	Origin	Insertion	Innervation
– Tibialis posterior	Lateral half of middle one-third of posterior surface of tibia, medial aspect of fibular head and proximal portion of body, interosseous membrane	Tuberosity of navicular and under surface of medial cuneiform, extension continues forward and lateral to intermediate and lateral cuneiforms and to plantar surfaces of bases of second to fourth metatarsals	Tibial N.

THE KNEE: AXIAL ANATOMY

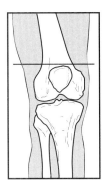

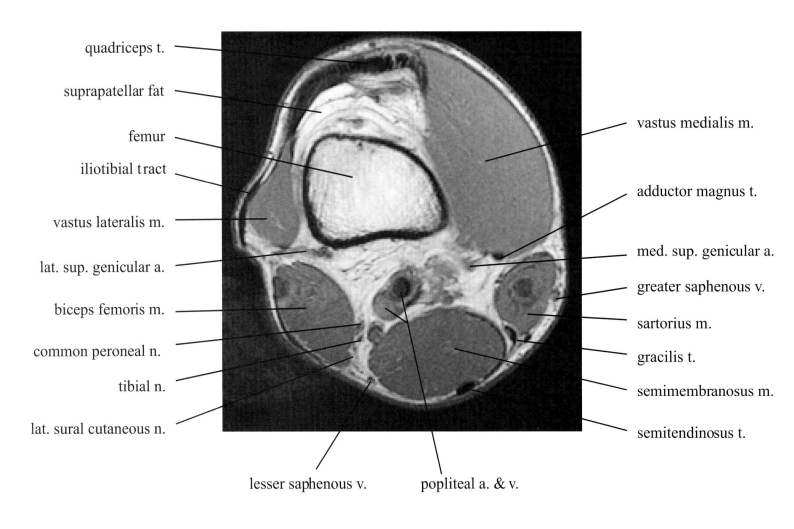

quadriceps t.

suprapatellar fat

femur

iliotibial tract

vastus lateralis m.

lat. sup. genicular a.

biceps femoris m.

common peroneal n.

tibial n.

lat. sural cutaneous n.

vastus medialis m.

adductor magnus t.

med. sup. genicular a.

greater saphenous v.

sartorius m.

gracilis t.

semimembranosus m.

semitendinosus t.

lesser saphenous v.   popliteal a. & v.

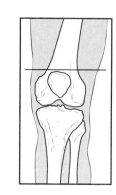

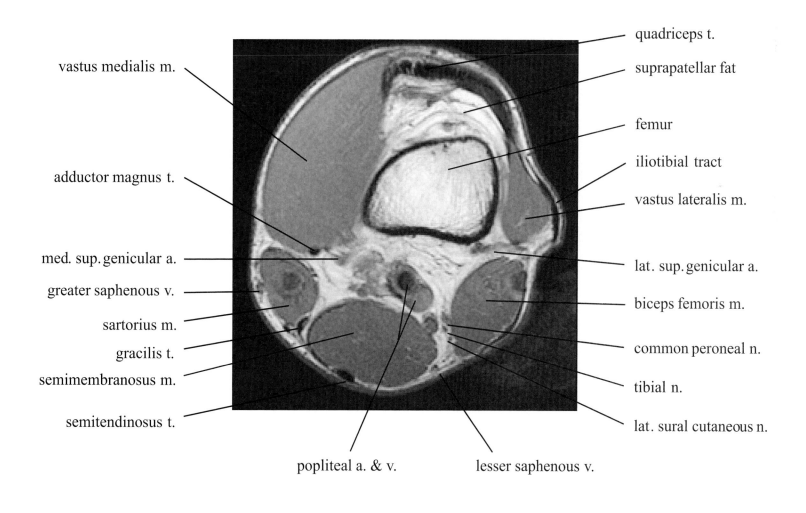

vastus medialis m.

adductor magnus t.

med. sup. genicular a.

greater saphenous v.

sartorius m.

gracilis t.

semimembranosus m.

semitendinosus t.

quadriceps t.

suprapatellar fat

femur

iliotibial tract

vastus lateralis m.

lat. sup. genicular a.

biceps femoris m.

common peroneal n.

tibial n.

lat. sural cutaneous n.

popliteal a. & v.

lesser saphenous v.

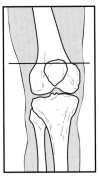

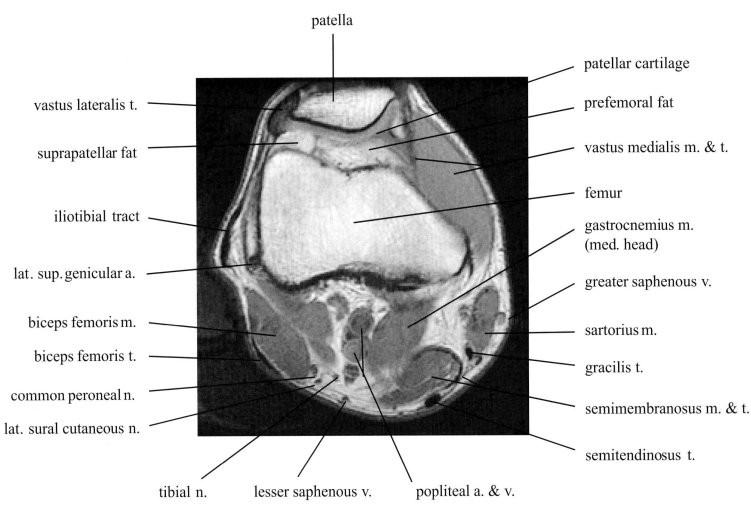

patella

patellar cartilage

vastus lateralis t.

prefemoral fat

suprapatellar fat

vastus medialis m. & t.

femur

iliotibial tract

gastrocnemius m. (med. head)

lat. sup. genicular a.

greater saphenous v.

biceps femoris m.

sartorius m.

biceps femoris t.

gracilis t.

common peroneal n.

semimembranosus m. & t.

lat. sural cutaneous n.

semitendinosus t.

tibial n.   lesser saphenous v.   popliteal a. & v.

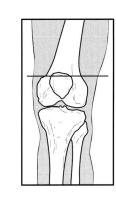

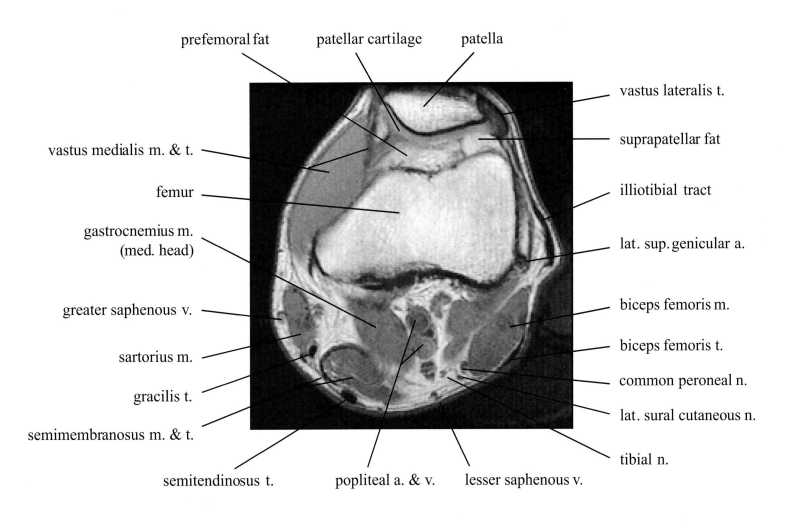

prefemoral fat

patellar cartilage

patella

vastus lateralis t.

suprapatellar fat

vastus medialis m. & t.

illiotibial tract

femur

lat. sup. genicular a.

gastrocnemius m. (med. head)

biceps femoris m.

greater saphenous v.

biceps femoris t.

sartorius m.

common peroneal n.

gracilis t.

lat. sural cutaneous n.

semimembranosus m. & t.

tibial n.

semitendinosus t.

popliteal a. & v.

lesser saphenous v.

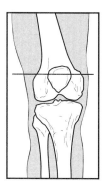

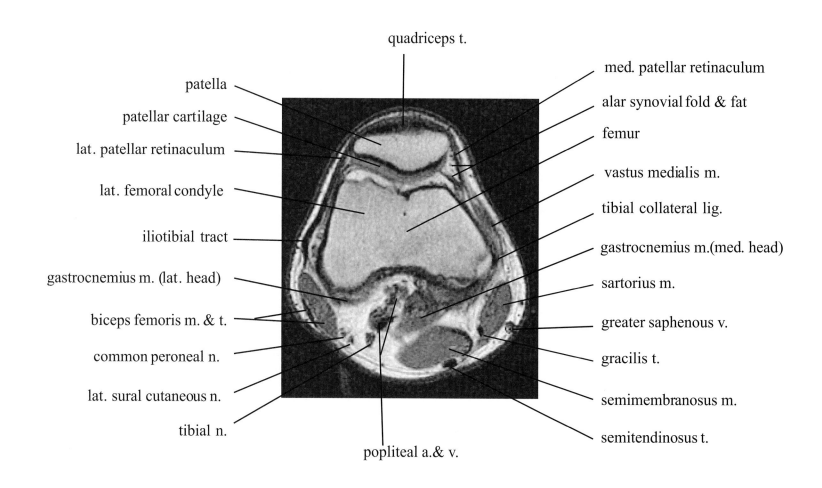

quadriceps t.

med. patellar retinaculum

patella

alar synovial fold & fat

patellar cartilage

femur

lat. patellar retinaculum

vastus medialis m.

lat. femoral condyle

tibial collateral lig.

iliotibial tract

gastrocnemius m.(med. head)

gastrocnemius m. (lat. head)

sartorius m.

biceps femoris m. & t.

greater saphenous v.

common peroneal n.

gracilis t.

lat. sural cutaneous n.

semimembranosus m.

tibial n.

semitendinosus t.

popliteal a.& v.

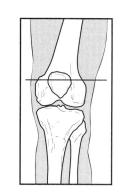

med. patellar retinaculum   quadriceps t.

alar synovial fat & fold

med. femoral condyle

vastus medialis m.

tibial collateral lig.

gastrocnemius m. (med. head)

sartorius m.

greater saphenous v.

gracilis t.

semimembranosus m.

semitendinosus t.   popliteal a. & v.

patella

patellar cartilage

lat. patellar retinaculum

lat. femoral condyle

iliotibial tract

gastrocnemius m. (lat. head)

biceps femoris m.

common peroneal n.

lat. sural cutaneous n.

tibial n.

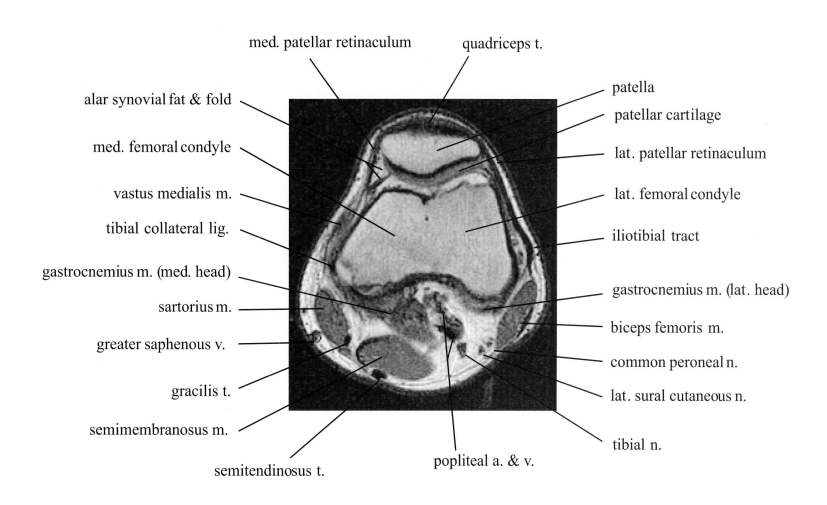

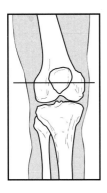

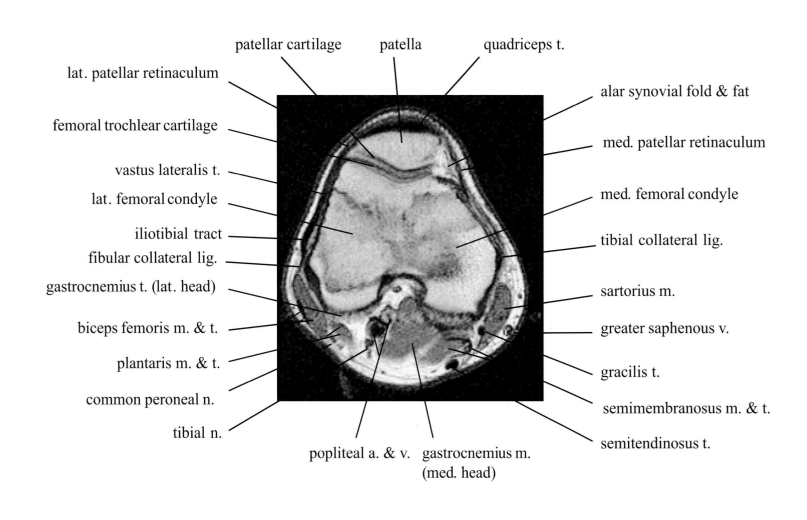

patellar cartilage   patella   quadriceps t.

lat. patellar retinaculum

femoral trochlear cartilage

vastus lateralis t.

lat. femoral condyle

iliotibial tract

fibular collateral lig.

gastrocnemius t. (lat. head)

biceps femoris m. & t.

plantaris m. & t.

common peroneal n.

tibial n.

alar synovial fold & fat

med. patellar retinaculum

med. femoral condyle

tibial collateral lig.

sartorius m.

greater saphenous v.

gracilis t.

semimembranosus m. & t.

semitendinosus t.

popliteal a. & v.   gastrocnemius m. (med. head)

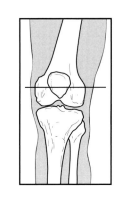

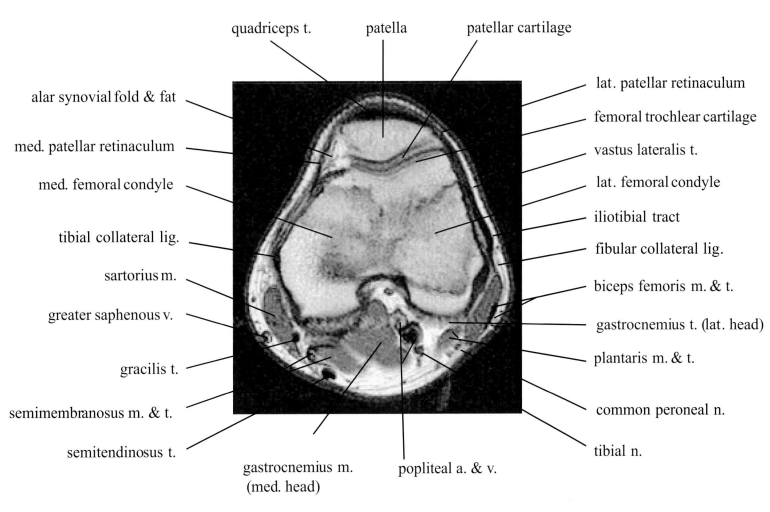

quadriceps t.

patella

patellar cartilage

alar synovial fold & fat

med. patellar retinaculum

med. femoral condyle

tibial collateral lig.

sartorius m.

greater saphenous v.

gracilis t.

semimembranosus m. & t.

semitendinosus t.

lat. patellar retinaculum

femoral trochlear cartilage

vastus lateralis t.

lat. femoral condyle

iliotibial tract

fibular collateral lig.

biceps femoris m. & t.

gastrocnemius t. (lat. head)

plantaris m. & t.

common peroneal n.

tibial n.

gastrocnemius m.
(med. head)

popliteal a. & v.

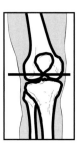

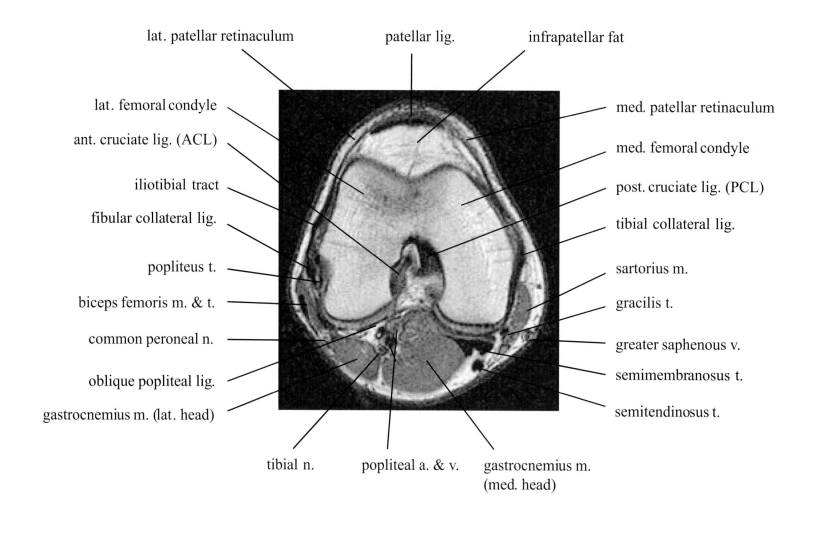

lat. patellar retinaculum

patellar lig.

infrapatellar fat

lat. femoral condyle

ant. cruciate lig. (ACL)

iliotibial tract

fibular collateral lig.

popliteus t.

biceps femoris m. & t.

common peroneal n.

oblique popliteal lig.

gastrocnemius m. (lat. head)

med. patellar retinaculum

med. femoral condyle

post. cruciate lig. (PCL)

tibial collateral lig.

sartorius m.

gracilis t.

greater saphenous v.

semimembranosus t.

semitendinosus t.

tibial n.

popliteal a. & v.

gastrocnemius m. (med. head)

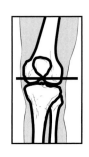

infrapatellar fat

patellar lig.

lat. patellar retinaculum

med. patellar retinaculum

med. femoral condyle

post. cruciate lig. (PCL)

tibial collateral lig.

sartorius m.

gracilis t.

greater saphenous v.

semimembranosus t.

semitendinosus t.

lat. femoral condyle

ant. cruciate lig. (ACL)

iliotibial tract

fibular collateral lig.

popliteus t.

biceps femoris m. & t.

common peroneal n.

oblique popliteal lig.

gastrocnemius m.
(lat. head)

gastrocnemius m.
(med. head)

popliteal a. & v.

tibial n.

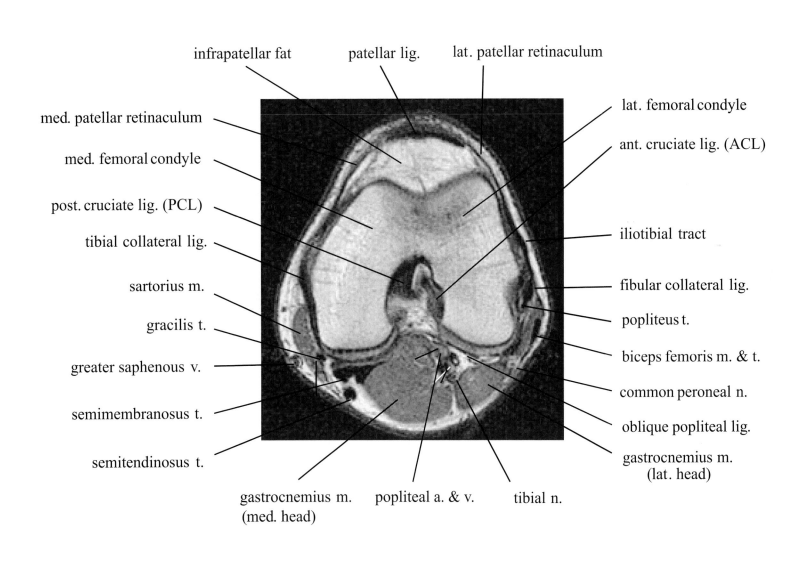

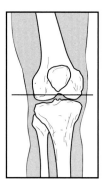

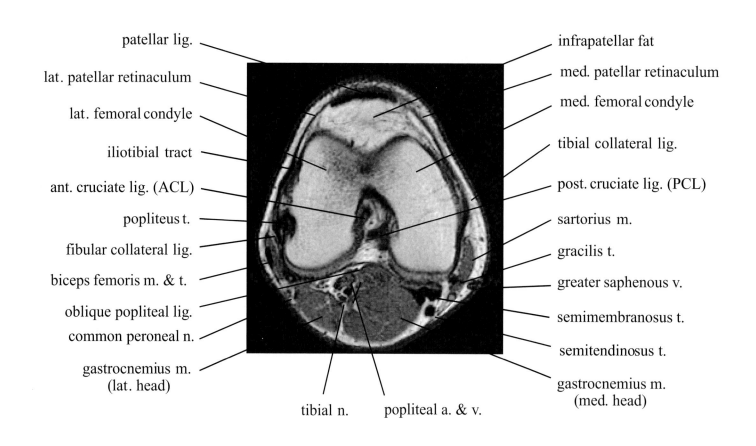

patellar lig.

lat. patellar retinaculum

lat. femoral condyle

iliotibial tract

ant. cruciate lig. (ACL)

popliteus t.

fibular collateral lig.

biceps femoris m. & t.

oblique popliteal lig.

common peroneal n.

gastrocnemius m.
(lat. head)

infrapatellar fat

med. patellar retinaculum

med. femoral condyle

tibial collateral lig.

post. cruciate lig. (PCL)

sartorius m.

gracilis t.

greater saphenous v.

semimembranosus t.

semitendinosus t.

gastrocnemius m.
(med. head)

tibial n.   popliteal a. & v.

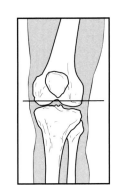

patellar lig.

med. patellar retinaculum

med. femoral condyle

tibial collateral lig.

post. cruciate lig. (PCL)

sartorius m.

gracilis t.

greater saphenous v.

semimembranosus t.

semitendinosus t.

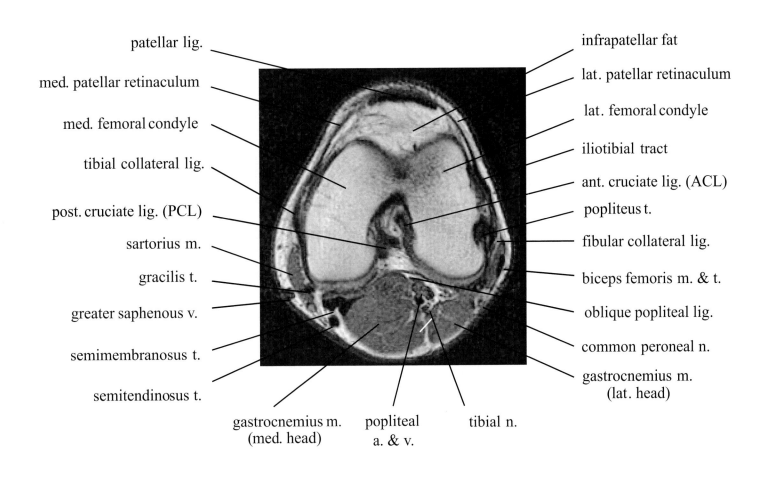

infrapatellar fat

lat. patellar retinaculum

lat. femoral condyle

iliotibial tract

ant. cruciate lig. (ACL)

popliteus t.

fibular collateral lig.

biceps femoris m. & t.

oblique popliteal lig.

common peroneal n.

gastrocnemius m.
(lat. head)

gastrocnemius m.
(med. head)

popliteal
a. & v.

tibial n.

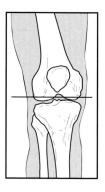

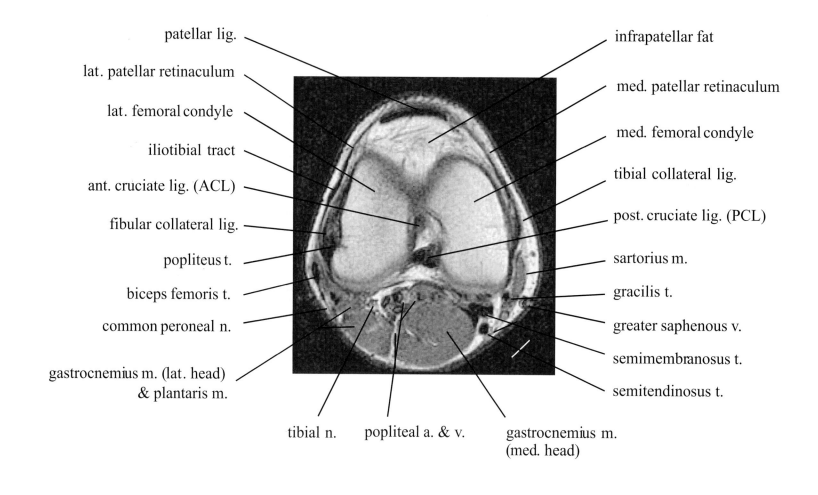

patellar lig.

lat. patellar retinaculum

lat. femoral condyle

iliotibial tract

ant. cruciate lig. (ACL)

fibular collateral lig.

popliteus t.

biceps femoris t.

common peroneal n.

gastrocnemius m. (lat. head)
& plantaris m.

infrapatellar fat

med. patellar retinaculum

med. femoral condyle

tibial collateral lig.

post. cruciate lig. (PCL)

sartorius m.

gracilis t.

greater saphenous v.

semimembranosus t.

semitendinosus t.

tibial n.   popliteal a. & v.   gastrocnemius m.
(med. head)

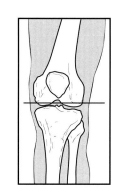

infrapatellar fat

med. patellar retinaculum

med. femoral condyle

tibial collateral lig.

post. cruciate lig. (PCL)

sartorius m.

gracilis t.

greater saphenous v.

semimembranosus t.

semitendinosus t.

patellar lig.

lat. patellar retinaculum

lat. femoral condyle

iliotibial tract

ant. cruciate lig. (ACL)

fibular collateral lig.

popliteus t.

biceps femoris t.

common peroneal n.

gastrocnemius m.
(lat. head) & plantaris m.

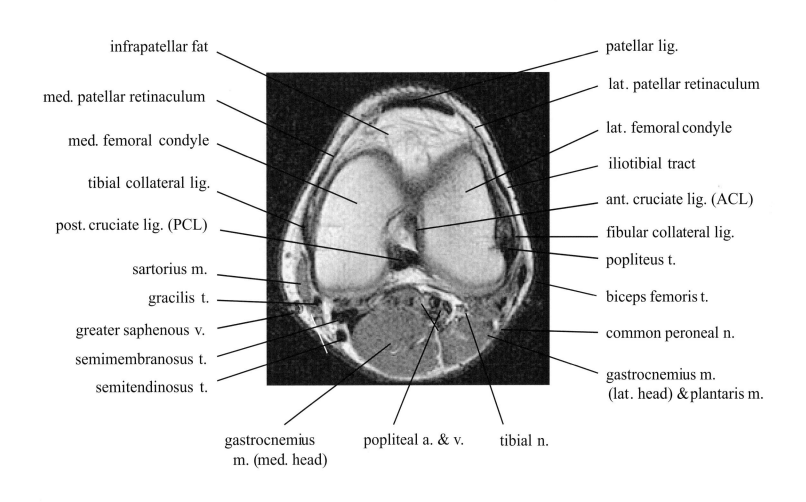

gastrocnemius
m. (med. head)

popliteal a. & v.

tibial n.

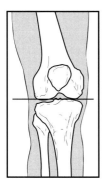

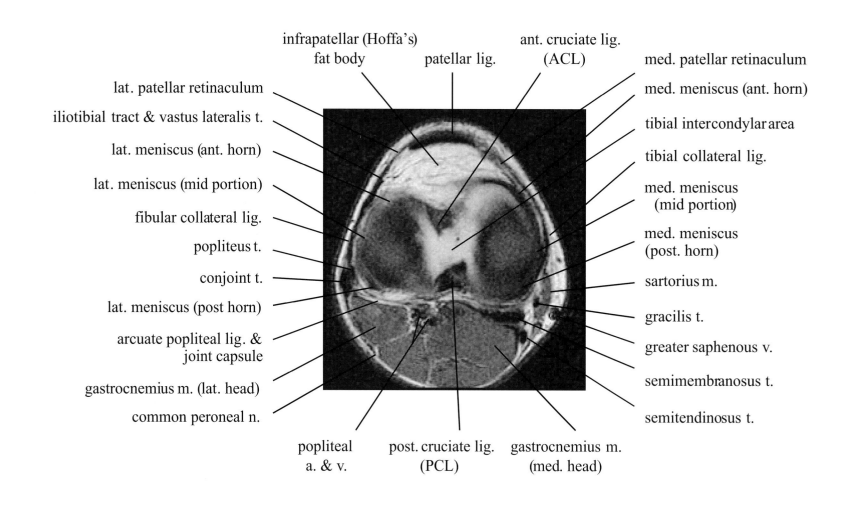

infrapatellar (Hoffa's)
fat body

patellar lig.

ant. cruciate lig.
(ACL)

med. patellar retinaculum

lat. patellar retinaculum

med. meniscus (ant. horn)

iliotibial tract & vastus lateralis t.

tibial intercondylar area

lat. meniscus (ant. horn)

tibial collateral lig.

lat. meniscus (mid portion)

med. meniscus
(mid portion)

fibular collateral lig.

med. meniscus
(post. horn)

popliteus t.

conjoint t.

sartorius m.

lat. meniscus (post horn)

gracilis t.

arcuate popliteal lig. &
joint capsule

greater saphenous v.

gastrocnemius m. (lat. head)

semimembranosus t.

common peroneal n.

semitendinosus t.

popliteal
a. & v.

post. cruciate lig.
(PCL)

gastrocnemius m.
(med. head)

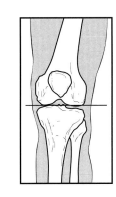

ant. cruciate lig.
(ACL)

patellar lig.

infrapatellar (Hoffa's)
fat body

med. patellar retinaculum

med. meniscus (ant. horn)

tibial intercondylar area

tibial collateral lig.

med. meniscus
(mid portion)

med. meniscus
(post. horn)

sartorius m.

gracilis t.

greater saphenous v.

semimembranosus t.

semitendinosus t.

lat. patellar retinaculum

iliotibial tract & vastus lateralis t.

lat. meniscus (ant. horn)

lat. meniscus (mid portion)

fibular collateral lig.

popliteus t.

conjoint t.

lat. meniscus (post horn)

arcuate popliteal lig. &
joint capsule

gastrocnemius m. (lat. head)

common peroneal n.

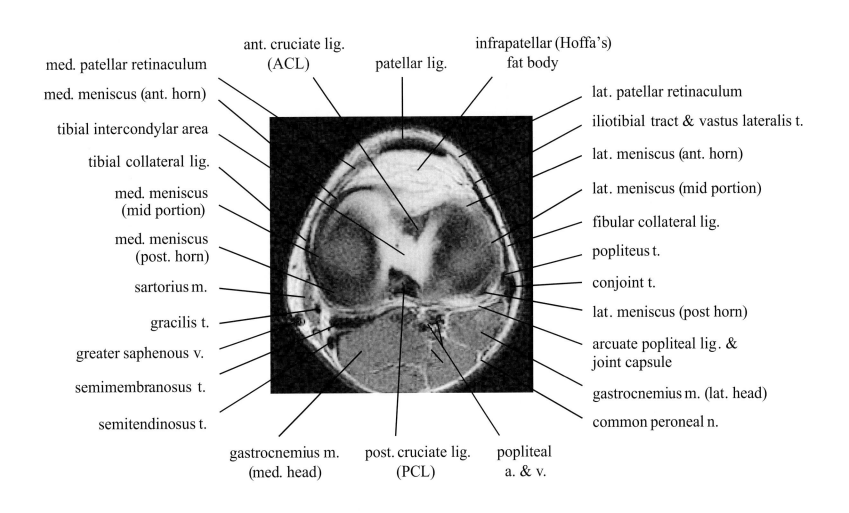

gastrocnemius m.
(med. head)

post. cruciate lig.
(PCL)

popliteal
a. & v.

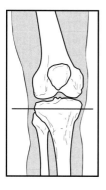

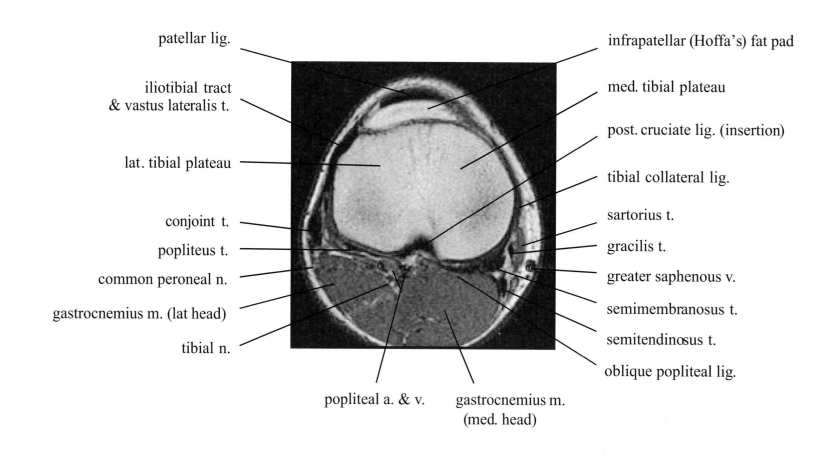

patellar lig.

iliotibial tract
& vastus lateralis t.

lat. tibial plateau

conjoint t.

popliteus t.

common peroneal n.

gastrocnemius m. (lat head)

tibial n.

infrapatellar (Hoffa's) fat pad

med. tibial plateau

post. cruciate lig. (insertion)

tibial collateral lig.

sartorius t.

gracilis t.

greater saphenous v.

semimembranosus t.

semitendinosus t.

oblique popliteal lig.

popliteal a. & v.   gastrocnemius m.
                        (med. head)

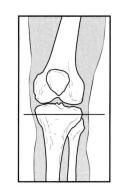

med. tibial plateau

post. cruciate lig. (insertion)

tibial collateral lig.

sartorius m.

gracilis t.

greater saphenous v.

semimembranosus t.

semitendinosus t.

oblique popliteal lig.

patellar lig.

infrapatellar (Hoffa's) fat pad

lat. tibial plateau

iliotibial tract &
vastus lateralis t.

conjoint t.

popliteus m.

common peroneal n.

gastrocnemius m.
(lat. head)

tibial n.

gastrocnemius m.
(med. head)

popliteal a. & v.

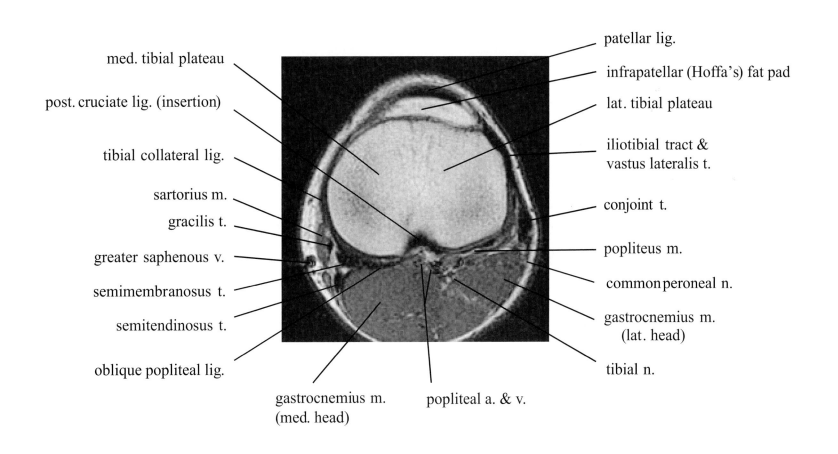

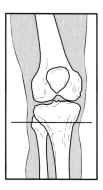

patellar lig.

tibia

sup. tibiofibular joint

conjoint t.

fibular head

soleus m.

ant. tibial a.

gastrocnemius m.
(lat. head)

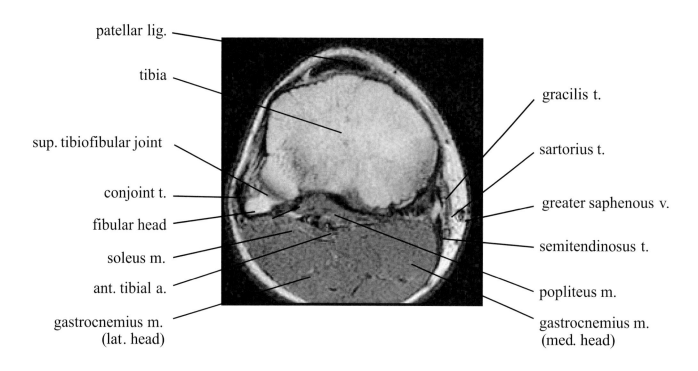

gracilis t.

sartorius t.

greater saphenous v.

semitendinosus t.

popliteus m.

gastrocnemius m.
(med. head)

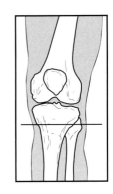

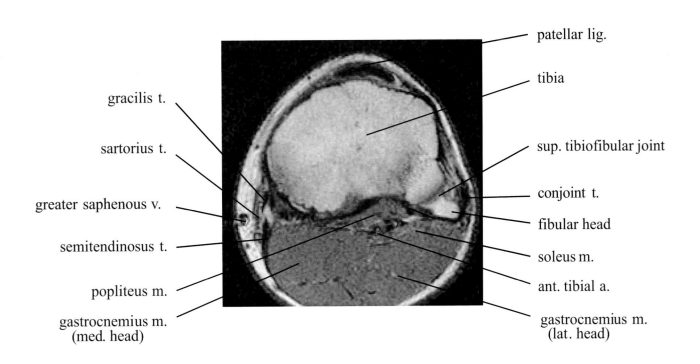

patellar lig.

tibia

sup. tibiofibular joint

conjoint t.

fibular head

soleus m.

ant. tibial a.

gastrocnemius m.
(lat. head)

gracilis t.

sartorius t.

greater saphenous v.

semitendinosus t.

popliteus m.

gastrocnemius m.
(med. head)

THE KNEE: SAGITTAL ANATOMY

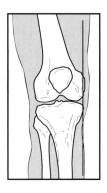

vastus medialis m. ——————

med. femoral condyle ——————

med. meniscus (ant. horn) ——————

med. tibial plateau ——————

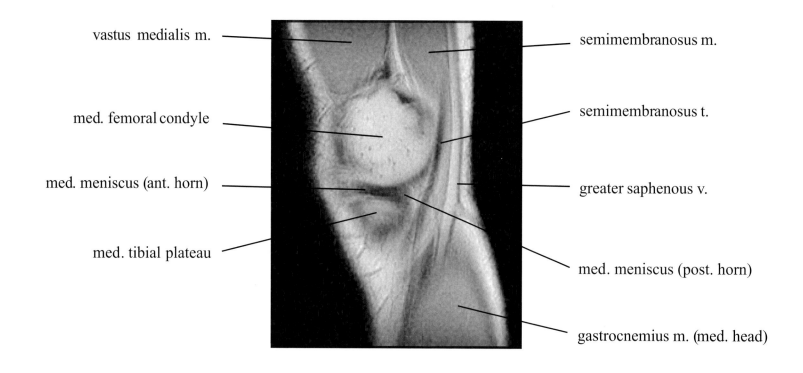

semimembranosus m.

semimembranosus t.

greater saphenous v.

med. meniscus (post. horn)

gastrocnemius m. (med. head)

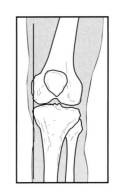

semimembranosus m. ⎯⎯⎯⎯⎯

semimembranosus t. ⎯⎯⎯⎯⎯

greater saphenous v. ⎯⎯⎯⎯⎯

med. meniscus (post. horn) ⎯⎯⎯⎯⎯

gastrocnemius m. (med. head) ⎯⎯⎯⎯⎯

vastus medialis m.

med. femoral condyle

med. meniscus (ant. horn)

med. tibial plateau

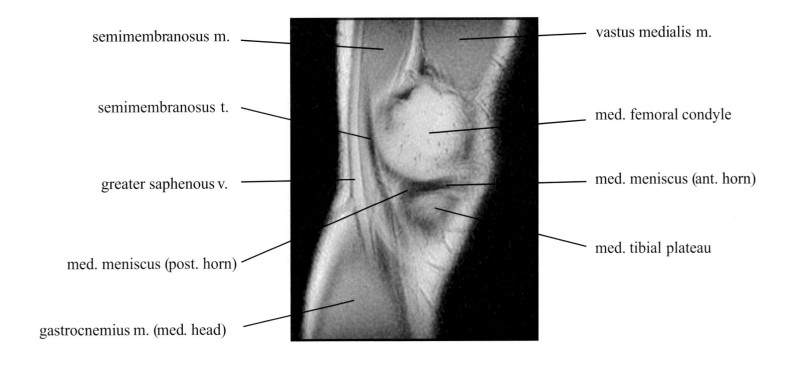

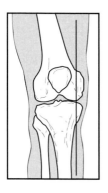

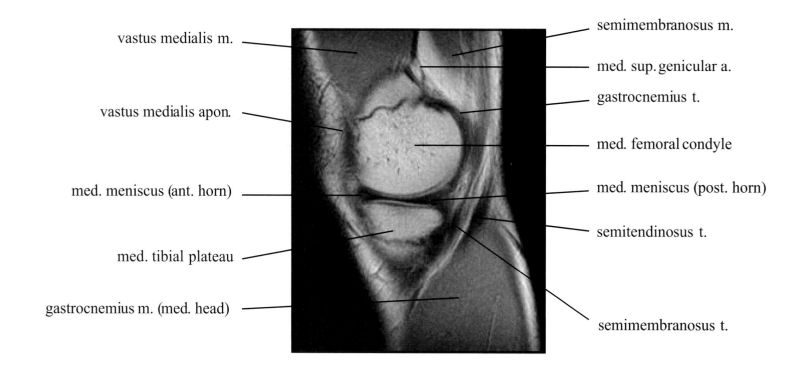

vastus medialis m.

vastus medialis apon.

med. meniscus (ant. horn)

med. tibial plateau

gastrocnemius m. (med. head)

semimembranosus m.

med. sup. genicular a.

gastrocnemius t.

med. femoral condyle

med. meniscus (post. horn)

semitendinosus t.

semimembranosus t.

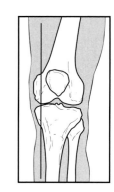

semimembranosus m.

med. sup. genicular a.

gastrocnemius t.

med. femoral condyle

med. meniscus (post. horn)

semitendinosus t.

semimembranosus t.

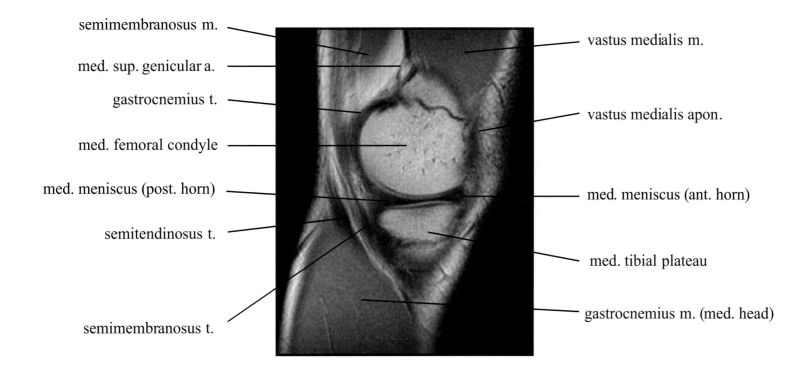

vastus medialis m.

vastus medialis apon.

med. meniscus (ant. horn)

med. tibial plateau

gastrocnemius m. (med. head)

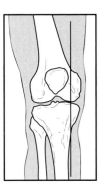

vastus medialis m.

vastus medialis apon.

med. femoral condyle

med. meniscus (ant. horn)

med. tibial plateau

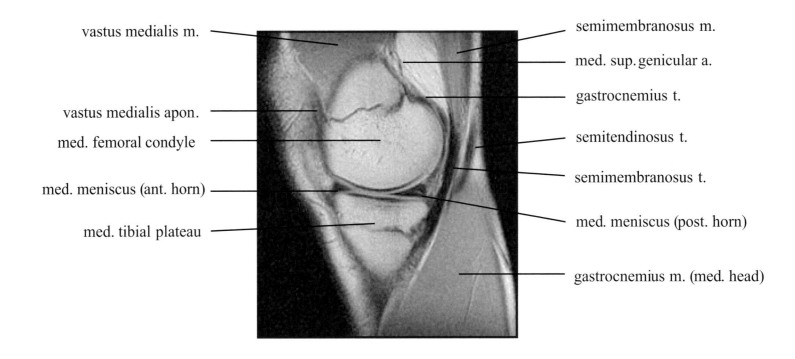

semimembranosus m.

med. sup. genicular a.

gastrocnemius t.

semitendinosus t.

semimembranosus t.

med. meniscus (post. horn)

gastrocnemius m. (med. head)

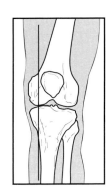

semimembranosus m. —

med. sup. genicular a. ———

gastrocnemius t. ———

semitendinosus t. ———

semimembranosus t. ———

med. meniscus (post. horn) ———

gastrocnemius m. (med. head) ———

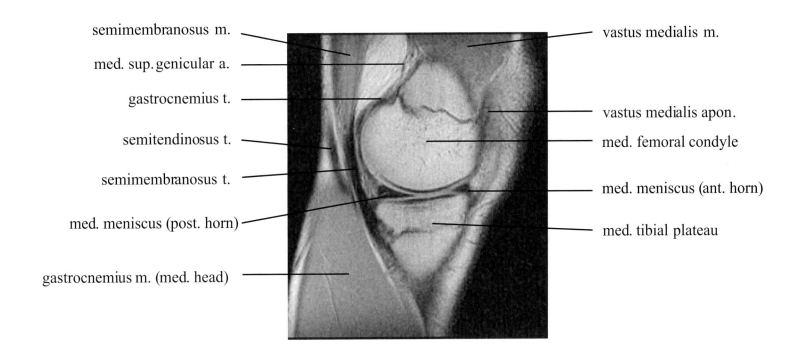

— vastus medialis m.

— vastus medialis apon.

— med. femoral condyle

— med. meniscus (ant. horn)

— med. tibial plateau

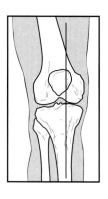

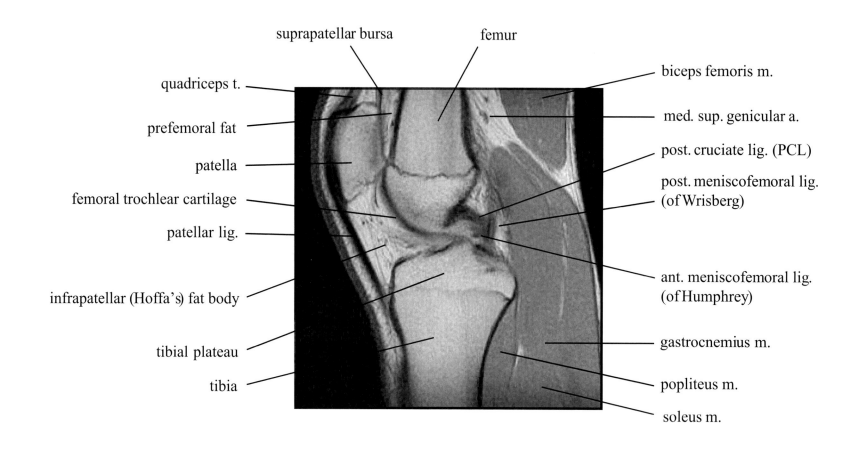

suprapatellar bursa

femur

quadriceps t.

prefemoral fat

patella

femoral trochlear cartilage

patellar lig.

infrapatellar (Hoffa's) fat body

tibial plateau

tibia

biceps femoris m.

med. sup. genicular a.

post. cruciate lig. (PCL)

post. meniscofemoral lig. (of Wrisberg)

ant. meniscofemoral lig. (of Humphrey)

gastrocnemius m.

popliteus m.

soleus m.

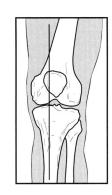

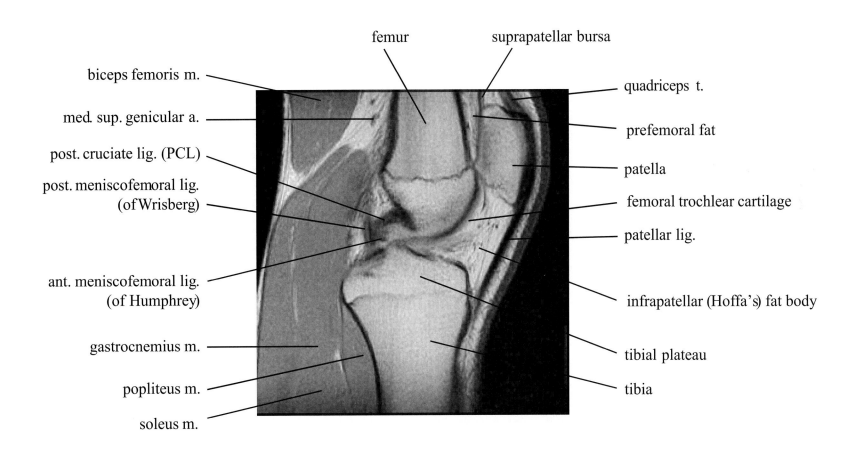

femur

suprapatellar bursa

biceps femoris m.

med. sup. genicular a.

post. cruciate lig. (PCL)

post. meniscofemoral lig.
(of Wrisberg)

ant. meniscofemoral lig.
(of Humphrey)

gastrocnemius m.

popliteus m.

soleus m.

quadriceps t.

prefemoral fat

patella

femoral trochlear cartilage

patellar lig.

infrapatellar (Hoffa's) fat body

tibial plateau

tibia

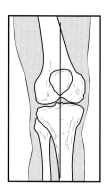

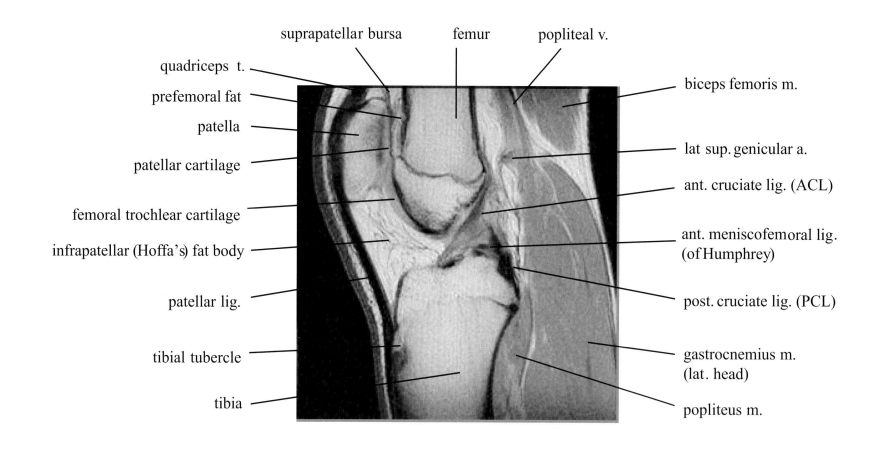

suprapatellar bursa

femur

popliteal v.

quadriceps t.

prefemoral fat

patella

patellar cartilage

femoral trochlear cartilage

infrapatellar (Hoffa's) fat body

patellar lig.

tibial tubercle

tibia

biceps femoris m.

lat sup. genicular a.

ant. cruciate lig. (ACL)

ant. meniscofemoral lig.
(of Humphrey)

post. cruciate lig. (PCL)

gastrocnemius m.
(lat. head)

popliteus m.

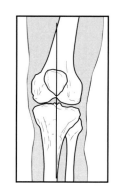

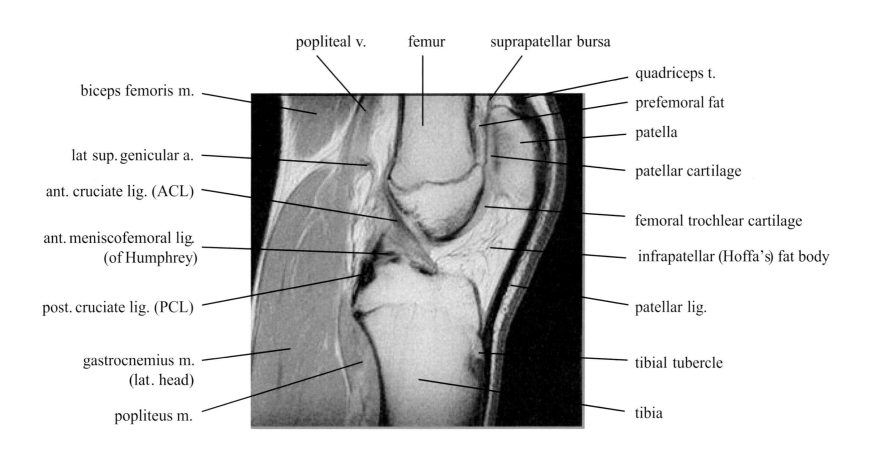

popliteal v.   femur   suprapatellar bursa

biceps femoris m.

lat sup. genicular a.

ant. cruciate lig. (ACL)

ant. meniscofemoral lig.
(of Humphrey)

post. cruciate lig. (PCL)

gastrocnemius m.
(lat. head)

popliteus m.

quadriceps t.

prefemoral fat

patella

patellar cartilage

femoral trochlear cartilage

infrapatellar (Hoffa's) fat body

patellar lig.

tibial tubercle

tibia

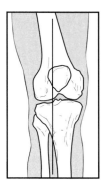

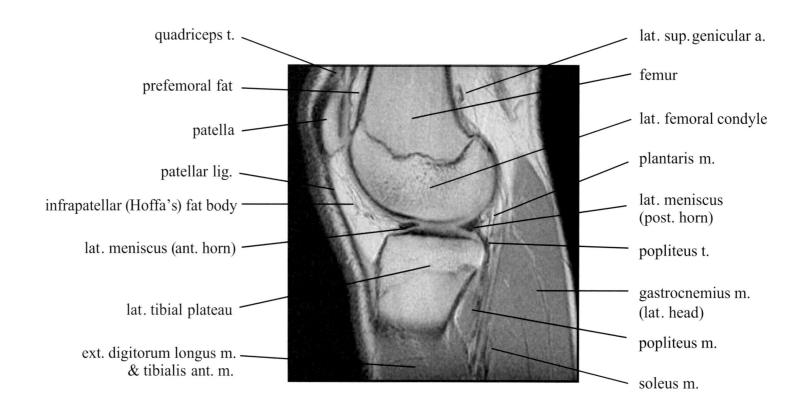

quadriceps t.

prefemoral fat

patella

patellar lig.

infrapatellar (Hoffa's) fat body

lat. meniscus (ant. horn)

lat. tibial plateau

ext. digitorum longus m.
& tibialis ant. m.

lat. sup. genicular a.

femur

lat. femoral condyle

plantaris m.

lat. meniscus
(post. horn)

popliteus t.

gastrocnemius m.
(lat. head)

popliteus m.

soleus m.

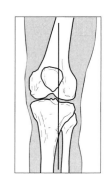

lat. sup. genicular a.

femur

lat. femoral condyle

plantaris m.

lat. meniscus
(post. horn)

popliteus t.

gastrocnemius m.
(lat. head)

popliteus m.

soleus m.

quadriceps t.

prefemoral fat

patella

patellar lig.

infrapatellar (Hoffa's) fat body

lat. meniscus (ant. horn)

lat. tibial plateau

ext. digitorum longus m.
& tibialis ant. m.

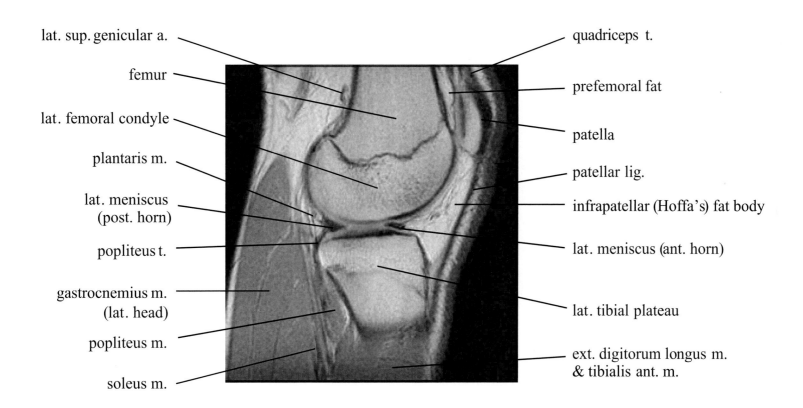

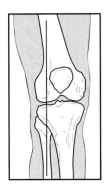

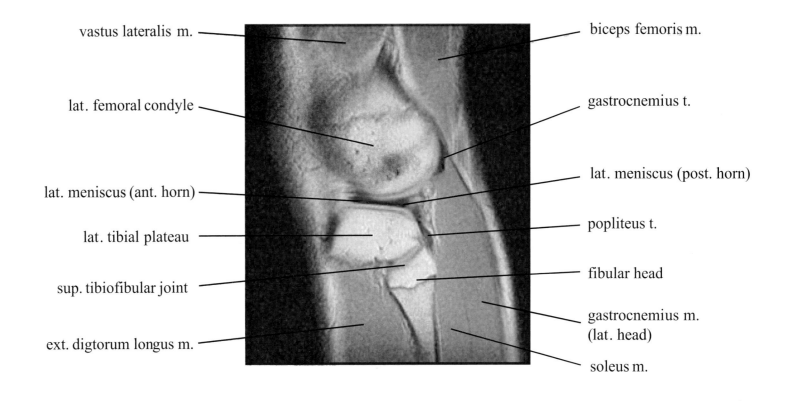

vastus lateralis m.

biceps femoris m.

lat. femoral condyle

gastrocnemius t.

lat. meniscus (post. horn)

lat. meniscus (ant. horn)

popliteus t.

lat. tibial plateau

fibular head

sup. tibiofibular joint

gastrocnemius m.
(lat. head)

ext. digtorum longus m.

soleus m.

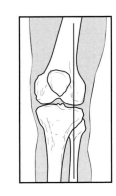

biceps femoris m.

vastus lateralis m.

gastrocnemius t.

lat. femoral condyle

lat. meniscus (post. horn)

lat. meniscus (ant. horn)

popliteus t.

lat. tibial plateau

fibular head

sup. tibiofibular joint

gastrocnemius m.
(lat. head)

ext. digtorum longus m.

soleus m.

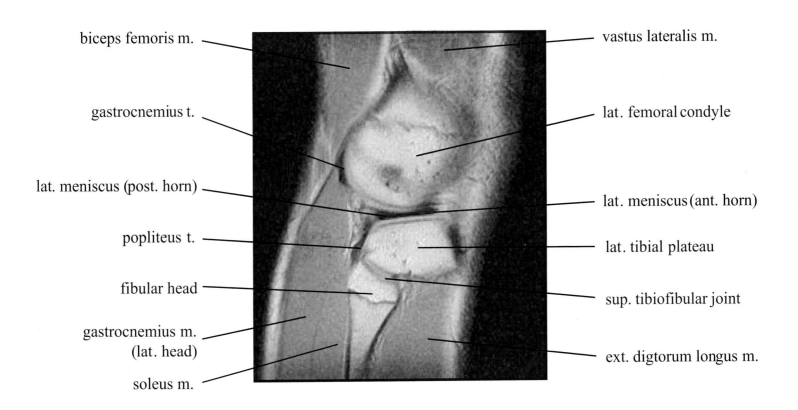

THE KNEE: CORONAL ANATOMY

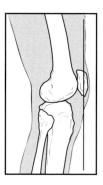

patella

lat patellar retinaculum

patellar lig.

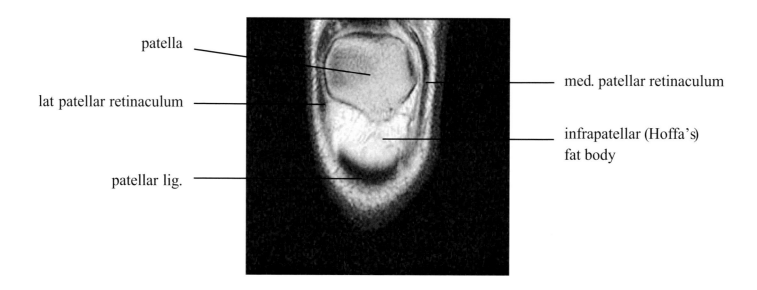

med. patellar retinaculum

infrapatellar (Hoffa's)
fat body

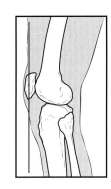

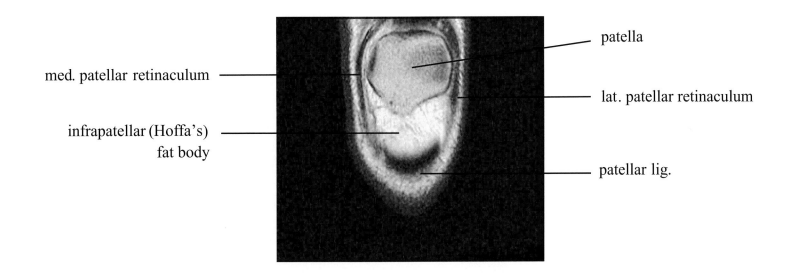

med. patellar retinaculum ——————

infrapatellar (Hoffa's)
fat body ——————

—————— patella

—————— lat. patellar retinaculum

—————— patellar lig.

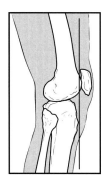

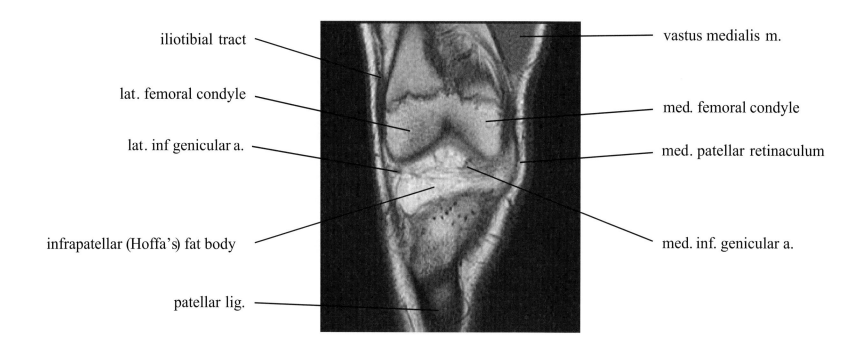

iliotibial tract

lat. femoral condyle

lat. inf genicular a.

infrapatellar (Hoffa's) fat body

patellar lig.

vastus medialis m.

med. femoral condyle

med. patellar retinaculum

med. inf. genicular a.

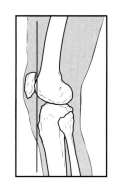

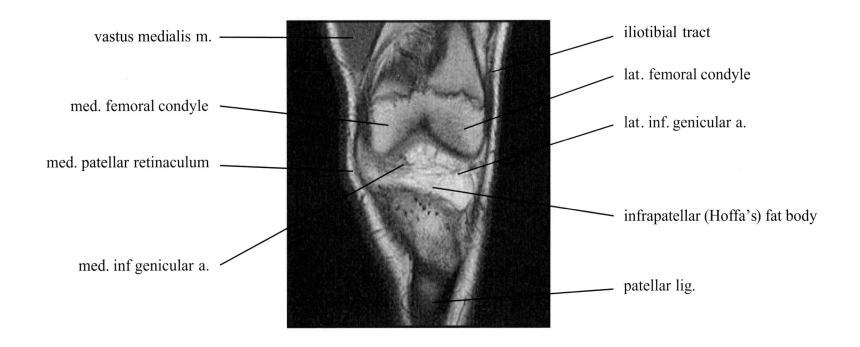

vastus medialis m.

iliotibial tract

med. femoral condyle

lat. femoral condyle

med. patellar retinaculum

lat. inf. genicular a.

med. inf genicular a.

infrapatellar (Hoffa's) fat body

patellar lig.

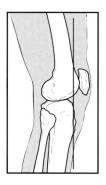

vastus lateralis m.

femur

lat. femoral condyle

infrapatellar (Hoffa's) fat body

iliotibial tract

transverse meniscal lig.

Gerdy's tubercle

lat. tibial plateau

peroneus longus m.

ext. digitorum longus m.

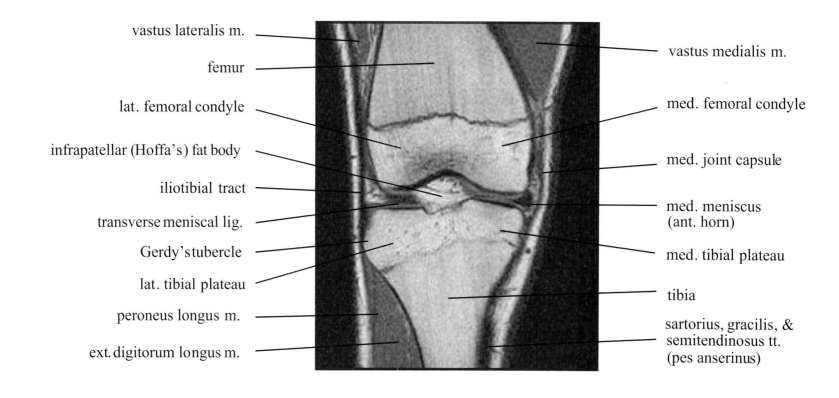

vastus medialis m.

med. femoral condyle

med. joint capsule

med. meniscus
(ant. horn)

med. tibial plateau

tibia

sartorius, gracilis, &
semitendinosus tt.
(pes anserinus)

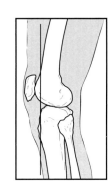

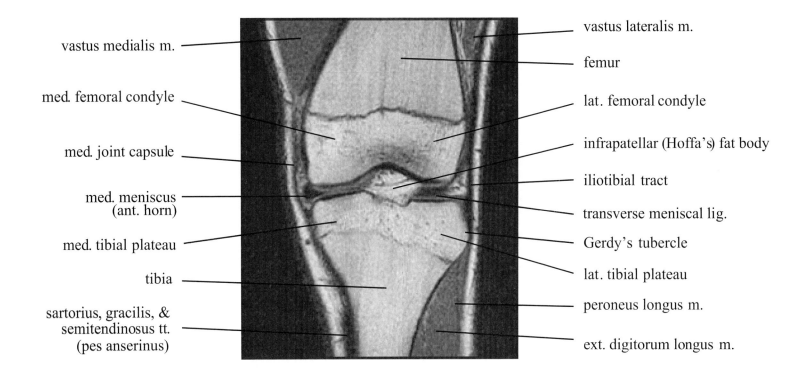

vastus medialis m.

med. femoral condyle

med. joint capsule

med. meniscus
(ant. horn)

med. tibial plateau

tibia

sartorius, gracilis, &
semitendinosus tt.
(pes anserinus)

vastus lateralis m.

femur

lat. femoral condyle

infrapatellar (Hoffa's) fat body

iliotibial tract

transverse meniscal lig.

Gerdy's tubercle

lat. tibial plateau

peroneus longus m.

ext. digitorum longus m.

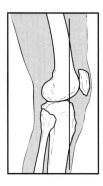

vastus lateralis m. —

lat. sup. genicular a. —

iliotibial tract —

lat. femoral condyle —

infrapatellar (Hoffa's) fat body —

lat. meniscus (ant. horn) —

transverse meniscal lig. —

peroneus longus m. —

ext. digitorum longus m. —

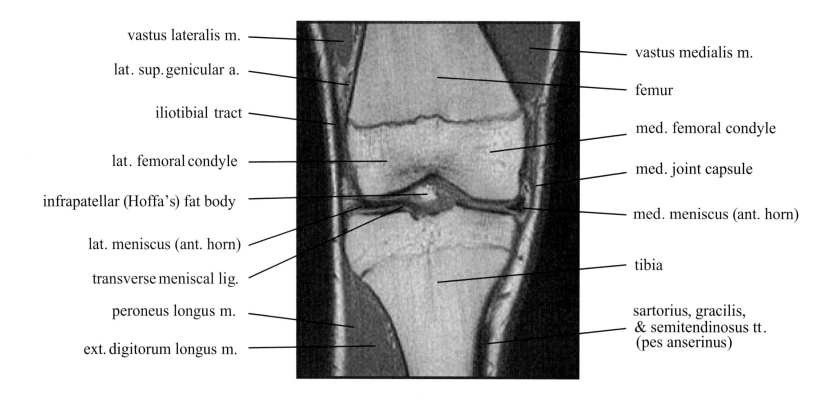

— vastus medialis m.

— femur

— med. femoral condyle

— med. joint capsule

— med. meniscus (ant. horn)

— tibia

— sartorius, gracilis,
& semitendinosus tt.
(pes anserinus)

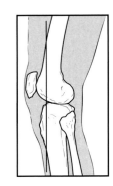

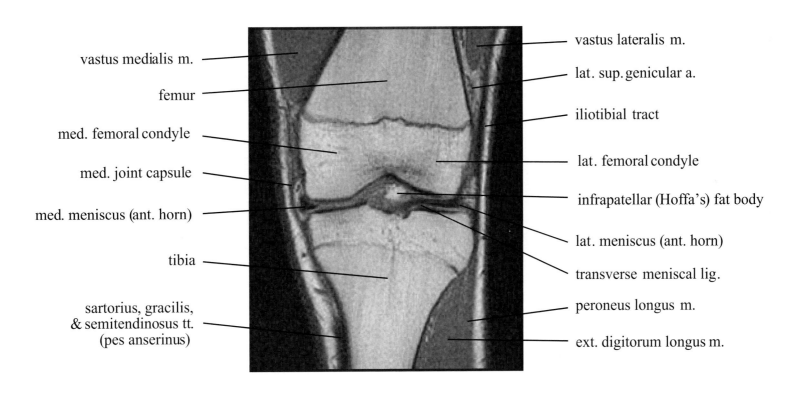

vastus medialis m.

femur

med. femoral condyle

med. joint capsule

med. meniscus (ant. horn)

tibia

sartorius, gracilis,
& semitendinosus tt.
(pes anserinus)

vastus lateralis m.

lat. sup. genicular a.

iliotibial tract

lat. femoral condyle

infrapatellar (Hoffa's) fat body

lat. meniscus (ant. horn)

transverse meniscal lig.

peroneus longus m.

ext. digitorum longus m.

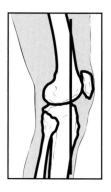

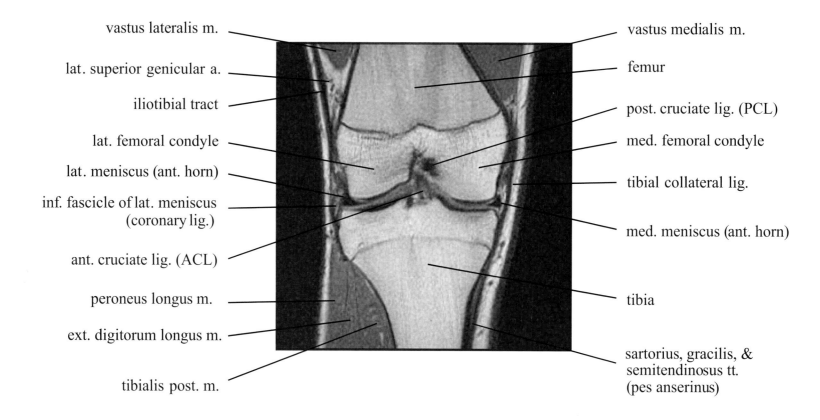

vastus lateralis m.

lat. superior genicular a.

iliotibial tract

lat. femoral condyle

lat. meniscus (ant. horn)

inf. fascicle of lat. meniscus
(coronary lig.)

ant. cruciate lig. (ACL)

peroneus longus m.

ext. digitorum longus m.

tibialis post. m.

vastus medialis m.

femur

post. cruciate lig. (PCL)

med. femoral condyle

tibial collateral lig.

med. meniscus (ant. horn)

tibia

sartorius, gracilis, &
semitendinosus tt.
(pes anserinus)

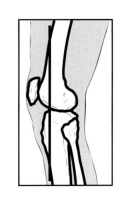

vastus medialis m.

femur

post. cruciate lig. (PCL)

med. femoral condyle

tibial collateral lig.

med. meniscus (ant. horn)

tibia

sartorius, gracilis, &
semitendinosus tt.
(pes anserinus)

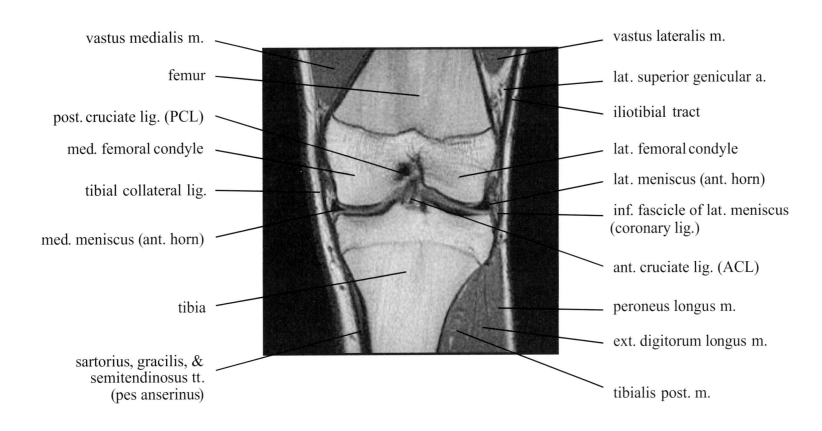

vastus lateralis m.

lat. superior genicular a.

iliotibial tract

lat. femoral condyle

lat. meniscus (ant. horn)

inf. fascicle of lat. meniscus
(coronary lig.)

ant. cruciate lig. (ACL)

peroneus longus m.

ext. digitorum longus m.

tibialis post. m.

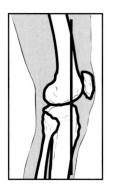

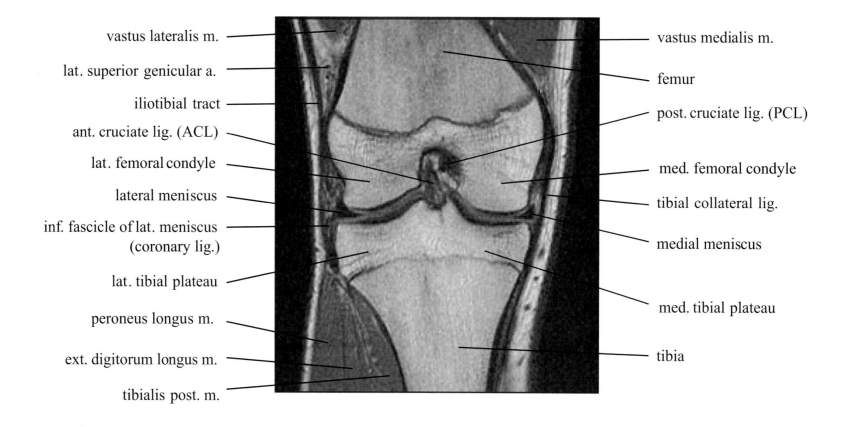

vastus lateralis m.

lat. superior genicular a.

iliotibial tract

ant. cruciate lig. (ACL)

lat. femoral condyle

lateral meniscus

inf. fascicle of lat. meniscus
(coronary lig.)

lat. tibial plateau

peroneus longus m.

ext. digitorum longus m.

tibialis post. m.

vastus medialis m.

femur

post. cruciate lig. (PCL)

med. femoral condyle

tibial collateral lig.

medial meniscus

med. tibial plateau

tibia

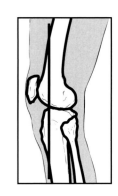

vastus medialis m. —————

femur ——

post. cruciate lig. (PCL) ——

med. femoral condyle ——

tibial collateral lig. ——

medial meniscus ——

med. tibial plateau ——

tibia ——

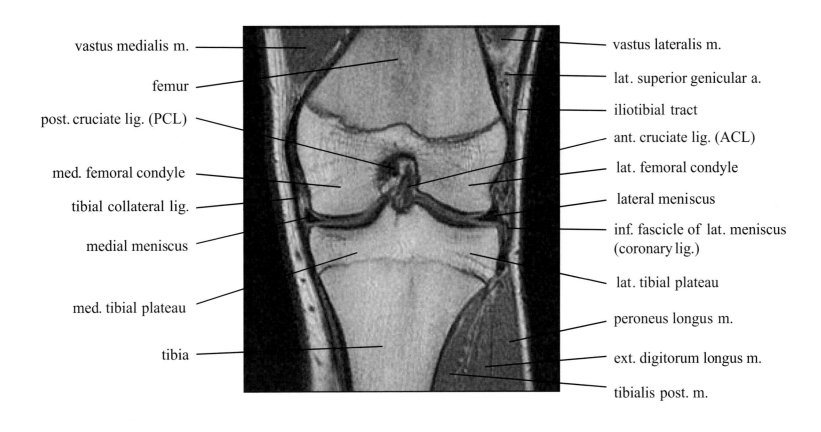

————— vastus lateralis m.

—— lat. superior genicular a.

—— iliotibial tract

—— ant. cruciate lig. (ACL)

—— lat. femoral condyle

—— lateral meniscus

—— inf. fascicle of lat. meniscus
    (coronary lig.)

—— lat. tibial plateau

—— peroneus longus m.

—— ext. digitorum longus m.

—— tibialis post. m.

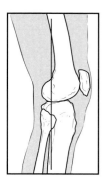

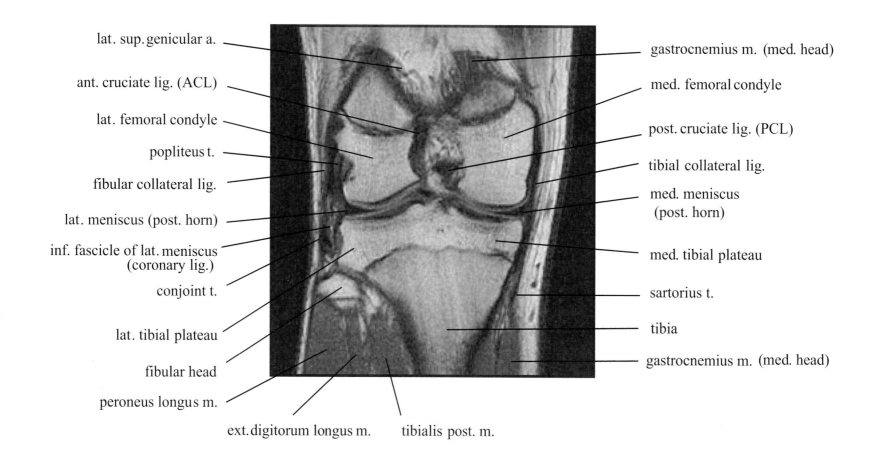

lat. sup. genicular a.

ant. cruciate lig. (ACL)

lat. femoral condyle

popliteus t.

fibular collateral lig.

lat. meniscus (post. horn)

inf. fascicle of lat. meniscus
(coronary lig.)

conjoint t.

lat. tibial plateau

fibular head

peroneus longus m.

ext. digitorum longus m.

tibialis post. m.

gastrocnemius m. (med. head)

med. femoral condyle

post. cruciate lig. (PCL)

tibial collateral lig.

med. meniscus
(post. horn)

med. tibial plateau

sartorius t.

tibia

gastrocnemius m. (med. head)

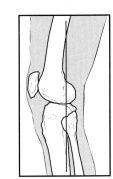

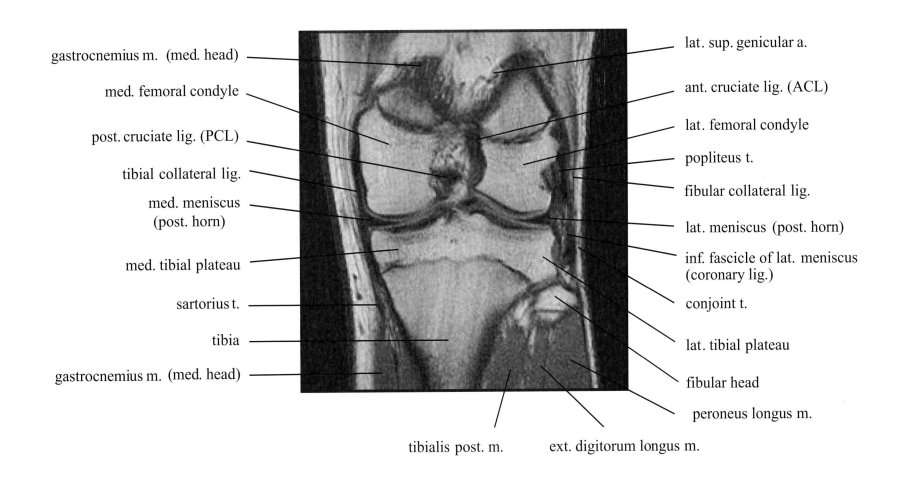

gastrocnemius m. (med. head)

med. femoral condyle

post. cruciate lig. (PCL)

tibial collateral lig.

med. meniscus
(post. horn)

med. tibial plateau

sartorius t.

tibia

gastrocnemius m. (med. head)

lat. sup. genicular a.

ant. cruciate lig. (ACL)

lat. femoral condyle

popliteus t.

fibular collateral lig.

lat. meniscus (post. horn)

inf. fascicle of lat. meniscus
(coronary lig.)

conjoint t.

lat. tibial plateau

fibular head

peroneus longus m.

tibialis post. m.   ext. digitorum longus m.

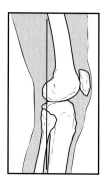

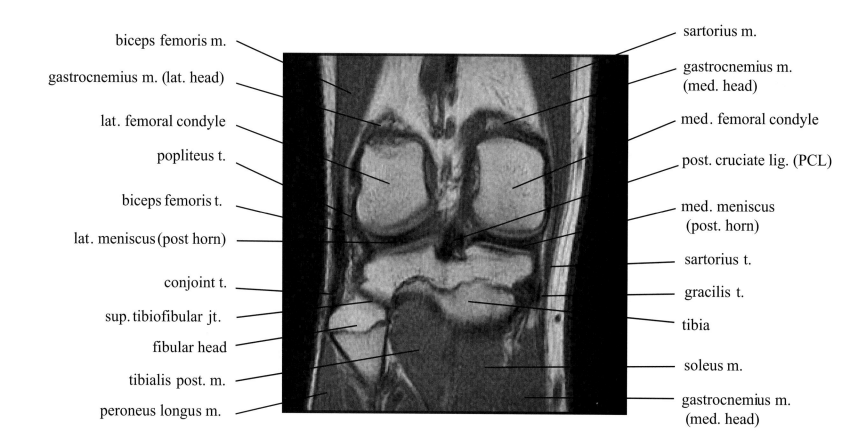

biceps femoris m.

gastrocnemius m. (lat. head)

lat. femoral condyle

popliteus t.

biceps femoris t.

lat. meniscus (post horn)

conjoint t.

sup. tibiofibular jt.

fibular head

tibialis post. m.

peroneus longus m.

sartorius m.

gastrocnemius m. (med. head)

med. femoral condyle

post. cruciate lig. (PCL)

med. meniscus (post. horn)

sartorius t.

gracilis t.

tibia

soleus m.

gastrocnemius m. (med. head)

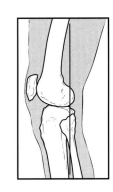

sartorius m.

gastrocnemius m.
(med. head)

med. femoral condyle

post. cruciate lig. (PCL)

med. meniscus
(post. horn)

sartorius t.

gracilis t.

tibia

soleus m.

gastrocnemius m.
(med. head)

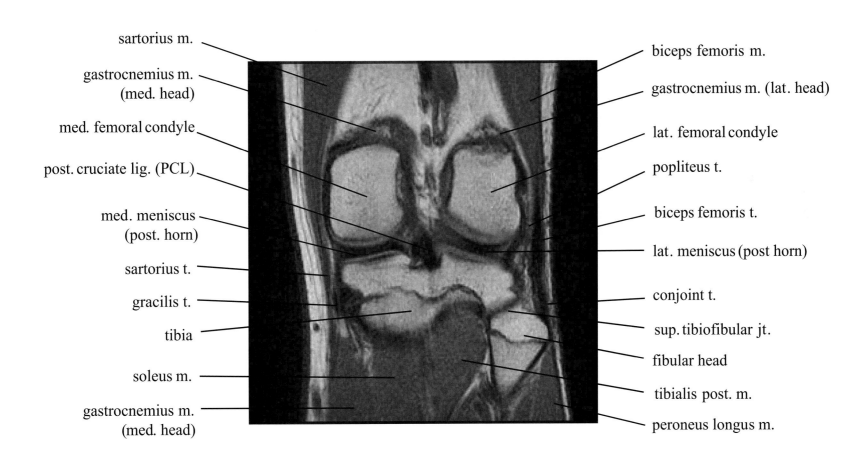

biceps femoris m.

gastrocnemius m. (lat. head)

lat. femoral condyle

popliteus t.

biceps femoris t.

lat. meniscus (post horn)

conjoint t.

sup. tibiofibular jt.

fibular head

tibialis post. m.

peroneus longus m.

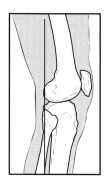

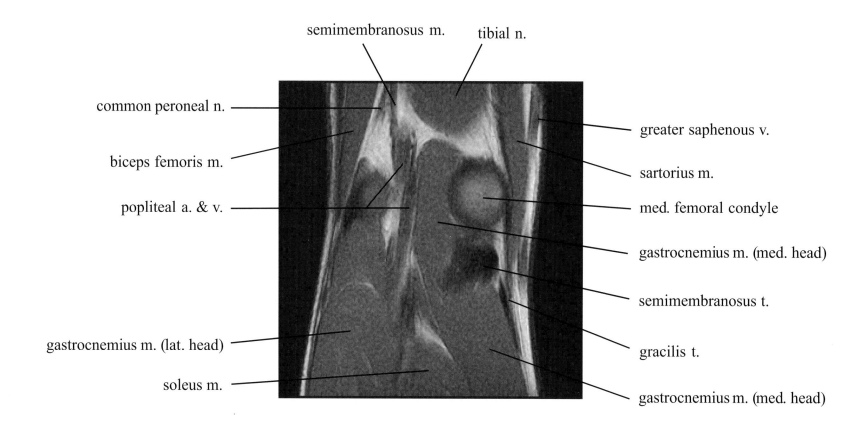

semimembranosus m.

tibial n.

common peroneal n.

biceps femoris m.

popliteal a. & v.

gastrocnemius m. (lat. head)

soleus m.

greater saphenous v.

sartorius m.

med. femoral condyle

gastrocnemius m. (med. head)

semimembranosus t.

gracilis t.

gastrocnemius m. (med. head)

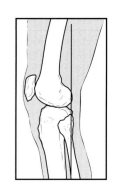

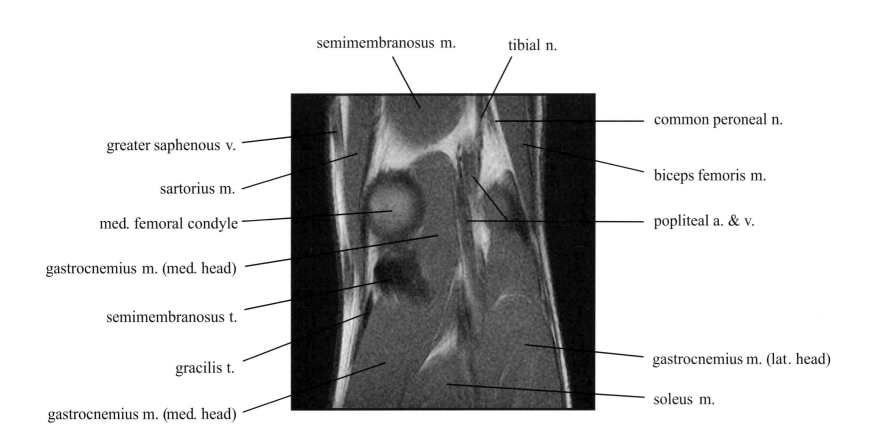

semimembranosus m.

tibial n.

common peroneal n.

greater saphenous v.

biceps femoris m.

sartorius m.

med. femoral condyle

popliteal a. & v.

gastrocnemius m. (med. head)

semimembranosus t.

gracilis t.

gastrocnemius m. (lat. head)

soleus m.

gastrocnemius m. (med. head)

THE LOWER EXTREMITY: AXIAL ANATOMY

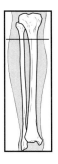

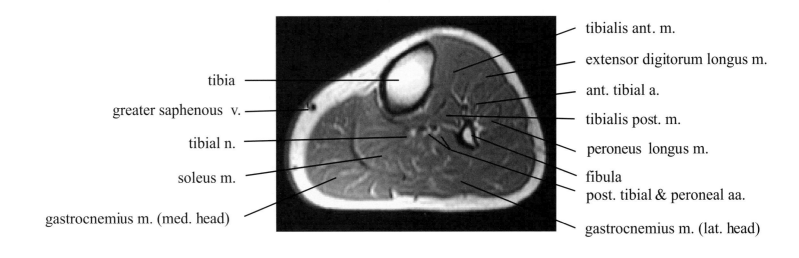

tibialis ant. m.

extensor digitorum longus m.

tibia

ant. tibial a.

greater saphenous v.

tibialis post. m.

tibial n.

peroneus longus m.

soleus m.

fibula

post. tibial & peroneal aa.

gastrocnemius m. (med. head)

gastrocnemius m. (lat. head)

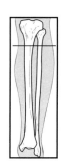

tibialis ant. m.

extensor digitorum longus m.

ant. tibial a.

tibialis post. m.

peroneus longus m.

fibula

post. tibial & peroneal aa.

gastrocnemius m. (lat. head)

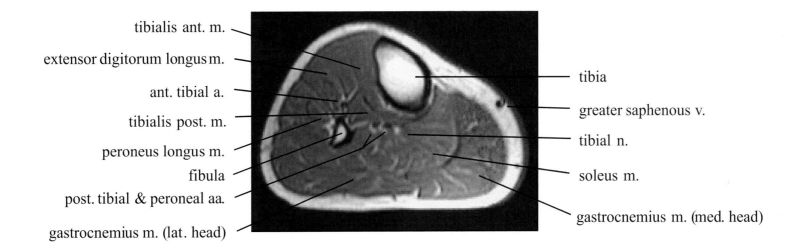

tibia

greater saphenous v.

tibial n.

soleus m.

gastrocnemius m. (med. head)

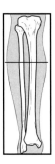

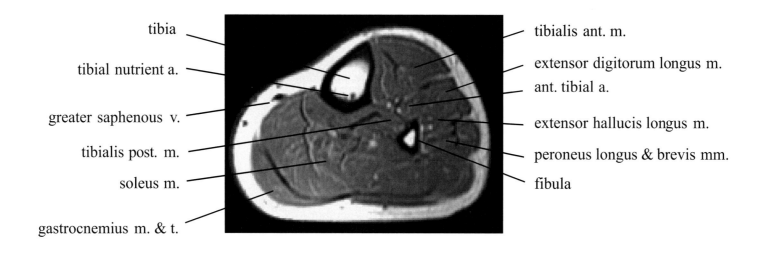

tibia

tibial nutrient a.

greater saphenous v.

tibialis post. m.

soleus m.

gastrocnemius m. & t.

tibialis ant. m.

extensor digitorum longus m.

ant. tibial a.

extensor hallucis longus m.

peroneus longus & brevis mm.

fibula

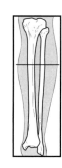

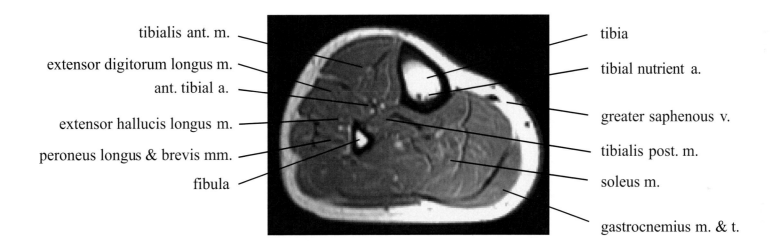

tibialis ant. m.

extensor digitorum longus m.

ant. tibial a.

extensor hallucis longus m.

peroneus longus & brevis mm.

fibula

tibia

tibial nutrient a.

greater saphenous v.

tibialis post. m.

soleus m.

gastrocnemius m. & t.

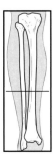

tibia

greater saphenous v.

flexor digitorum longus m.

tibialis post. m.

soleus m.

gastrocnemius t.

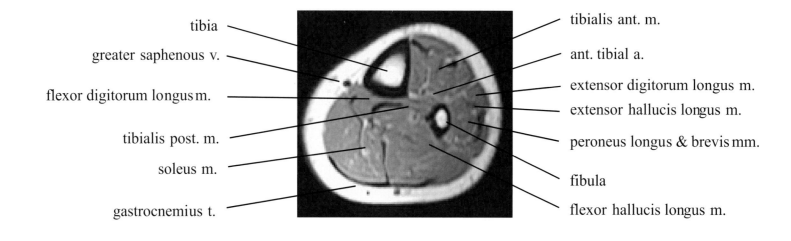

tibialis ant. m.

ant. tibial a.

extensor digitorum longus m.

extensor hallucis longus m.

peroneus longus & brevis mm.

fibula

flexor hallucis longus m.

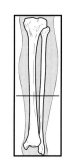

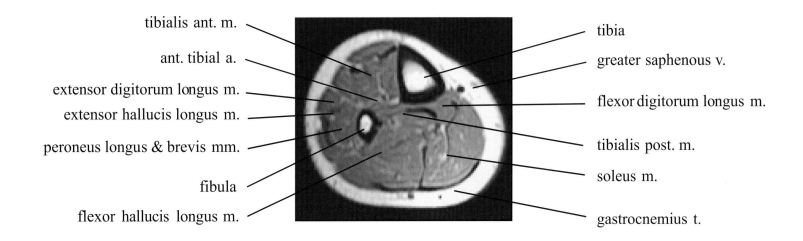

tibialis ant. m.

ant. tibial a.

extensor digitorum longus m.

extensor hallucis longus m.

peroneus longus & brevis mm.

fibula

flexor hallucis longus m.

tibia

greater saphenous v.

flexor digitorum longus m.

tibialis post. m.

soleus m.

gastrocnemius t.

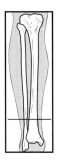

tibia

greater saphenous v.

flexor digitorum longus m. & t.

tibialis post. m.

soleus m.

gastrocnemius t.

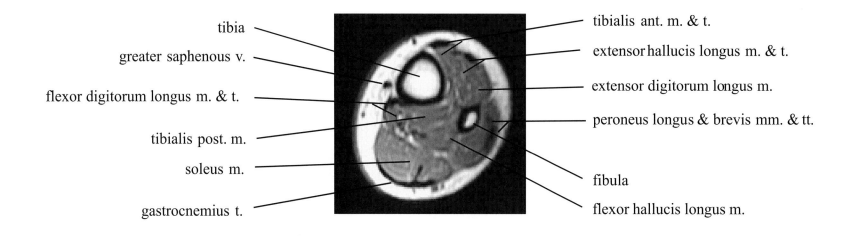

tibialis ant. m. & t.

extensor hallucis longus m. & t.

extensor digitorum longus m.

peroneus longus & brevis mm. & tt.

fibula

flexor hallucis longus m.

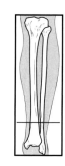

tibialis ant. m. & t.

extensor hallucis longus m. & t.

extensor digitorum longus m.

peroneus longus & brevis mm. & tt.

fibula

flexor hallucis longus m.

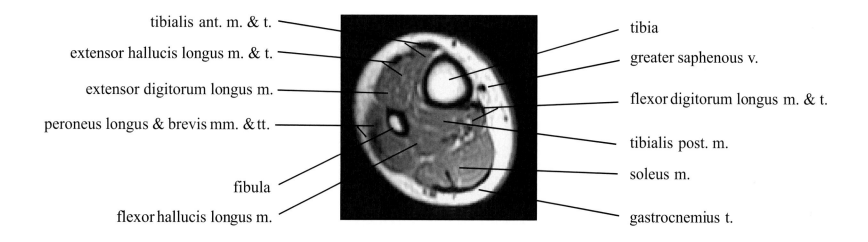

tibia

greater saphenous v.

flexor digitorum longus m. & t.

tibialis post. m.

soleus m.

gastrocnemius t.

THE LOWER EXTREMITY: SAGITTAL ANATOMY

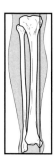

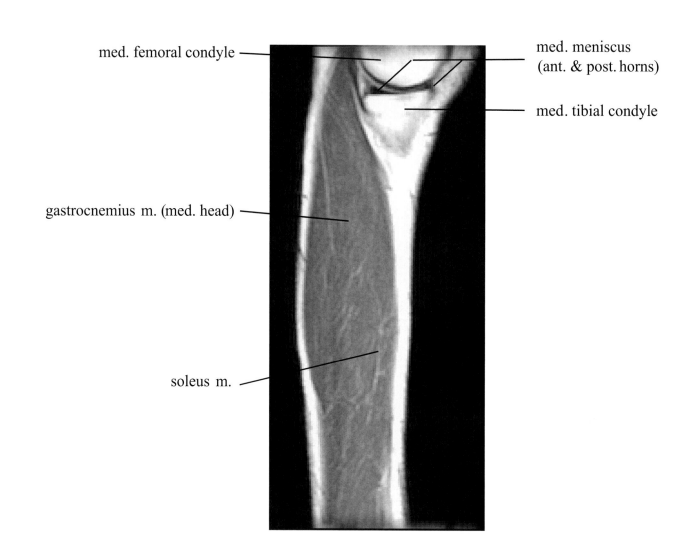

med. femoral condyle ——

med. meniscus
(ant. & post. horns)

med. tibial condyle

gastrocnemius m. (med. head) ——

soleus m. ——

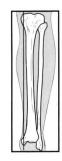

med. meniscus
(ant. & post. horns)

med. tibial condyle

med. femoral condyle

gastrocnemius m. (med. head)

soleus m.

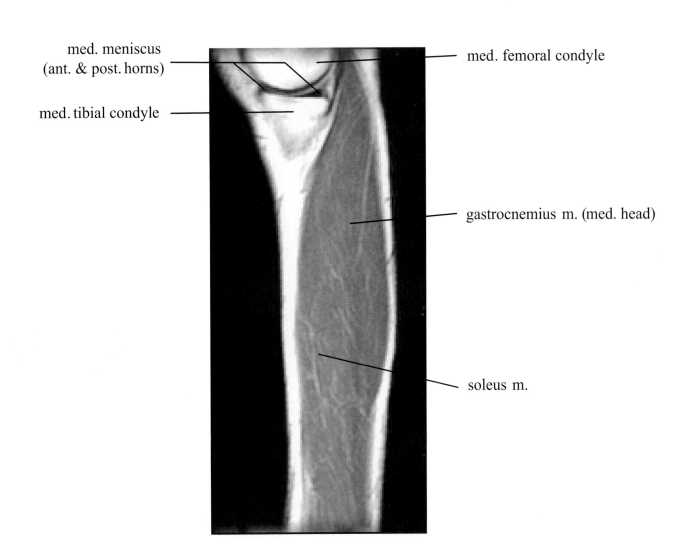

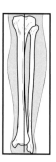

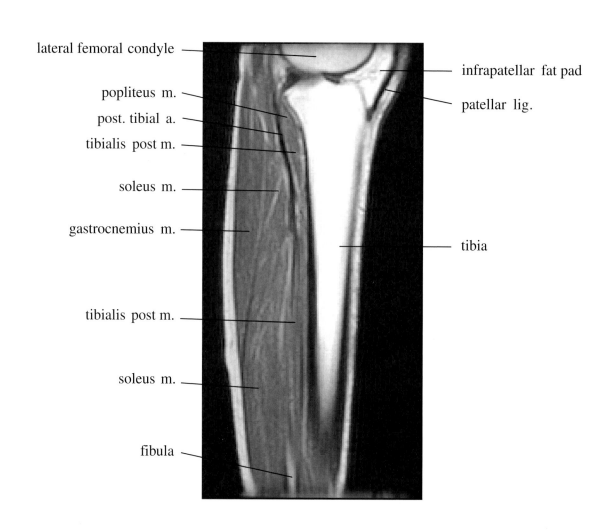

lateral femoral condyle

popliteus m.

post. tibial a.

tibialis post m.

soleus m.

gastrocnemius m.

tibialis post m.

soleus m.

fibula

infrapatellar fat pad

patellar lig.

tibia

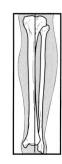

infrapatellar fat pad

patellar lig.

tibia

lateral femoral condyle

popliteus m.

post. tibial a.

tibialis post m.

soleus m.

gastrocnemius m.

tibialis post m.

soleus m.

fibula

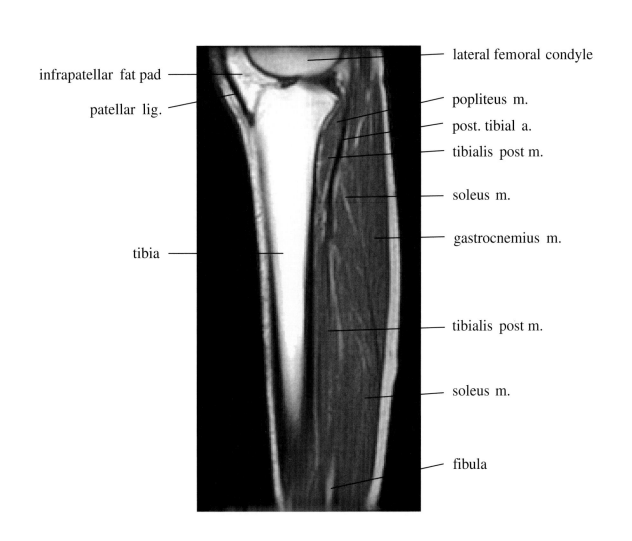

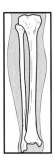

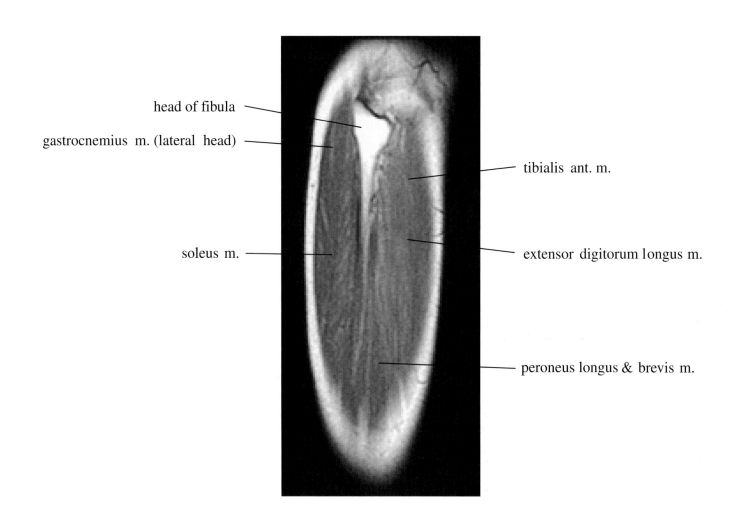

head of fibula

gastrocnemius m. (lateral head)

tibialis ant. m.

soleus m.

extensor digitorum longus m.

peroneus longus & brevis m.

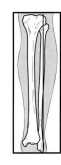

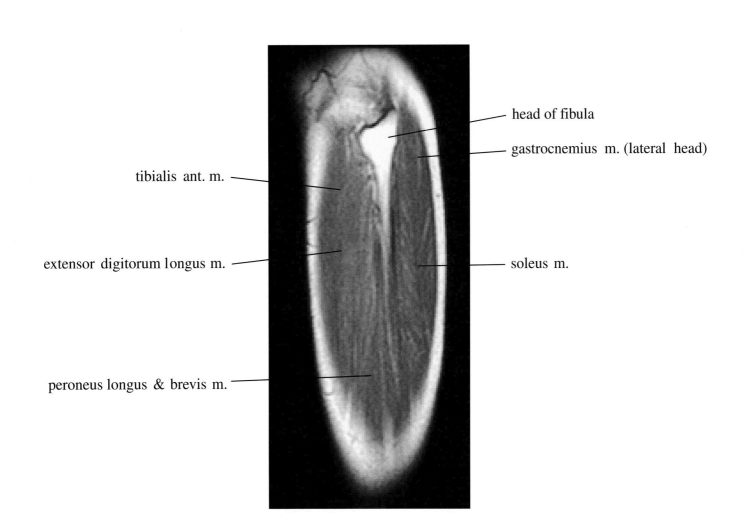

head of fibula

gastrocnemius m. (lateral head)

tibialis ant. m.

extensor digitorum longus m.

soleus m.

peroneus longus & brevis m.

THE LOWER EXTREMITY: CORONAL ANATOMY

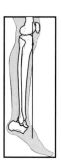

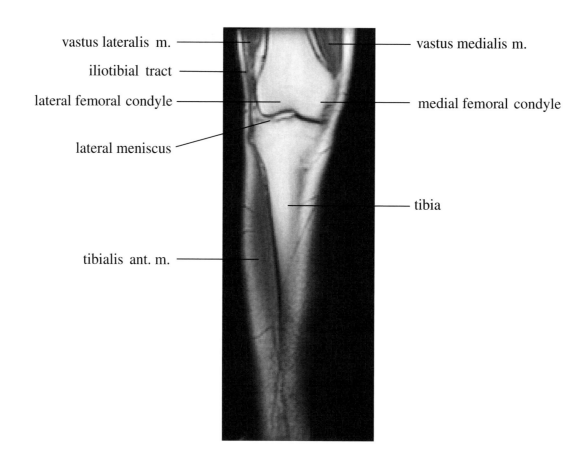

vastus lateralis m.

iliotibial tract

lateral femoral condyle

lateral meniscus

tibialis ant. m.

vastus medialis m.

medial femoral condyle

tibia

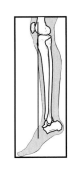

vastus medialis m. —————

————— vastus lateralis m.

————— iliotibial tract

medial femoral condyle —————

————— lateral femoral condyle

————— lateral meniscus

tibia —————

————— tibialis ant. m.

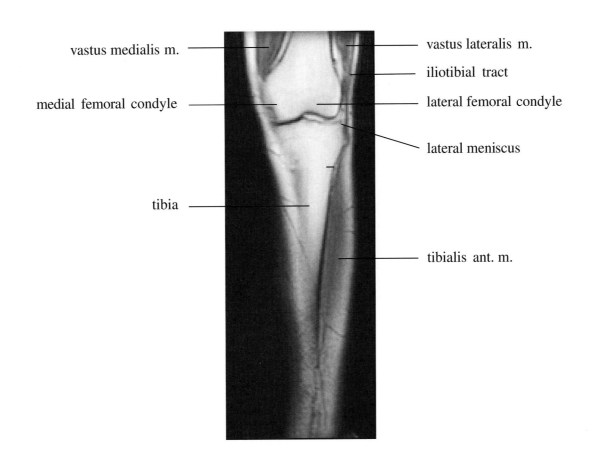

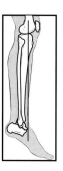

lateral femoral condyle ———————   ——————— medial femoral condyle

tibia

tibialis ant. m. ———————

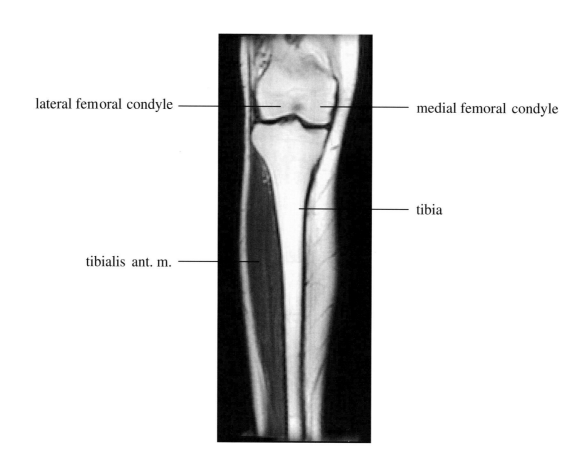

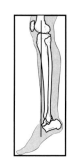

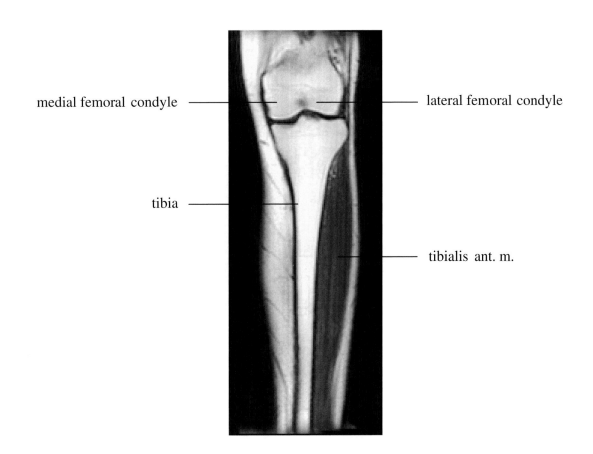

medial femoral condyle ——————————   ———————— lateral femoral condyle

tibia ——————————   ———————— tibialis ant. m.

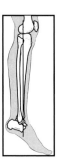

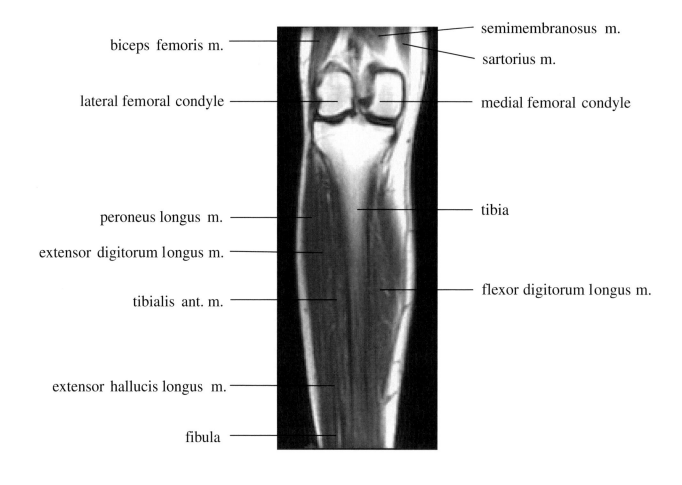

biceps femoris m.

semimembranosus m.

sartorius m.

lateral femoral condyle

medial femoral condyle

peroneus longus m.

tibia

extensor digitorum longus m.

tibialis ant. m.

flexor digitorum longus m.

extensor hallucis longus m.

fibula

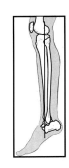

semimembranosus m.

sartorius m.

medial femoral condyle

tibia

flexor digitorum longus m.

biceps femoris m.

lateral femoral condyle

peroneus longus m.

extensor digitorum longus m.

tibialis ant. m.

extensor hallucis longus m.

fibula

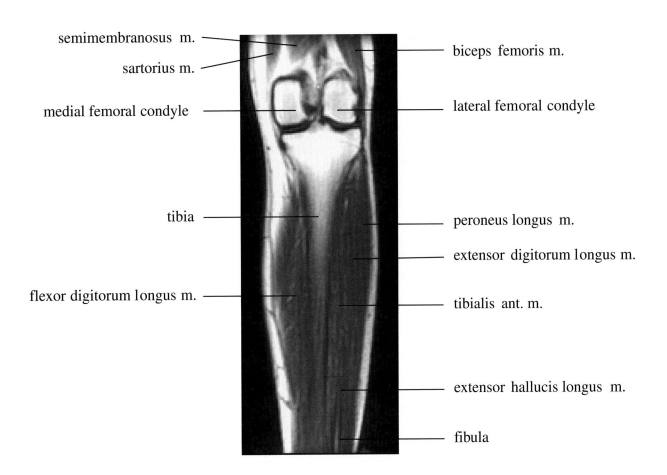

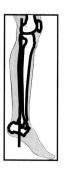

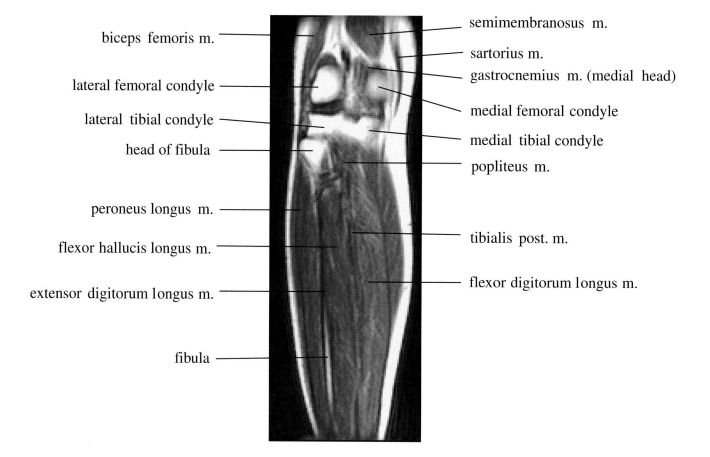

biceps femoris m.

lateral femoral condyle

lateral tibial condyle

head of fibula

peroneus longus m.

flexor hallucis longus m.

extensor digitorum longus m.

fibula

semimembranosus m.

sartorius m.

gastrocnemius m. (medial head)

medial femoral condyle

medial tibial condyle

popliteus m.

tibialis post. m.

flexor digitorum longus m.

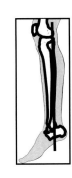

semimembranosus m.

sartorius m.

gastrocnemius m. (medial head)

medial femoral condyle

medial tibial condyle

popliteus m.

tibialis post. m.

flexor digitorum longus m.

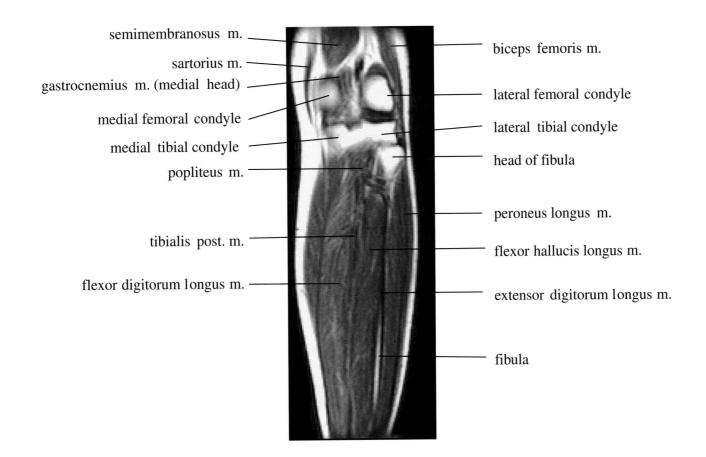

biceps femoris m.

lateral femoral condyle

lateral tibial condyle

head of fibula

peroneus longus m.

flexor hallucis longus m.

extensor digitorum longus m.

fibula

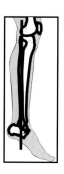

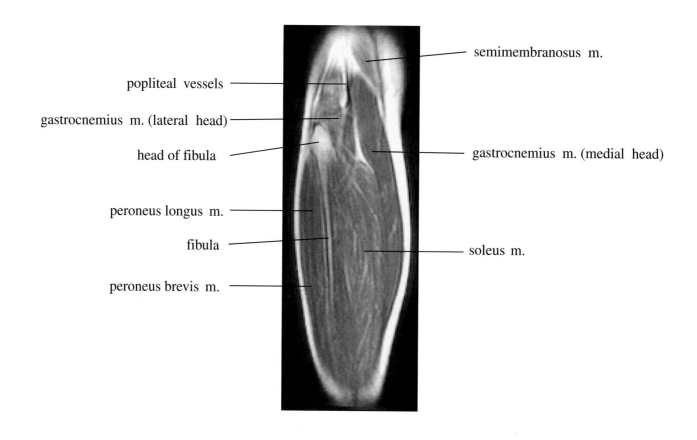

semimembranosus m.

popliteal vessels

gastrocnemius m. (lateral head)

head of fibula

gastrocnemius m. (medial head)

peroneus longus m.

fibula

soleus m.

peroneus brevis m.

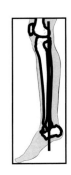

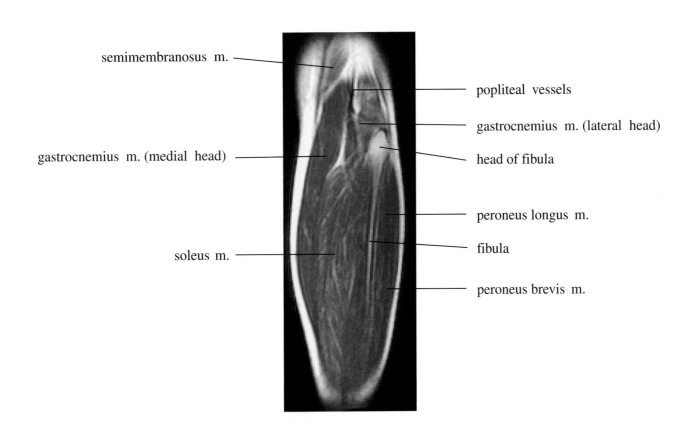

semimembranosus m.

popliteal vessels

gastrocnemius m. (lateral head)

gastrocnemius m. (medial head)

head of fibula

peroneus longus m.

soleus m.

fibula

peroneus brevis m.

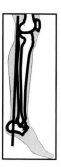

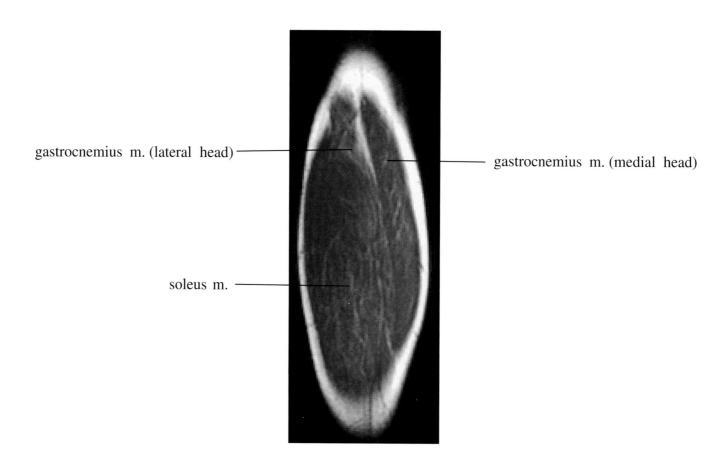

gastrocnemius m. (lateral head) ———

——— gastrocnemius m. (medial head)

soleus m. ———

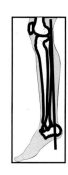

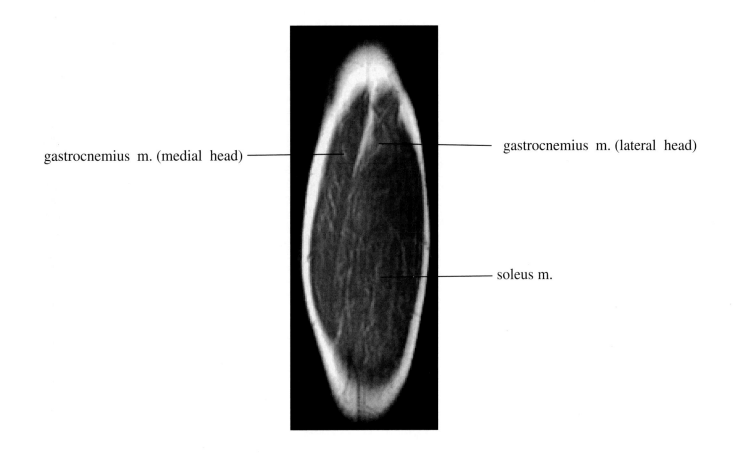

gastrocnemius m. (medial head) ——— ——— gastrocnemius m. (lateral head)

——— soleus m.

7

THE ANKLE AND FOOT

Interest in MR imaging of the ankle and foot has been increasing in recent years. The most common reason for MR imaging of the foot and ankle is for evaluation of suspected injuries to the tendons, ligaments, or chondroosseous structures, particularly osteochondrosis dissecans of the talus. Other common indications for the study include suspected tarsal coalition, suspected stress fractures (fatigue fractures and insufficiency fractures), evaluation of the neuropathic foot in diabetes, evaluation of Morton's neuroma, and preoperative evaluation of suspected soft-tissue infection of osteomyelitis. Less common rationales for the MR imaging study include suspected plantar fasciitis, suspected soft-tissue ganglions, and evaluation of the patient with arthritis.

PRACTICAL PROTOCOL CONSIDERATIONS

MR imaging of the foot and ankle can be performed with the same extremity coils that are used for imaging of the knee or with dedicated extremity surface coils such as the quadrature or phased array coils. Either of these coils can give diagnostic images. The patient is placed in the supine position with the foot comfortably positioned in the coil and the toes up. In general, small fields of view (10–12 cm) are used. Ten 3–4 mm slices with 0.5- to 1-mm interslice gaps are used.

Occasionally, the patient may be imaged with the foot in plantar flexion to decrease the curvature of the peroneal tendons and minimize the "magic angle" effect. When necessary, oblique axial and coronal planes may also be employed to visualize the obliquely oriented ligaments of the ankle. Intravenous gadolinium is used mainly for the evaluation of solid masses or suspected infection.

Menu of Protocols: Ankle and Foot

Plane	Pulse Sequence	FA (degrees)	TR (msec)	TE (msec)	TI (msec)	FOV (cm)	Matrix (256X-)	ST/G (mm)	NEX	Comments
Localizer (transaxial)	SE		500	min		20	192	4/1	1	Either is acceptable
Localizer (coronal)	SE		300	20		24	192	5/1	0.5	
Localizer (sagittal)	SE		300	min		18	128	5/1	1	
Transaxial	SE, double echo		2000	20/80		12	128	3–4/1	2	Either is acceptable
Transaxial	FSE, double echo		6000	17/102		14–15	256	4/0.5	1	
Transaxial	FSE, FS		5200	70		14	256	5/1	2	
Coronal	FSE, FS		3000	20		12	128	3–4/1	2	Either is acceptable
Coronal	FSE, double echo		6000	17/102		15	128	4/0.5	2	
Coronal	SE		300	min		12–14	192	3/1.5	2	
Sagittal	SE		600	20		12	128	3/1	2	Either is acceptable
Sagittal	FMPIR		5500	18	150	15–16	256	4/0.5	2	
Sagittal	FSE, double echo		4000	20/100		12–14	192	3/1	2	
Sagittal	SE, double echo		2000	20/80		16	192	3/1	1–2	
Sagittal	3D FRE, SPGR, FS	30	45	15		12–14	192	1.5/0	1	
Pre-GAD (axial, coronal, sagittal)	SE (±FS)		600	20		12–14	192	3/1	2	Depends on site of abnormality— intravenous GAD for tumors, cysts, infection
Post-GAD (axial, coronal, sagittal)	SE (±FS)		600	20		12–14	192	3/1	2	Depends on site of abnormality— intravenous GAD for tumors, cysts, infection

MAJOR OSTEOCHONDRAL STRUCTURES/LANDMARKS

Ankle

- Distal tibia
  - Tibial articular cartilage
  - Medial malleolus
  - Posterior malleolus
  - Fibular notch

- Distal fibula
  - Lateral malleolus
  - Fossa of lateral malleolus

Foot

- Talus
  - Head
  - Neck
  - Trochlea
  - Posterior process
  - Medial tubercle
  - Lateral tubercle
- Calcaneus
  - Tuberosity
  - Medial process
  - Lateral process
  - Sustentaculum tali
- Navicular
  - Navicular tuberosity
- Cuboid
- Cuneiforms
  - Lateral
  - Intermediate
  - Medial
- Metatarsals
  - Base
  - Shaft
  - Head
- Proximal phalanges (I–V)
  - Base
  - Head
  - Tuberosity (V)

- Middle phalanges
- Distal phalanges
  - Base
  - Tuberosity (tuft)
- Sesamoid bones (variable)

MAJOR LIGAMENTS/TENDONS/BURSAE

Ligaments

- Tibiofibular joint
  - Anterior tibiofibular
  - Posterior tibiofibular
- Lateral collateral ligamentous complex
  - Anterior talofibular
  - Calcaneofibular
  - Posterior talofibular
- Deltoid (medial)
  - Superficial
    - Anterior tibiotalar
    - Tibionavicular
    - Tibiocalcaneal
    - Posterior tibiofalar
  - Deep
    - Anterior tibiotalar
    - Posterior tibiotalar
- Interosseous talocalacaneal
- Dorsal talonavicular
- Bifurcate
  - Calcaneonavicular portion
  - Calcaneocuboid portion
- Dorsal cuboideonavicular
- Dorsal cuneonavicular

- Dorsal intercuneiform
- Dorsal tarsometatarsal
- Dorsal metatarsal
- Dorsal cuneocuboid
- Dorsal calcaneocuboid
- Plantar calcaneonavicular
- Plantar cuboideonavicular
- Plantar cuneonavicular
- Plantar calcaneocuboid
- Plantar tarsometatarsal
- Deep transverse metatarsal
- Plantar ligaments (plates)

Tendons

- Anterior tendons (under superior and inferior extensor retinaculae)
  - Extensor digitorum longus
  - Extensor hallucis longus
  - Tibialis anterior
- Medial tendons (under flexor retinaculum)
  - Flexor hallucis longus
  - Flexor digitorum longus
  - Tibialis posterior
- Lateral tendons
  - Peroneus brevis
  - Peroneus longus
- Posterior tendons
  - Achilles tendon (largest tendon in body)
- Peroneus tertius

Bursae

- Retrocalcaneal (pre-Achilles)

MAJOR MUSCLES

(See lower limb)

ORIGIN/INSERTION/INNERVATION OF MAJOR MUSCLES

(See lower limb)

FOOT

Muscle	Origin	Insertion	Innervation
Interosseous			
– Dorsal interosseous (I, II)	From the sides of metatarsals (I, II)	Same sides of bases of proximal phalanges (I, II)	Deep branch of lateral plantar N.
– Dorsal interosseous (III, IV)	From the sides of metatarsals (III, IV)	Lateral sides of bases of proximal phalanges (III, IV)	Deep branch of lateral plantar N.
– Plantar interosseous	Bases of medial sides of metatarsals (III, IV, V)	Medial sides of proximal phalanges (III, IV, V)	Deep branch of lateral plantar N.
Great Toe Intrinsic Muscles			
– Abductor hallucis	Medial process of calcaneal tuberosity flexor retinaculum, intermuscular septum	Medial aspect of base of proximal phalanx of first toe	Lateral plantar N.

(continued)

ORIGIN/INSERTION/INNERVATION OF MAJOR MUSCLES (*CONTINUED*)

Muscle	Origin	Insertion	Innervation
– Abductor hallucis brevis			
• Medial belly	Plantar aspect of cuboid and lateral cuneiform, tibialis anterior tendon, medial first metatarsal	Blends with abductor hallucis to insert on medial aspect of base of proximal phalanx of first toe	Lateral plantar N.
• Lateral belly	Plantar aspect of cuboid and lateral cuneiform, tibialis anterior tendon, medial first metatarsal	Lateral side of base of proximal phalanx of first toe	Lateral plantar N.

Fifth Toe Intrinsic Muscles

Muscle	Origin	Insertion	Innervation
– Abductor digiti minimi	Lateral and medial processes of calcaneus, intermuscular septum, lateral plantar fascia	Lateral side of proximal phalanx of fifth toe	Lateral plantar N.
– Flexor digiti minimi brevis	Tuberosity of cuboid, base of fifth metatarsal, peroneus longus tendon sheath	Base of proximal phalanx of fifth toe	Superficial branch of lateral plantar N.
– Opponeus digiti minimi (variably present)	Tuberosity of cuboid, peroneus longus tendon sheath	Lateral surface of fifth metatarsal	Superficial branch of lateral plantar N. or branch of nerve to flexor digiti minimi brevis

(continued)

ORIGIN/INSERTION/INNERVATION OF MAJOR MUSCLES (*CONTINUED*)

Muscle	*Origin*	*Insertion*	*Innervation*
– Extensor digitorum brevis	Lateral and superior calcaneal surfaces and inferior extensor retinaculum	Base of first metatarsal (extensor hallucis brevis), base of second proximal phalanx, bases of remaining middle phalanges	Deep peroneal N.
– Flexor digitorum brevis	Medial process of calcaneus, plantar aponeurosis, intermuscular septum	Pass superficial to long flexor, divide to form opening on proximal phalanx of toes through which long flexor tendons pass, then insert onto base of middle phalanx	Lateral plantar N.
– Quadratus plantae (accessory to long digital flexor)			
• Lateral head	Lateral border of plantar surface of calcaneus and from long plantar ligament	Tendon of flexor digitorum longus muscle	Lateral plantar N.
• Medial head	Medial surface of calcaneus and medial border of long plantar ligament	Tendon of flexor digitorum longus muscle	Lateral plantar N.

(*continued*)

ORIGIN/INSERTION/INNERVATION OF MAJOR MUSCLES (*CONTINUED*)

Muscle	*Origin*	*Insertion*	*Innervation*
• Lumbricals	Four tendons of flexor digitorum longus muscle	Medial surface of extensor expansion over lateral four toes	Lateral plantar N.

THE ANKLE: AXIAL ANATOMY

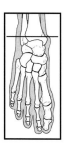

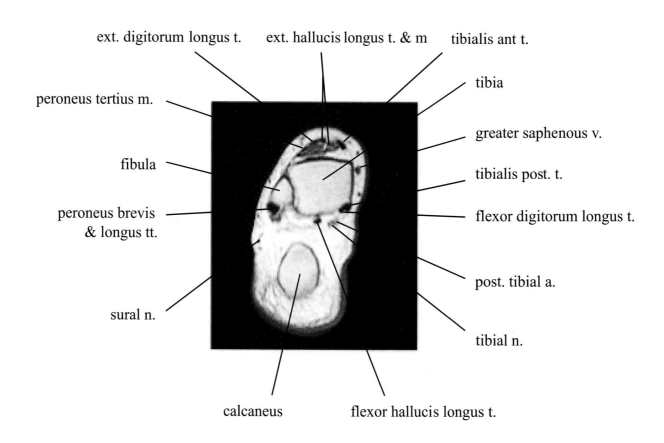

ext. digitorum longus t.

ext. hallucis longus t. & m

tibialis ant t.

tibia

peroneus tertius m.

greater saphenous v.

fibula

tibialis post. t.

peroneus brevis
& longus tt.

flexor digitorum longus t.

post. tibial a.

sural n.

tibial n.

calcaneus

flexor hallucis longus t.

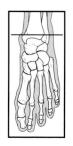

tibialis ant t.   ext. hallucis longus t. & m.   ext. digitorum longus t.

tibia

peroneus tertius m.

greater saphenous v.

fibula

tibialis post. t.

flexor digitorum longus t.

peroneus longus
& brevis tt.

post. tibial a.

sural n.

tibial n.

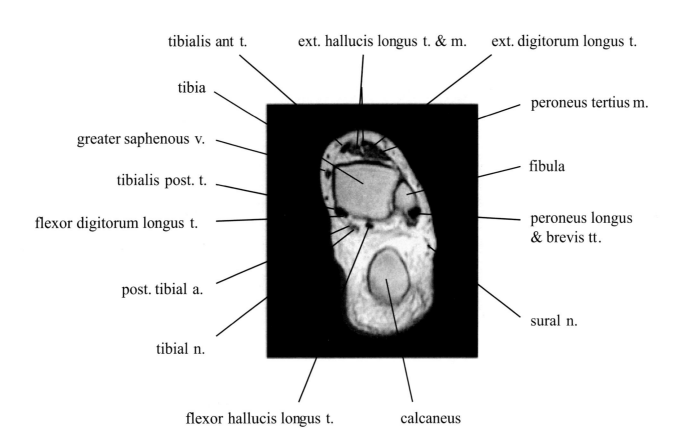

flexor hallucis longus t.   calcaneus

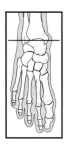

ext. digitorum longus t.   ant. tibial a.   ext. hallucis longus t. & m.

peroneus tertius m.

ant. tibiofibular jt.

tibiotalar jt.

fibula

peroneus longus
& brevis tt.

sural n.

tibialis ant t.

tibia

greater saphenous v.

tibialis post. t.

flex. digitorum longus t.

post. tibial a.

tibial n.

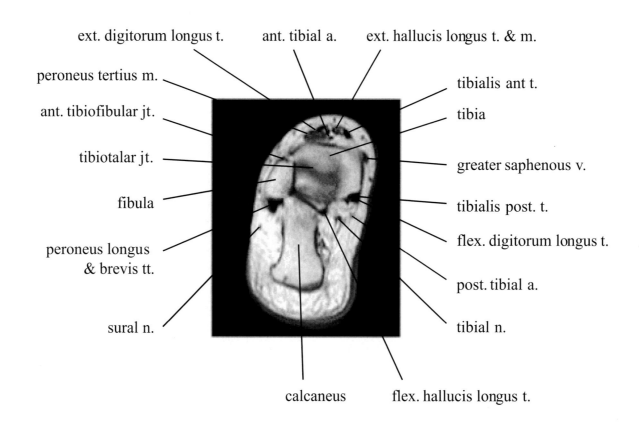

calcaneus   flex. hallucis longus t.

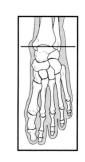

ext. hallucis longus t. & m.

ant. tibial a.

ext. digitorum longus t.

tibialis ant t.

peroneus tertius m.

tibia

ant. tibiofibular jt.

greater saphenous v.

tibiotalar jt.

tibialis post. t.

fibula

flex. digitorum longus t.

post. tibial a.

peroneus longus
& brevis tt.

tibial n.

sural n.

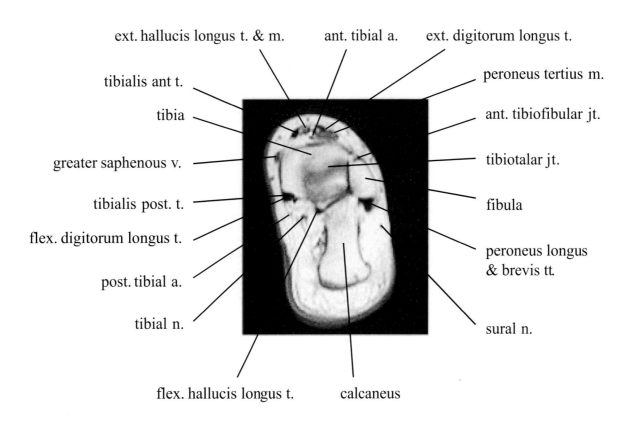

flex. hallucis longus t.

calcaneus

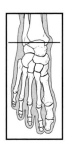

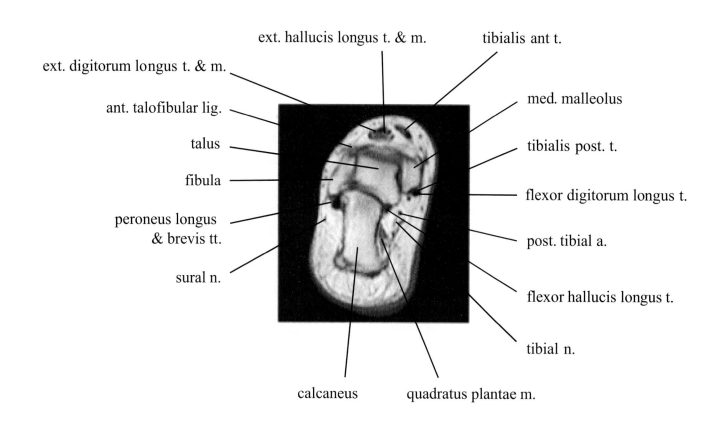

ext. hallucis longus t. & m.

tibialis ant t.

ext. digitorum longus t. & m.

ant. talofibular lig.

med. malleolus

talus

tibialis post. t.

fibula

flexor digitorum longus t.

peroneus longus
& brevis tt.

post. tibial a.

sural n.

flexor hallucis longus t.

tibial n.

calcaneus

quadratus plantae m.

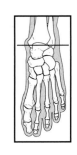

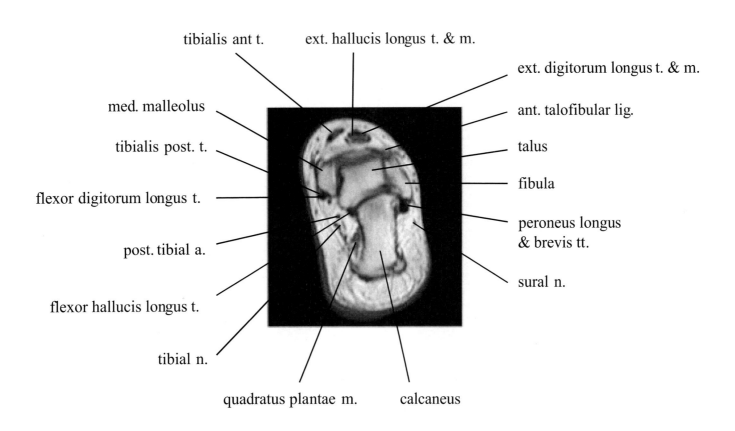

tibialis ant t.

ext. hallucis longus t. & m.

ext. digitorum longus t. & m.

med. malleolus

ant. talofibular lig.

tibialis post. t.

talus

flexor digitorum longus t.

fibula

post. tibial a.

peroneus longus
& brevis tt.

flexor hallucis longus t.

sural n.

tibial n.

quadratus plantae m.

calcaneus

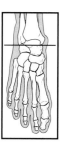

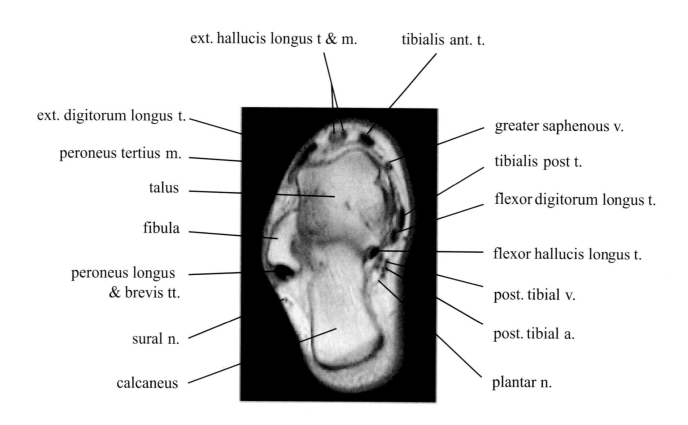

ext. hallucis longus t & m.

tibialis ant. t.

ext. digitorum longus t.

peroneus tertius m.

talus

fibula

peroneus longus
& brevis tt.

sural n.

calcaneus

greater saphenous v.

tibialis post t.

flexor digitorum longus t.

flexor hallucis longus t.

post. tibial v.

post. tibial a.

plantar n.

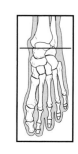

tibialis ant. t.

ext. hallucis longus t. & m

greater saphenous v.

ext. digitorum longus t.

tibialis post t.

peroneus tertius m.

flexor digitorum longus t.

talus

flexor hallucis longus t.

fibula

post. tibial v.

peroneus longus
& brevis tt.

post. tibial a.

sural n.

plantar n.

calcaneus

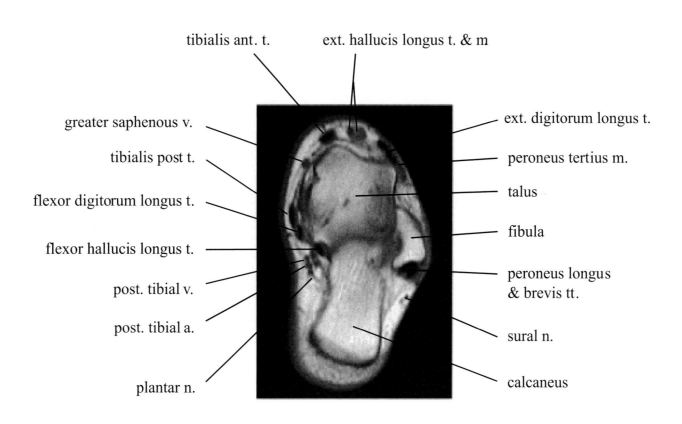

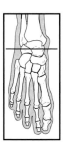

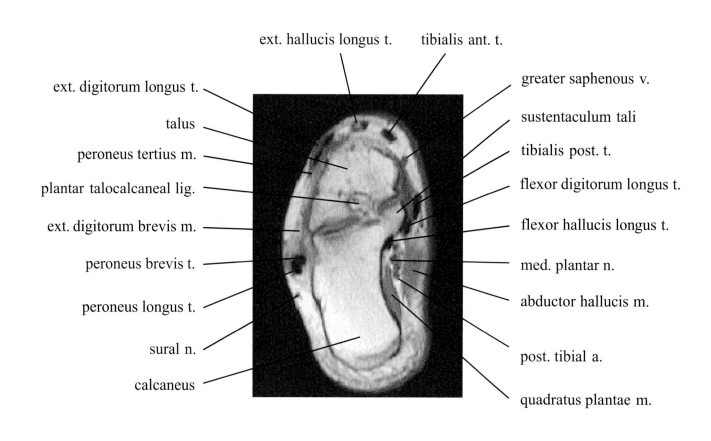

ext. hallucis longus t.   tibialis ant. t.

ext. digitorum longus t.

greater saphenous v.

talus

sustentaculum tali

peroneus tertius m.

tibialis post. t.

plantar talocalcaneal lig.

flexor digitorum longus t.

ext. digitorum brevis m.

flexor hallucis longus t.

peroneus brevis t.

med. plantar n.

peroneus longus t.

abductor hallucis m.

sural n.

post. tibial a.

calcaneus

quadratus plantae m.

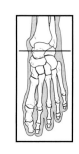

tibialis ant. t.   ext. hallucis longus t.

greater saphenous v.

sustentaculum tali

tibialis post. t.

flexor digitorum longus t.

flexor hallucis longus t.

med. plantar n.

abductor hallucis m.

post. tibial a.

quadratus plantae m.

ext. digitorum longus t.

talus

peroneus tertius m.

plantar talocalcaneal lig.

ext. digitorum brevis m.

peroneus brevis t.

peroneus longus t.

sural n.

calcaneus

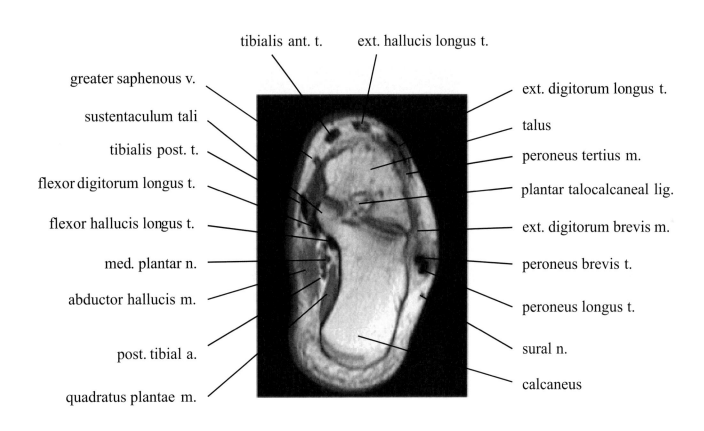

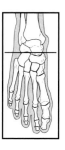

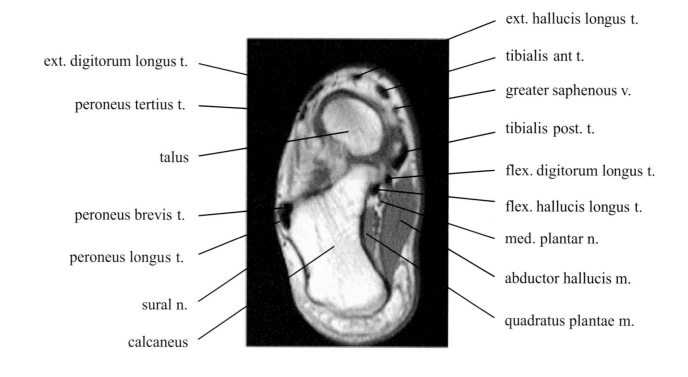

ext. digitorum longus t.

peroneus tertius t.

talus

peroneus brevis t.

peroneus longus t.

sural n.

calcaneus

ext. hallucis longus t.

tibialis ant t.

greater saphenous v.

tibialis post. t.

flex. digitorum longus t.

flex. hallucis longus t.

med. plantar n.

abductor hallucis m.

quadratus plantae m.

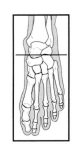

ext. hallucis longus t.

tibialis ant t.

greater saphenous v.

tibialis post. t.

flex. digitorum longus t.

flex. hallucis longus t.

med. plantar n.

abductor hallucis m.

quadratus plantae m.

ext. digitorum longus t.

peroneus tertius t.

talus

peroneus brevis t.

peroneus longus t.

sural n.

calcaneus

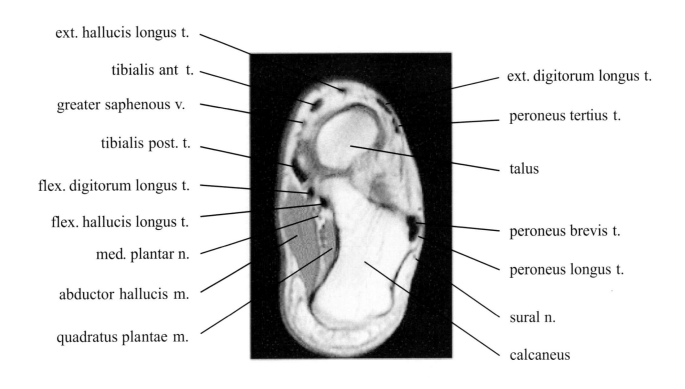

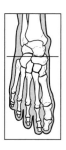

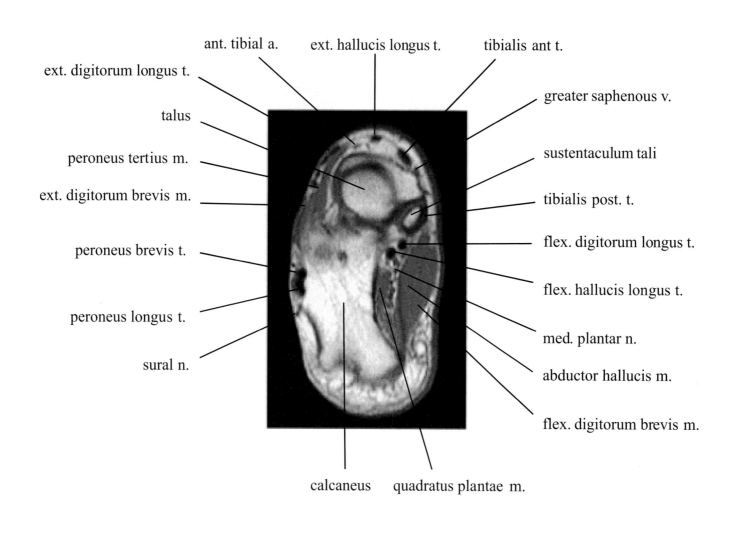

ant. tibial a.

ext. hallucis longus t.

tibialis ant t.

ext. digitorum longus t.

talus

peroneus tertius m.

ext. digitorum brevis m.

peroneus brevis t.

peroneus longus t.

sural n.

greater saphenous v.

sustentaculum tali

tibialis post. t.

flex. digitorum longus t.

flex. hallucis longus t.

med. plantar n.

abductor hallucis m.

flex. digitorum brevis m.

calcaneus   quadratus plantae m.

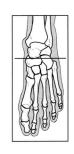

tibialis ant. t.

ext. hallucis longus t.

ant. tibial a.

greater saphenous v.

ext. digitorum longus t.

sustentaculum tali

talus

tibialis post. t.

peroneus tertius m.

flexor digitorum longus t.

ext. digitorum brevis m.

flexor hallucis longus t.

peroneus brevis t.

med. plantar n.

abductor hallucis m.

peroneus longus t.

flexor digitorum brevis m.

sural n.

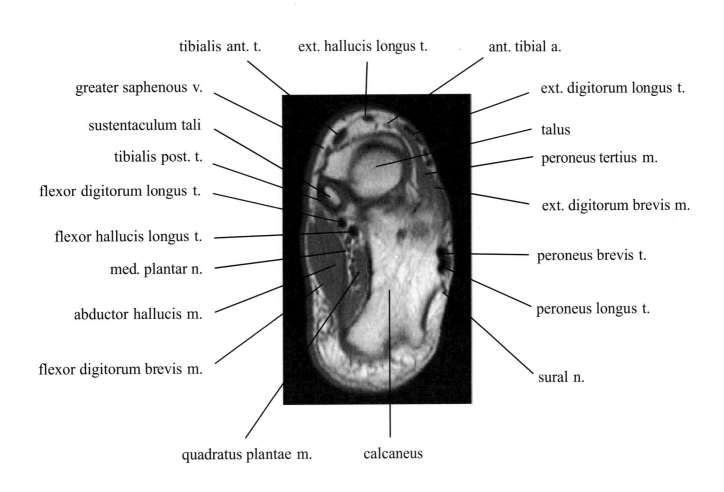

quadratus plantae m.

calcaneus

THE ANKLE: SAGITTAL ANATOMY

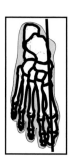

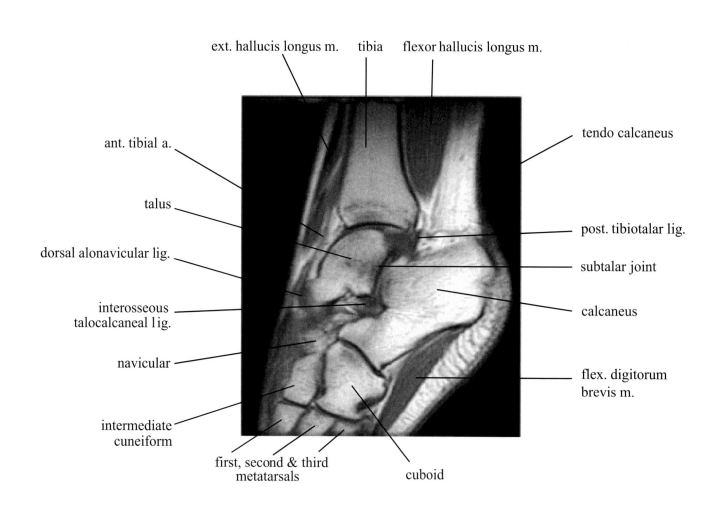

ext. hallucis longus m.   tibia   flexor hallucis longus m.

ant. tibial a.

tendo calcaneus

talus

post. tibiotalar lig.

dorsal alonavicular lig.

subtalar joint

interosseous
talocalcaneal lig.

calcaneus

navicular

flex. digitorum
brevis m.

intermediate
cuneiform

first, second & third
metatarsals

cuboid

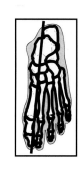

flexor hallucis longus m.   tibia   ext. hallucis longus m.

tendo calcaneus

ant. tibial a.

post. tibiotalar lig.

talus

subtalar joint

dorsal
talonavicular lig.

calcaneus

interosseous
talocalcaneal lig.

navicular

flex. digitorum
brevis m.

cuneiform
intermediate

cuboid

third, second& first
metatarsals

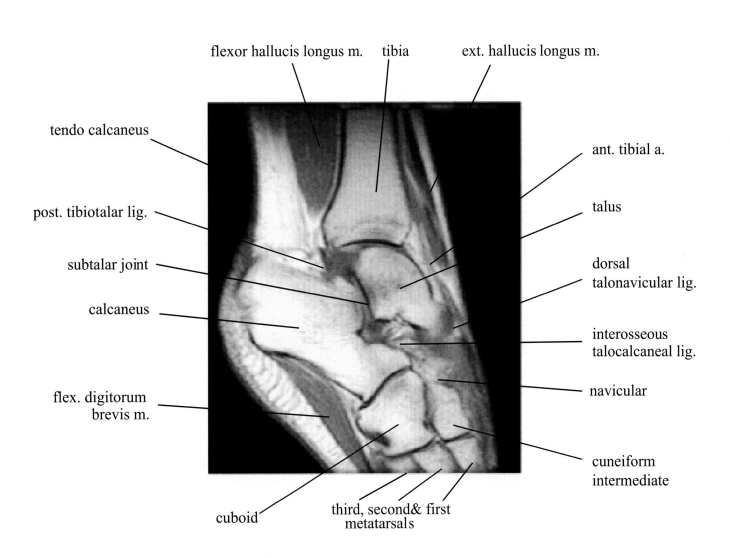

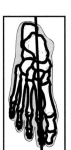

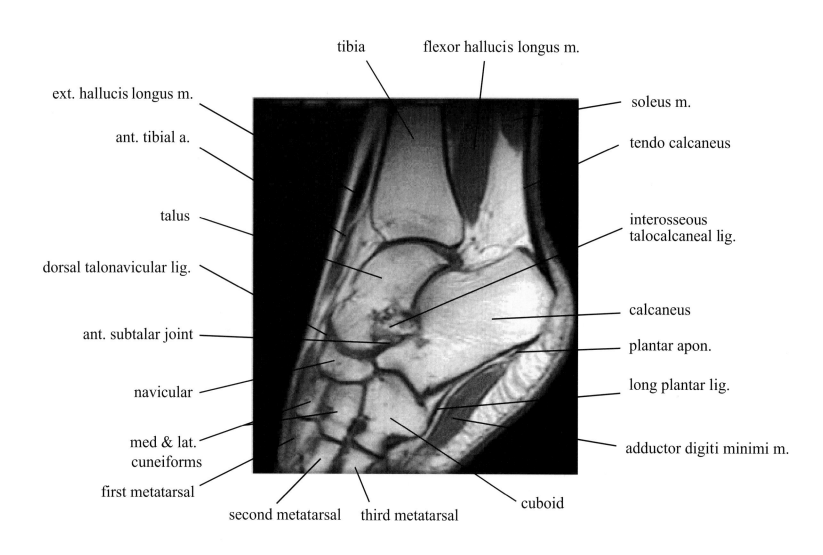

tibia

flexor hallucis longus m.

ext. hallucis longus m.

soleus m.

ant. tibial a.

tendo calcaneus

talus

interosseous
talocalcaneal lig.

dorsal talonavicular lig.

ant. subtalar joint

calcaneus

plantar apon.

navicular

long plantar lig.

med & lat.
cuneiforms

adductor digiti minimi m.

first metatarsal

cuboid

second metatarsal   third metatarsal

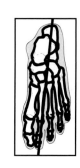

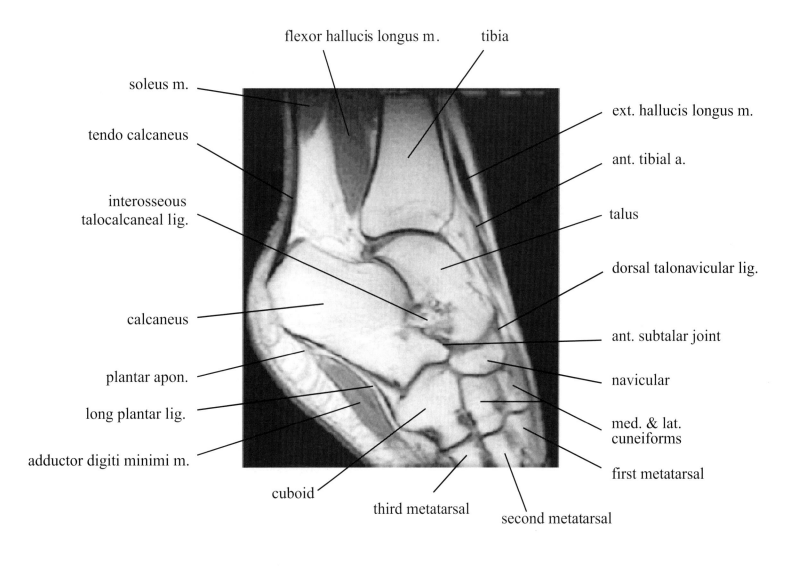

flexor hallucis longus m.

tibia

soleus m.

ext. hallucis longus m.

tendo calcaneus

ant. tibial a.

interosseous
talocalcaneal lig.

talus

dorsal talonavicular lig.

calcaneus

ant. subtalar joint

plantar apon.

navicular

long plantar lig.

med. & lat.
cuneiforms

adductor digiti minimi m.

first metatarsal

cuboid

third metatarsal

second metatarsal

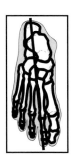

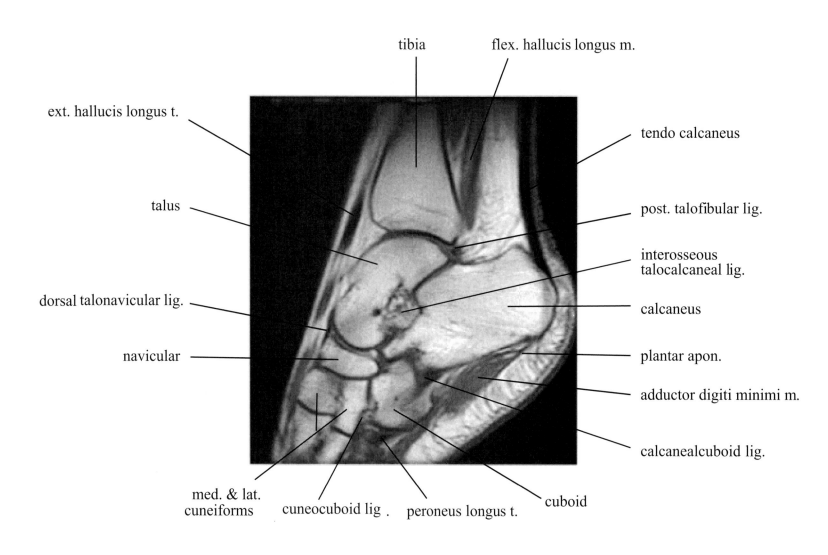

tibia

flex. hallucis longus m.

ext. hallucis longus t.

tendo calcaneus

talus

post. talofibular lig.

interosseous
talocalcaneal lig.

dorsal talonavicular lig.

calcaneus

navicular

plantar apon.

adductor digiti minimi m.

calcanealcuboid lig.

med. & lat.
cuneiforms

cuneocuboid lig .

peroneus longus t.

cuboid

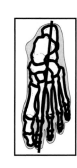

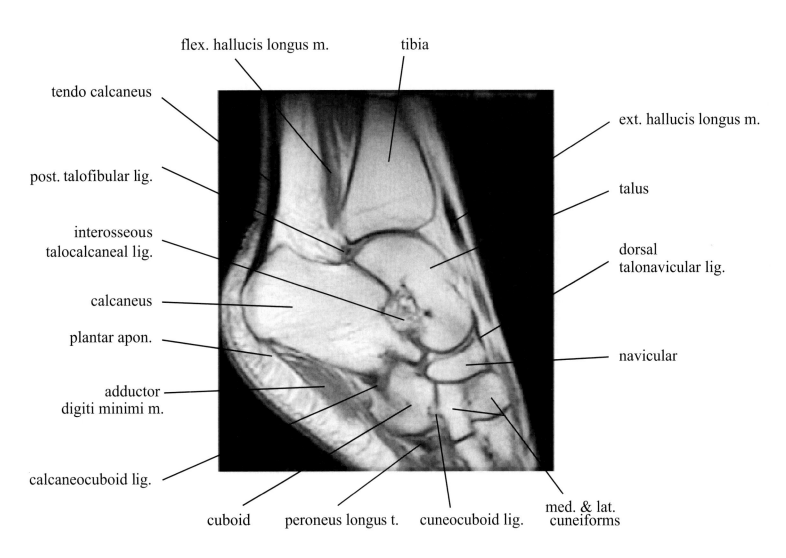

flex. hallucis longus m.

tibia

tendo calcaneus

ext. hallucis longus m.

post. talofibular lig.

talus

interosseous
talocalcaneal lig.

dorsal
talonavicular lig.

calcaneus

plantar apon.

navicular

adductor
digiti minimi m.

calcaneocuboid lig.

cuboid

peroneus longus t.

cuneocuboid lig.

med. & lat.
cuneiforms

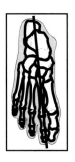

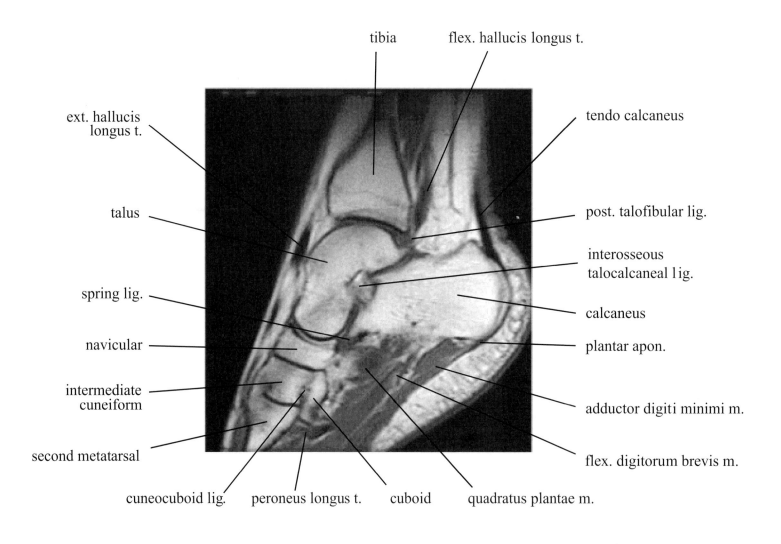

tibia

flex. hallucis longus t.

ext. hallucis
    longus t.

tendo calcaneus

talus

post. talofibular lig.

interosseous
    talocalcaneal lig.

spring lig.

calcaneus

navicular

plantar apon.

intermediate
    cuneiform

adductor digiti minimi m.

second metatarsal

flex. digitorum brevis m.

cuneocuboid lig.   peroneus longus t.   cuboid   quadratus plantae m.

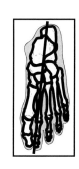

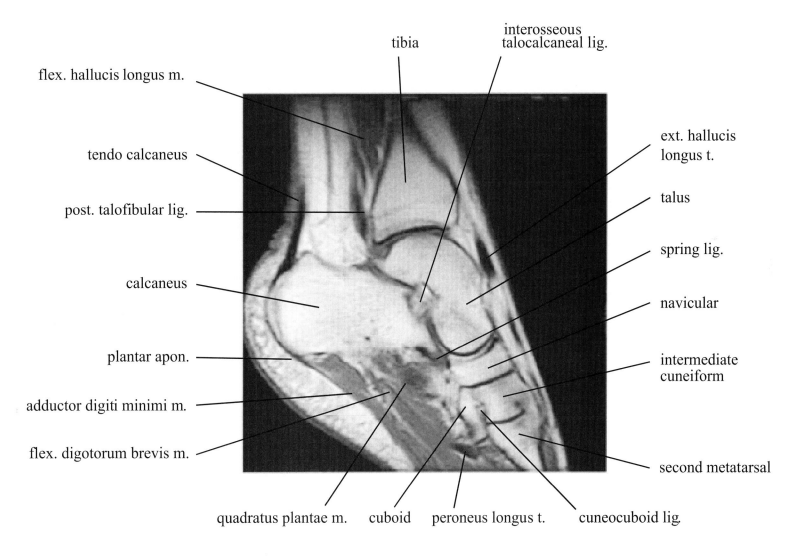

flex. hallucis longus m.

tendo calcaneus

post. talofibular lig.

calcaneus

plantar apon.

adductor digiti minimi m.

flex. digotorum brevis m.

tibia

interosseous
talocalcaneal lig.

ext. hallucis
longus t.

talus

spring lig.

navicular

intermediate
cuneiform

second metatarsal

quadratus plantae m.   cuboid   peroneus longus t.   cuneocuboid lig.

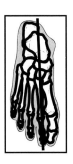

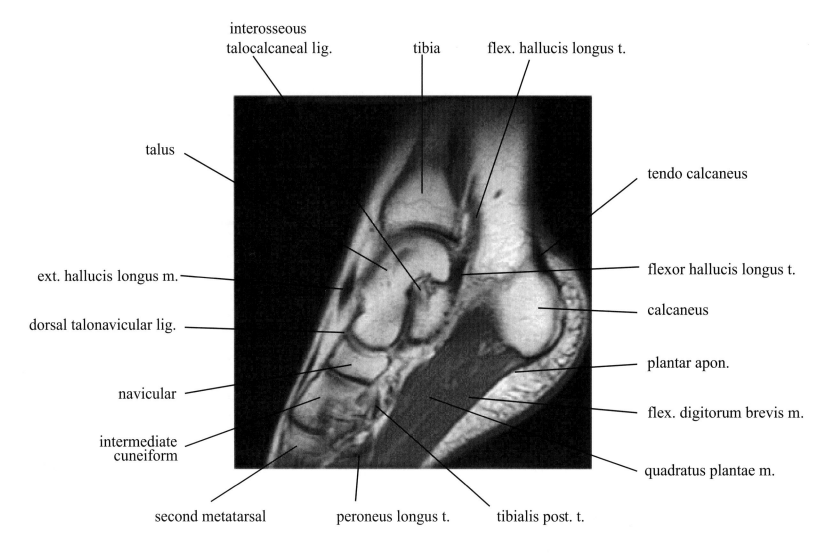

interosseous
talocalcaneal lig.

tibia

flex. hallucis longus t.

talus

tendo calcaneus

ext. hallucis longus m.

flexor hallucis longus t.

dorsal talonavicular lig.

calcaneus

navicular

plantar apon.

intermediate
cuneiform

flex. digitorum brevis m.

quadratus plantae m.

second metatarsal

peroneus longus t.

tibialis post. t.

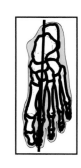

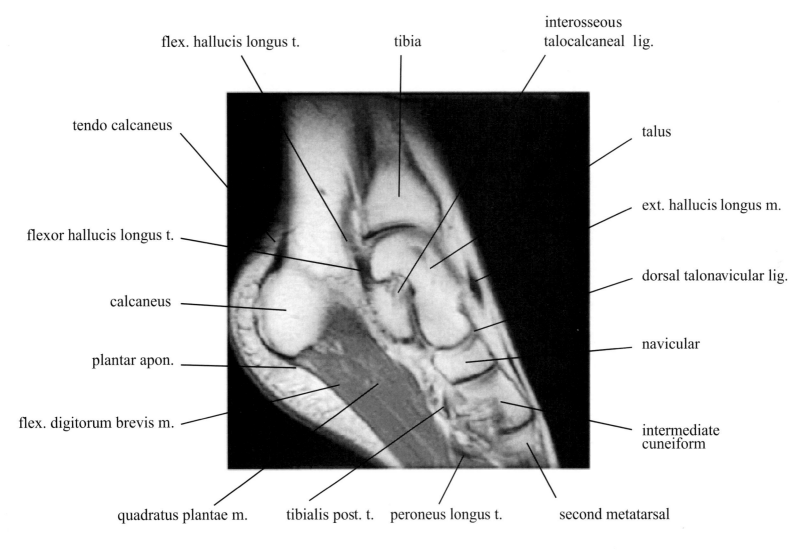

flex. hallucis longus t.

tibia

interosseous
talocalcaneal lig.

tendo calcaneus

talus

flexor hallucis longus t.

ext. hallucis longus m.

calcaneus

dorsal talonavicular lig.

plantar apon.

navicular

flex. digitorum brevis m.

intermediate
cuneiform

quadratus plantae m.

tibialis post. t.

peroneus longus t.

second metatarsal

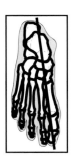

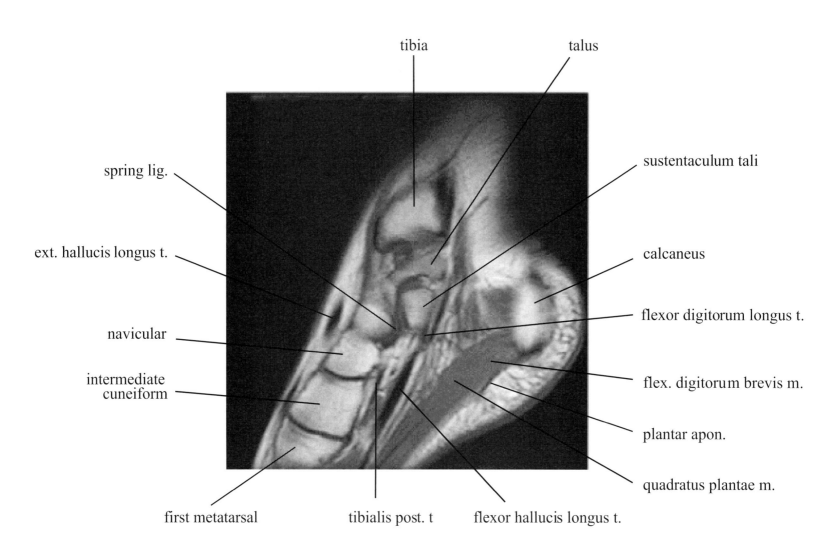

tibia

talus

spring lig.

sustentaculum tali

ext. hallucis longus t.

calcaneus

navicular

flexor digitorum longus t.

intermediate
cuneiform

flex. digitorum brevis m.

plantar apon.

quadratus plantae m.

first metatarsal

tibialis post. t

flexor hallucis longus t.

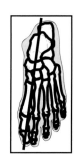

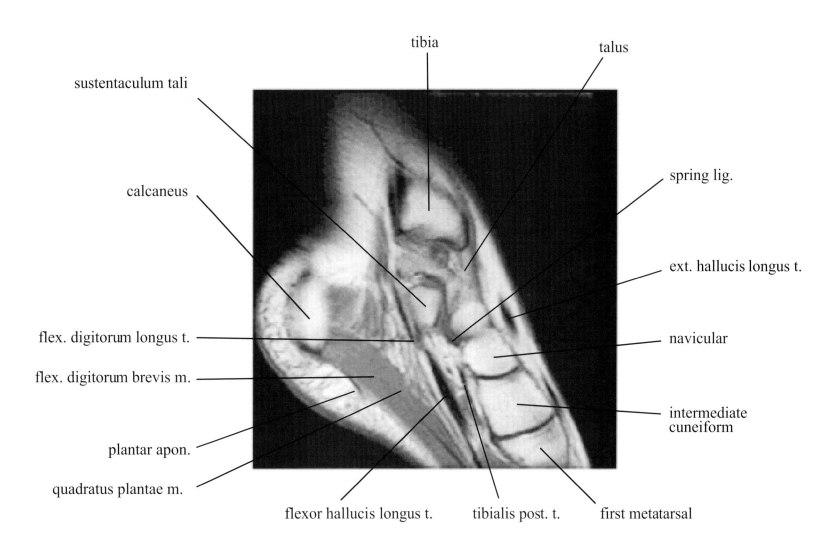

tibia

talus

sustentaculum tali

spring lig.

calcaneus

ext. hallucis longus t.

flex. digitorum longus t.

navicular

flex. digitorum brevis m.

intermediate
cuneiform

plantar apon.

quadratus plantae m.

flexor hallucis longus t.

tibialis post. t.

first metatarsal

THE ANKLE: CORONAL ANATOMY

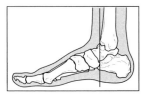

ext. hallucis longus t.

peroneus tertius t.

talus

ext. digitorum brevis m.

cuboid

lat. cuneiform

tibialis ant. t.

calcaneus

abductor hallucis m.

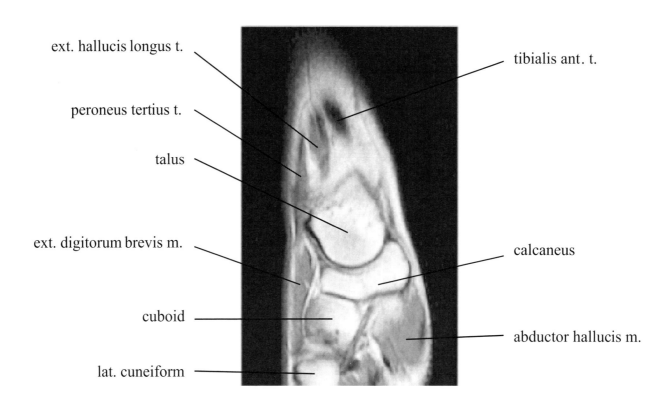

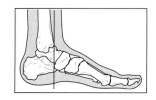

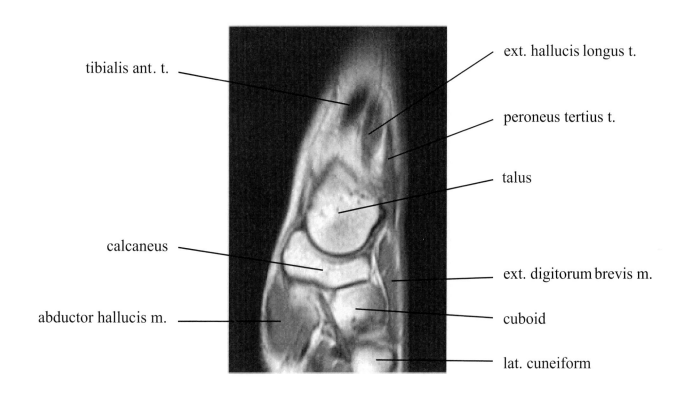

tibialis ant. t.

ext. hallucis longus t.

peroneus tertius t.

talus

calcaneus

ext. digitorum brevis m.

abductor hallucis m.

cuboid

lat. cuneiform

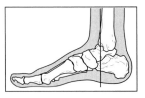

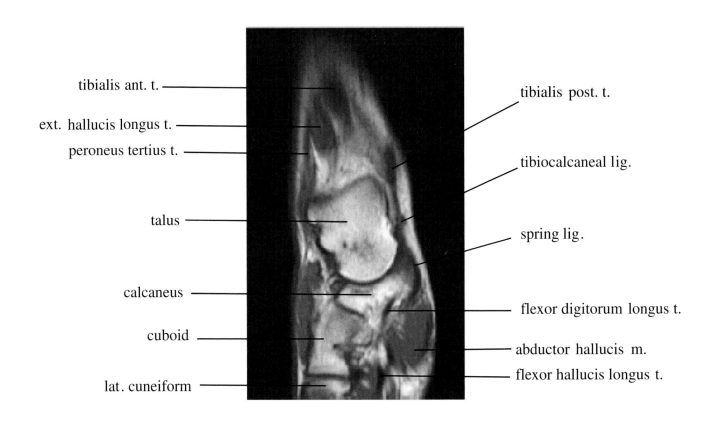

tibialis ant. t. ——————

ext. hallucis longus t. ——————

peroneus tertius t. ——————

talus ——————

calcaneus ——————

cuboid ——————

lat. cuneiform ——————

tibialis post. t.

tibiocalcaneal lig.

spring lig.

flexor digitorum longus t.

abductor hallucis m.

flexor hallucis longus t.

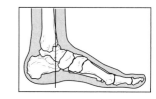

tibialis ant. t.

ext. hallucis longus t.

tibialis post. t

peroneus tertius t.

tibiocalcaneal lig.

spring lig.

talus

calcaneus

flex. digitorum longus t.

cuboid

abductor hallucis m.

lat. cuneiform

flexor hallucis longus t.

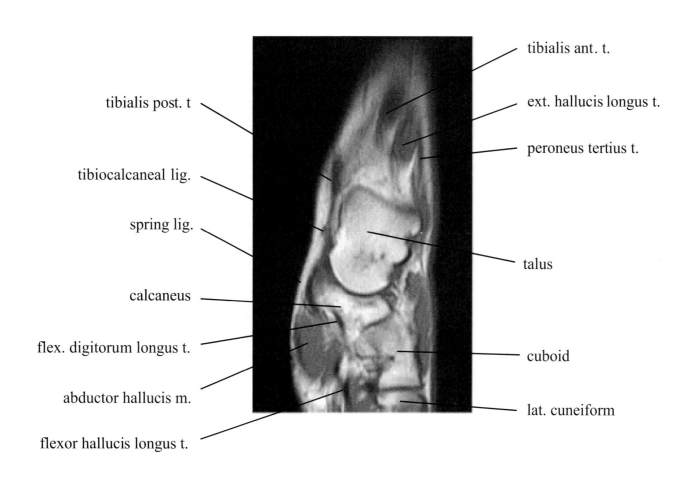

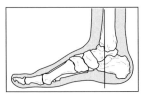

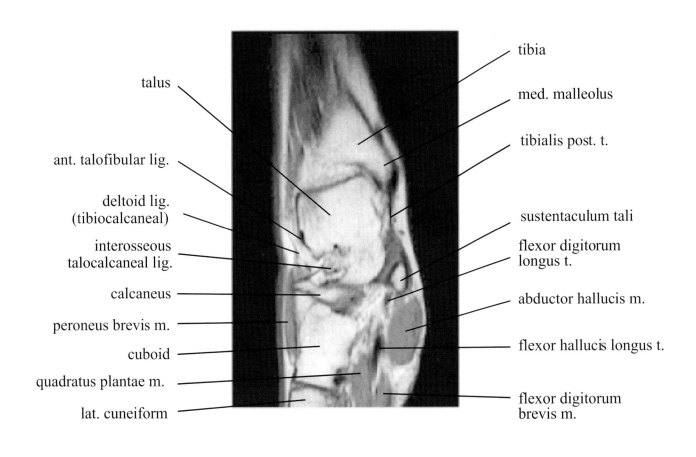

talus

ant. talofibular lig.

deltoid lig.
(tibiocalcaneal)

interosseous
talocalcaneal lig.

calcaneus

peroneus brevis m.

cuboid

quadratus plantae m.

lat. cuneiform

tibia

med. malleolus

tibialis post. t.

sustentaculum tali

flexor digitorum
longus t.

abductor hallucis m.

flexor hallucis longus t.

flexor digitorum
brevis m.

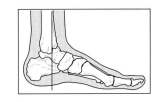

tibia

talus

med. malleolus

ant. talofibular lig.

tibialis post. t.

deltoid lig.
(tibiocalcaneal)

interosseous
talocalcaneal lig.

sustentaculum tali

calcaneus

flexor digitorum longus t.

peroneus brevis m.

abductor hallucis m.

cuboid

flexor hallucis longus t.

quadratus plantae m.

lat. cuneiform

flexor digitorum brevis m.

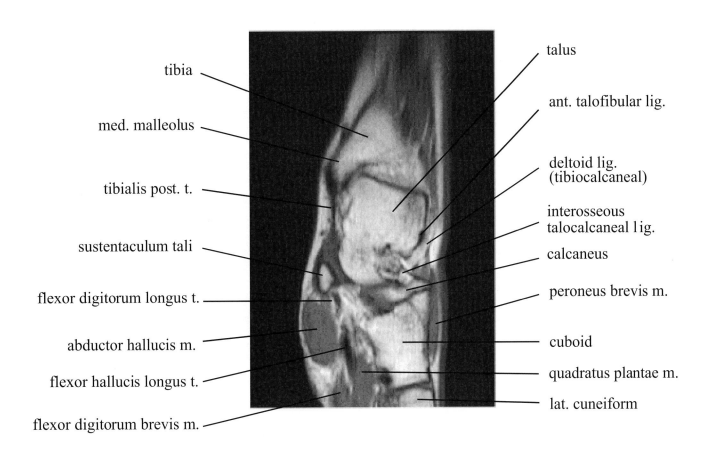

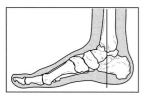

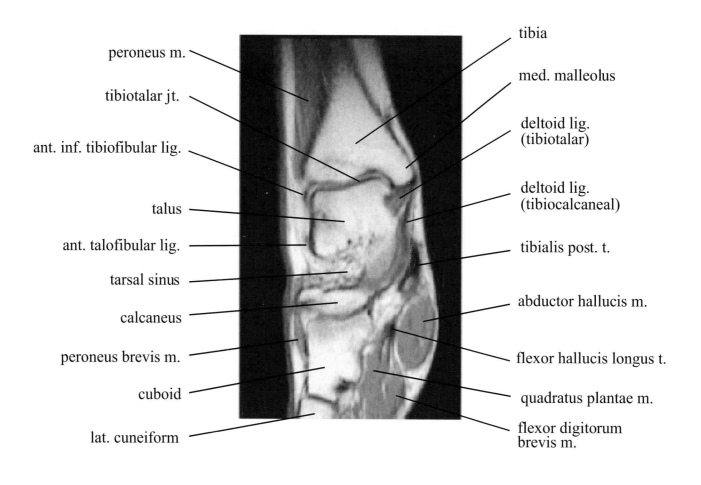

peroneus m.

tibiotalar jt.

ant. inf. tibiofibular lig.

talus

ant. talofibular lig.

tarsal sinus

calcaneus

peroneus brevis m.

cuboid

lat. cuneiform

tibia

med. malleolus

deltoid lig.
(tibiotalar)

deltoid lig.
(tibiocalcaneal)

tibialis post. t.

abductor hallucis m.

flexor hallucis longus t.

quadratus plantae m.

flexor digitorum
brevis m.

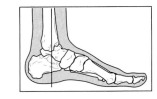

tibia

med. malleolus

deltoid lig.
(tibiotalar)

deltoid lig.
(tibiocalcaneal)

tibialis post. t.

abductor hallucis m.

flexor hallucis longus t.

peroneus m.

tibiotalar jt.

ant. inf. tibiofibular lig.

talus

ant. talofibular lig.

tarsal sinus

calcaneus

peroneus brevis m.

cuboid

lat. cuneiform

flexor digitorum
brevis m.

quadratus plantae m.

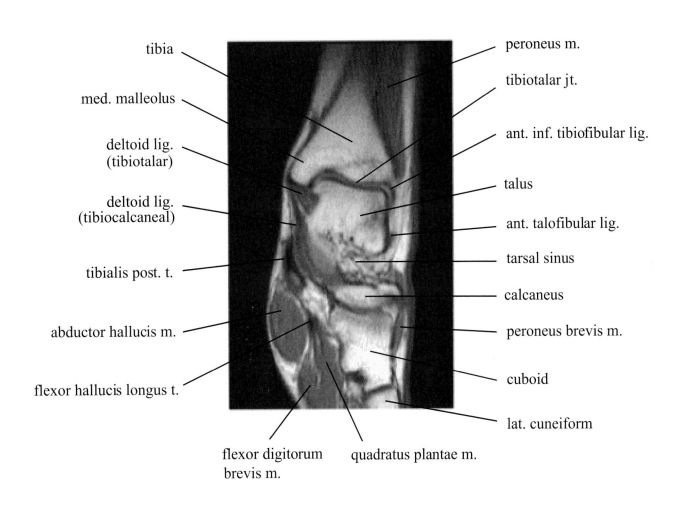

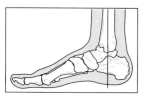

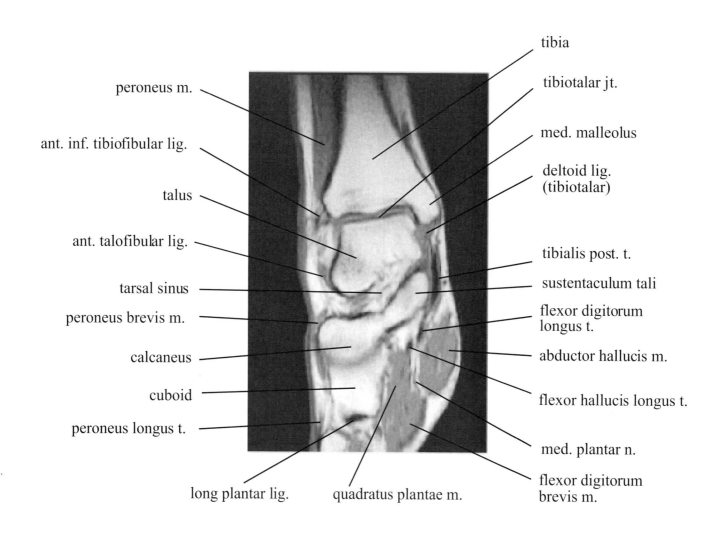

peroneus m.

ant. inf. tibiofibular lig.

talus

ant. talofibular lig.

tarsal sinus

peroneus brevis m.

calcaneus

cuboid

peroneus longus t.

long plantar lig.   quadratus plantae m.

tibia

tibiotalar jt.

med. malleolus

deltoid lig.
(tibiotalar)

tibialis post. t.

sustentaculum tali

flexor digitorum
longus t.

abductor hallucis m.

flexor hallucis longus t.

med. plantar n.

flexor digitorum
brevis m.

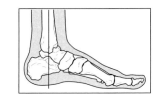

tibiotalar jt.

tibia

med. malleolus

peroneus m.

deltoid lig.
(tibiotalar)

ant. inf. tibiofibular lig.

talus

tibialis post. t.

ant. talofibular lig.

sustentaculum tali

tarsal sinus

flexor digitorum
longus t.

peroneus brevis m.

calcaneus

abductor hallucis m.

cuboid

flexor hallucis longus t.

peroneus longus t.

med. plantar n.

long plantar lig.

flexor digitorum
brevis m.

quadratus plantae m.

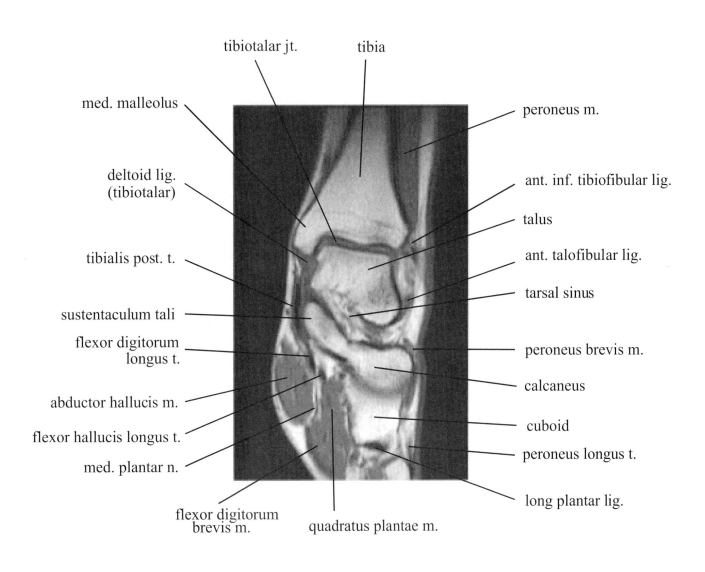

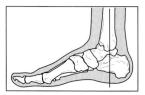

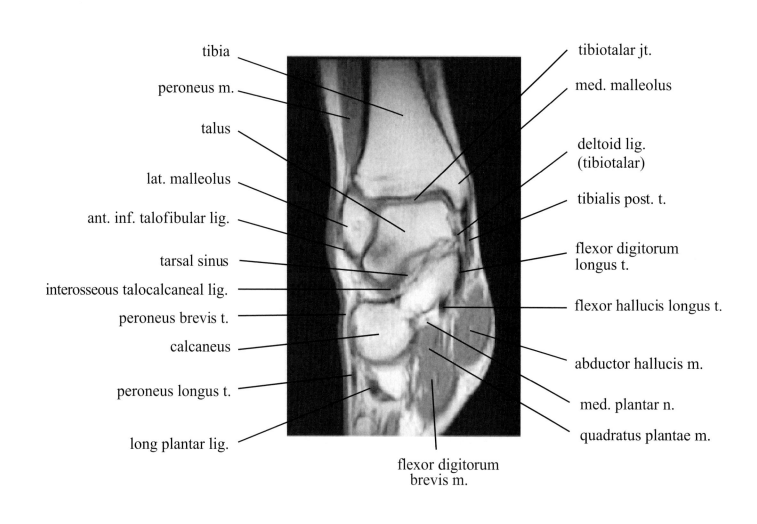

tibia

peroneus m.

talus

lat. malleolus

ant. inf. talofibular lig.

tarsal sinus

interosseous talocalcaneal lig.

peroneus brevis t.

calcaneus

peroneus longus t.

long plantar lig.

tibiotalar jt.

med. malleolus

deltoid lig.
(tibiotalar)

tibialis post. t.

flexor digitorum
longus t.

flexor hallucis longus t.

abductor hallucis m.

med. plantar n.

quadratus plantae m.

flexor digitorum
brevis m.

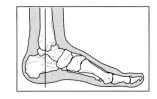

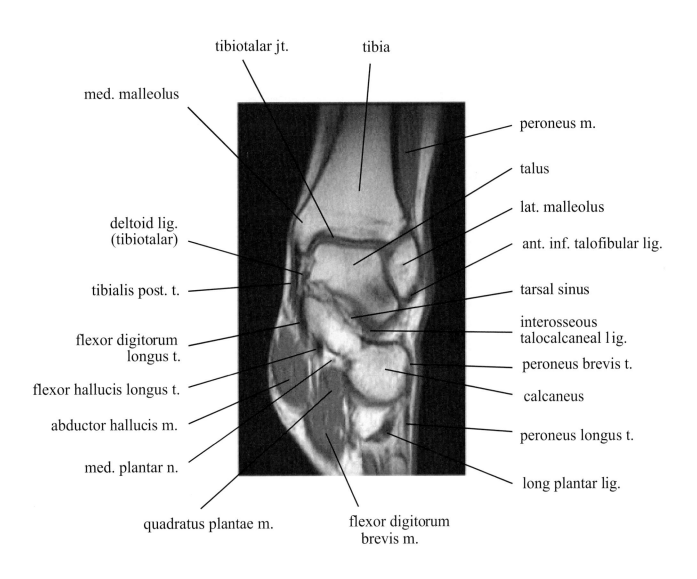

tibiotalar jt.

tibia

med. malleolus

peroneus m.

talus

lat. malleolus

deltoid lig.
(tibiotalar)

ant. inf. talofibular lig.

tibialis post. t.

tarsal sinus

interosseous
talocalcaneal lig.

flexor digitorum
longus t.

peroneus brevis t.

flexor hallucis longus t.

calcaneus

abductor hallucis m.

peroneus longus t.

med. plantar n.

long plantar lig.

quadratus plantae m.

flexor digitorum
brevis m.

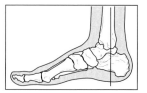

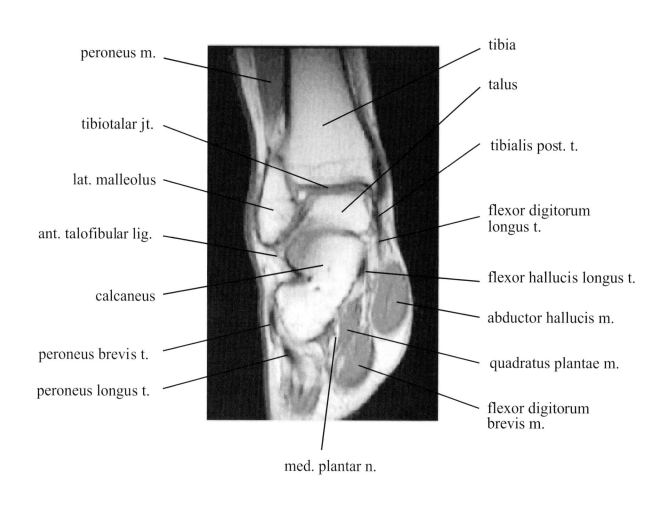

peroneus m.

tibiotalar jt.

lat. malleolus

ant. talofibular lig.

calcaneus

peroneus brevis t.

peroneus longus t.

tibia

talus

tibialis post. t.

flexor digitorum
longus t.

flexor hallucis longus t.

abductor hallucis m.

quadratus plantae m.

flexor digitorum
brevis m.

med. plantar n.

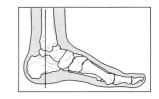

tibia

talus

tibialis post. t.

flexor digitorum longus t.

flexor hallucis longus t.

abductor hallucis m.

quadratus plantae m.

peroneus m.

tibiotalar jt.

lat. malleolus

calcaneus

ant. talofibular lig.

peroneus brevis t.

peroneus longus t.

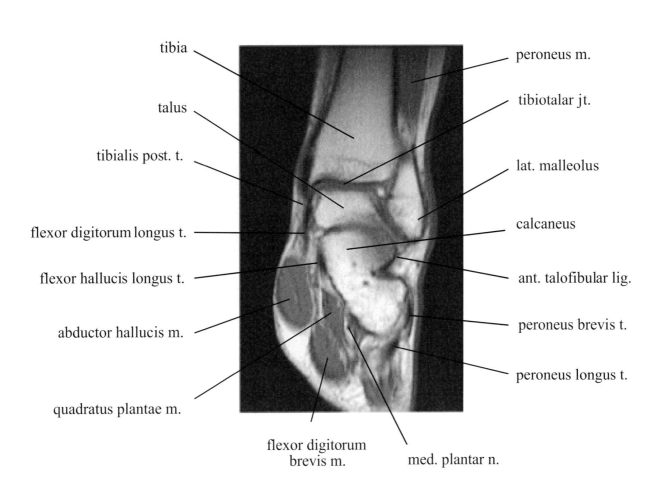

flexor digitorum
brevis m.

med. plantar n.

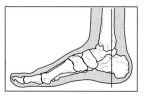

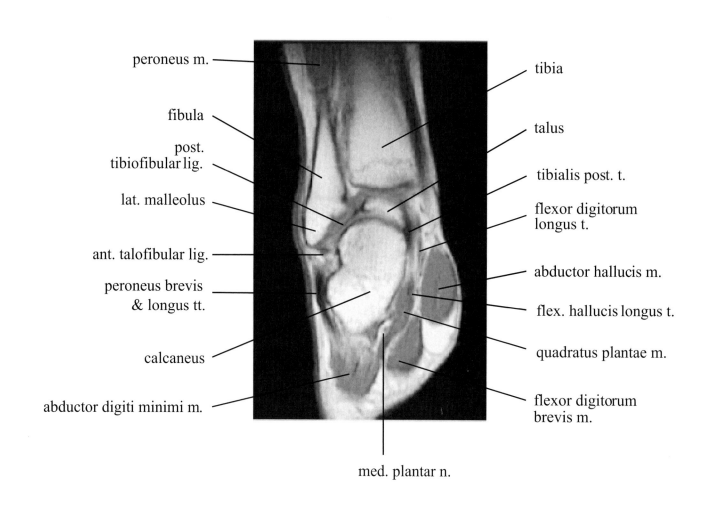

peroneus m.

fibula

post.
tibiofibular lig.

lat. malleolus

ant. talofibular lig.

peroneus brevis
& longus tt.

calcaneus

abductor digiti minimi m.

tibia

talus

tibialis post. t.

flexor digitorum
longus t.

abductor hallucis m.

flex. hallucis longus t.

quadratus plantae m.

flexor digitorum
brevis m.

med. plantar n.

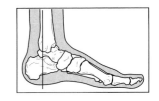

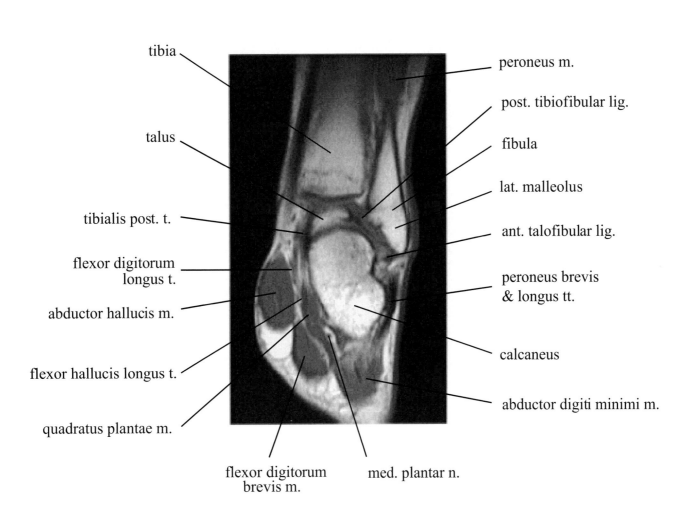

tibia

talus

tibialis post. t.

flexor digitorum
longus t.

abductor hallucis m.

flexor hallucis longus t.

quadratus plantae m.

flexor digitorum
brevis m.

med. plantar n.

peroneus m.

post. tibiofibular lig.

fibula

lat. malleolus

ant. talofibular lig.

peroneus brevis
& longus tt.

calcaneus

abductor digiti minimi m.

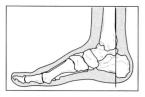

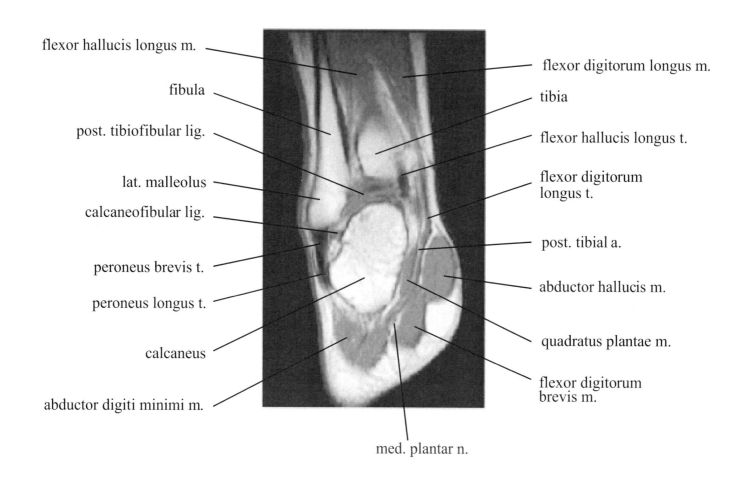

flexor hallucis longus m.

fibula

post. tibiofibular lig.

lat. malleolus

calcaneofibular lig.

peroneus brevis t.

peroneus longus t.

calcaneus

abductor digiti minimi m.

flexor digitorum longus m.

tibia

flexor hallucis longus t.

flexor digitorum longus t.

post. tibial a.

abductor hallucis m.

quadratus plantae m.

flexor digitorum brevis m.

med. plantar n.

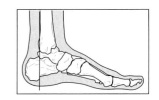

flexor digitorum longus m.

tibia

flexor hallucis longus t.

flexor digitorum
longus t.

post. tibial a.

abductor hallucis m.

quadratus plantae m.

flexor hallucis longus m.

fibula

post. tibiofibular lig.

lat. malleolus

calcaneofibular lig.

peroneus brevis t.

peroneus longus t.

calcaneus

abductor digiti minimi m.

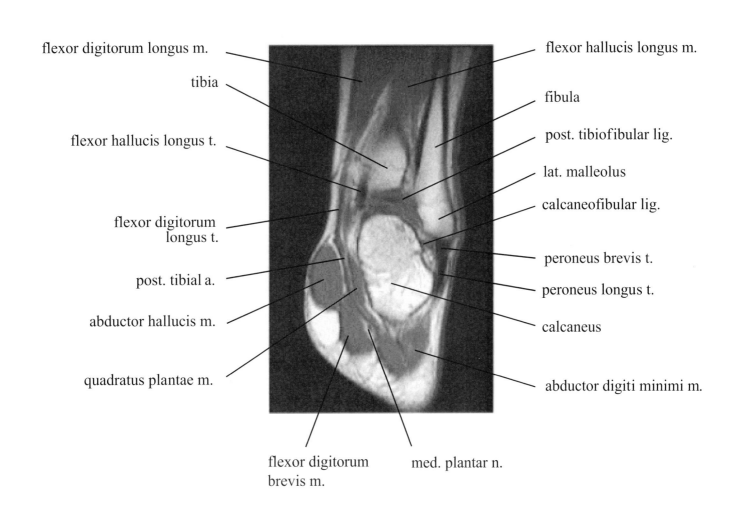

flexor digitorum
brevis m.

med. plantar n.

8

THE LUMBAR SPINE

MR images of the lumbar spine are often interpreted by neuroradiologists at academic institutions. However, this anatomic region is becoming increasingly important for the imager interpreting musculoskeletal scans. A large number of orthopaedists specialize in spine abnormalities, and it is important for the musculoskeletal radiologist to be able to communicate with them. The lumbar spine is included in this atlas for the sake of completeness, since many other atlases do not cover this anatomic region.

By far, the major indication for MR imaging of the lumbar spine is suspected degenerative disk disease. Evaluation consists of a search for disk protrusions, disk herniations, extruded disks, or secondary features of degenerative disease such as spinal stenosis. The patient who has undergone back surgery is also a candidate for MR imaging when there is suspicion of a recurrent disk herniation or complications from the surgery such as fractures or infection.

MR imaging is often used in the setting of acute trauma to evaluate the sequelae of injury and is an alternative to CT myelography.

Finally, lumbar spine imaging is performed for suspected infection, bleeding, primary tumors of the spinal column, and congenital disease.

PRACTICAL PROTOCOL CONSIDERATIONS

The patient is imaged while lying in the supine position. A variety of coils may be used, but the most common ones are coils with planar surfaces, quadrature coils, or the multicoil phased array design. The advantage of the phased array coil is that the areas of interest can be changed without changing the patient's position.

Cardiac gating or respiratory gating may be useful in some patients.

Menu of Protocols: Lumbar Spine

Plane	Pulse Sequence	FA (degrees)	TR (msec)	TE (msec)	TI (msec)	FOV (cm)	Matrix (256X-)	ST/G (mm)	NEX	Comments
Localizer (coronal)	SE		200	min		30	128	20/0	1	
Sagittal	SE		600	16		30	256	4/1	4	Either is acceptable
Sagittal	SE		3000	17		30	256	4/1	2	
Sagittal	SE		4000	102		30	256	4/1	2	
Sagittal	FSE, FS, double echo		3000	14/98		30	256	4/1	2	
Oblique transaxial	SE		4000	VAR		22	192	4/1	2	(Repeat pre- and
Oblique transaxial	SE		550	min		20	192	5/1	2	post-GAD)—for
Oblique transaxial	FSE		4500	102		16	192	5/2	2	postoperative pa-tients

MAJOR OSTEOCHONDRAL STRUCTURES/LANDMARKS

Lumbar Spine

- Vertebral bodies
- Intervertebral disk
- Posterior elements
  - Pedicle
  - Transverse process
  - Lamina
  - Spinous process
  - Superior articular facet (process)
  - Inferior articular facet (process)
- Sacrum
  - Promontory
  - Sacral foramen (anterior/posterior)
- Coccyx (with its fused segments)

MAJOR LIGAMENTS/TENDONS/BURSAE

Ligaments

- Anterior longitudinal
- Ligamentum flava
- Supraspinal (connect tips of spinous processes)
- Interspinal
- Sacroiliac (across sacroiliac joint)
  - Ventral
  - Interosseous
  - Short/long dorsal
- Sacrotuberous (sacrum to ischial tuberosity)
- Sacrospinal (sacrum to ischial spine)
- Iliolumbar (lumbar spine to superior ilium)

Tendons

Bursae

MAJOR MUSCLES

Deep Muscles

- Erector spinae
  - Longissimus
  - Iliocostalis lumborum
  - Spinalis
- Interspinal
- Intertransverse

Transversospinal Muscles

• Multifidus

• Rotares

• Quadratus lumborum

• Psoas

Other Muscles [Visibility on MR Images of the Lumbar Spine Depends on Field of View (FOV)]

• Serratus posterior inferior

• Latissimus dorsi

• Transverse abdominal

• Internal abdominal oblique

• External abdominal oblique

ORIGIN/INSERTION/INNERVATION OF MAJOR MUSCLES

Psoas, iliacus, pyriformis, gluteus maximus, gluteus medius (see Hips and Thigh)

Muscle	Origin	Insertion	Innervation
• Erector spinae	Common origin—posterior sacral surface, posterior iliac crest, lumbar spine spinous processes		
– Iliocostalis lumborum	Crest of ilium	Angles of lower six or seven ribs	Dorsal rami of spinal N.
– Longissimus		Lower nine or 10 ribs	Dorsal rami of spinal N.
– Spinalis	Last two thoracic and first two lumbar vertebrae	Spinous processes between fourth and eighth thoracic vertebrae	Dorsal rami of spinal N.
– Interspinal	Spinous process of vertebral body	Adjacent spinous process	Dorsal ramus of spinal N.

(continued)

ORIGIN/INSERTION/INNERVATION OF MAJOR MUSCLES (*CONTINUED*)

Muscle	*Origin*	*Insertion*	*Innervation*
– Intertransverse	Transverse process of vertebral body	Adjacent transverse process	Dorsal ramus of spinal N.
• Transversospinal muscle			
– Multifidus	Posterior surface of sacrum	Spinous processes of all vertebrae	Dorsal ramus of spinal N.
– Rotares	Posterior surface of sacrum	Adjacent or second spinous process	Dorsal ramus of spinal N.

THE LUMBAR SPINE: AXIAL ANATOMY

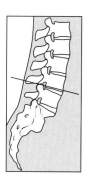

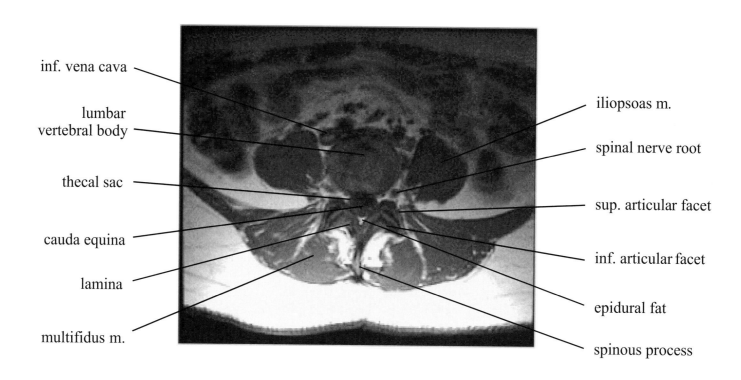

inf. vena cava

lumbar
vertebral body

thecal sac

cauda equina

lamina

multifidus m.

iliopsoas m.

spinal nerve root

sup. articular facet

inf. articular facet

epidural fat

spinous process

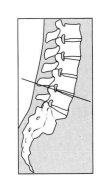

iliopsoas m.

spinal nerve root

retroperitoneal fat

iliac wing

cauda equina

ant. longitudinal lig.

intervertebral disc

sup. articular facet

inf. articular facet

multifidus m.

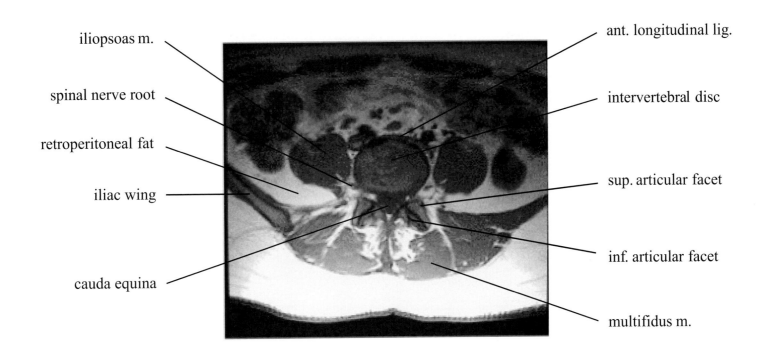

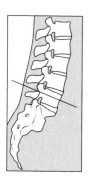

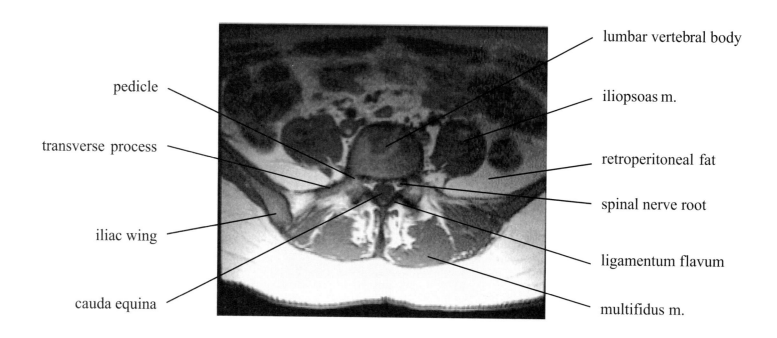

pedicle

transverse process

iliac wing

cauda equina

lumbar vertebral body

iliopsoas m.

retroperitoneal fat

spinal nerve root

ligamentum flavum

multifidus m.

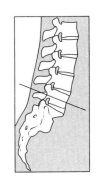

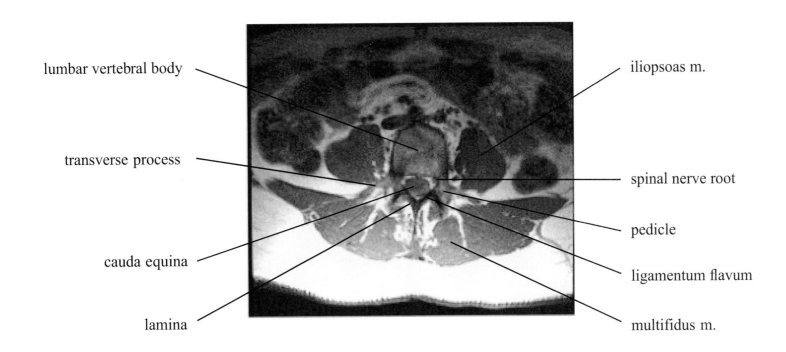

lumbar vertebral body

transverse process

cauda equina

lamina

iliopsoas m.

spinal nerve root

pedicle

ligamentum flavum

multifidus m.

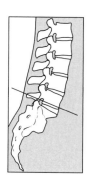

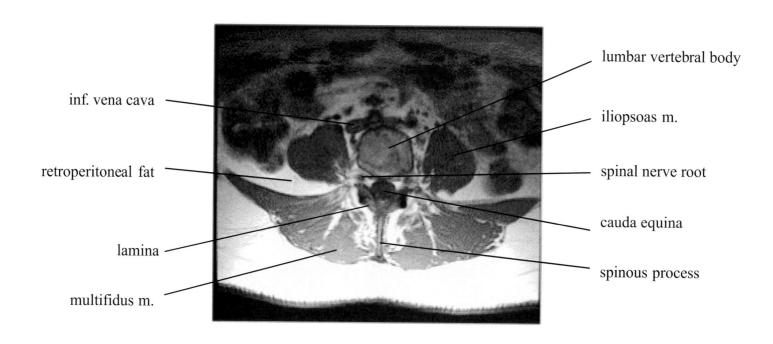

inf. vena cava

retroperitoneal fat

lamina

multifidus m.

lumbar vertebral body

iliopsoas m.

spinal nerve root

cauda equina

spinous process

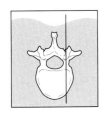

Lumbar Spine:
Sagittal Anatomy

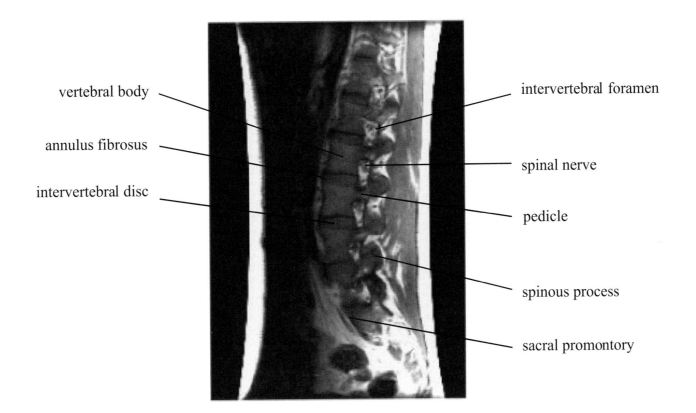

vertebral body

annulus fibrosus

intervertebral disc

intervertebral foramen

spinal nerve

pedicle

spinous process

sacral promontory

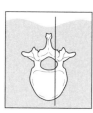

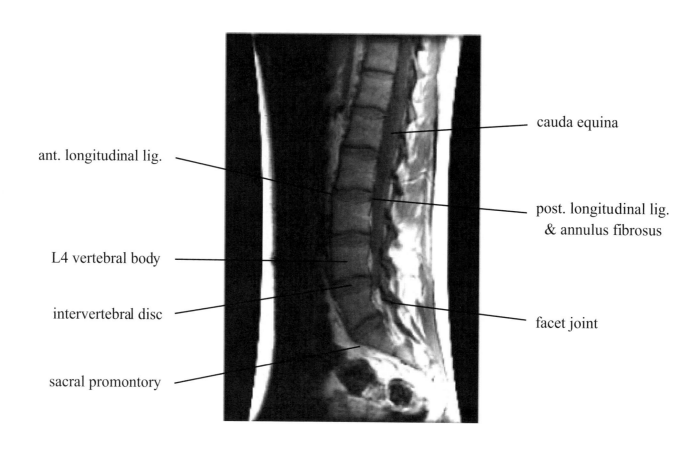

ant. longitudinal lig.

L4 vertebral body

intervertebral disc

sacral promontory

cauda equina

post. longitudinal lig.
 & annulus fibrosus

facet joint

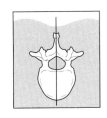

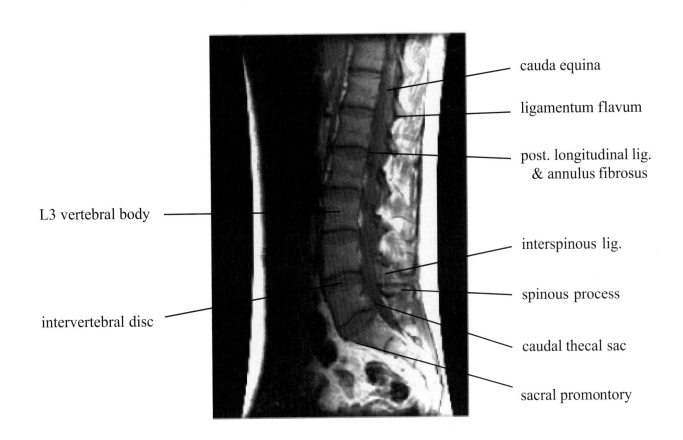

cauda equina

ligamentum flavum

post. longitudinal lig.
    & annulus fibrosus

L3 vertebral body

interspinous lig.

spinous process

intervertebral disc

caudal thecal sac

sacral promontory

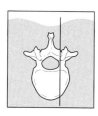

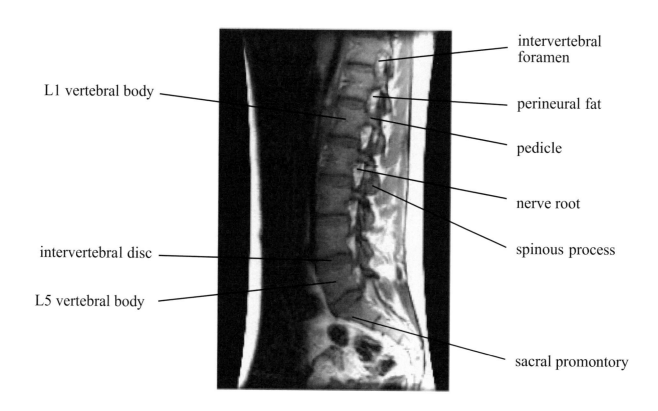

L1 vertebral body

intervertebral disc

L5 vertebral body

intervertebral foramen

perineural fat

pedicle

nerve root

spinous process

sacral promontory

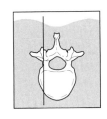

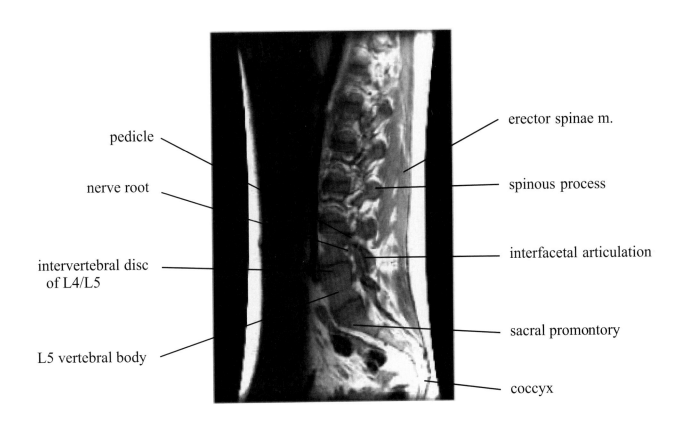

pedicle

nerve root

intervertebral disc
of L4/L5

L5 vertebral body

erector spinae m.

spinous process

interfacetal articulation

sacral promontory

coccyx

WORKS CONSULTED

El-Khoury GY, Bergman RA, Montgomery WJ, eds. *Sectional anatomy by MRI,* 2nd edition. New York: Churchill-Livingston, 1995.

Kneeland JB, ed. Update in musculoskeletal MR imaging. *Radiol Clin North Am* 1997; 35.

Netter FH. *The Ciba Collection of Medical Illustrations, Vol. 8. Musculoskeletal System, Part I, Anatomy, physiology, and metabolic disorders.* Summit, NJ: Ciba-Geigy Corp, 1987.

Resnick D, Kang HS, eds. *Internal derangements of joints—emphasis on MR imaging.* Philadelphia: WB Saunders Co, 1997.

Stoller DW, ed. *Magnetic resonance imaging in orthopaedics and sports medicine,* 2nd edition. Philadelphia: Lippincott-Raven Publishers, 1997.

Subject Index